ARCHITECTONICS OF THE CEREBRAL CORTEX

International Brain Research Organization
Monograph Series
Volume 3

INTERNATIONAL BRAIN RESEARCH
ORGANIZATION MONOGRAPH SERIES

SERIES EDITOR: MARY A. B. BRAZIER

INTERNATIONAL BRAIN RESEARCH
ORGANIZATION MONOGRAPH SERIES
Volume 3

Architectonics of
the Cerebral Cortex

Edited by

Mary A. B. Brazier
Brain Research Institute
University of California Los Angeles
Los Angeles, California

Hellmuth Petsche
Neurophysiologisches Institut
der Universität Wien
Wien, Austria

Raven Press ■ New York

Raven Press, 1140 Avenue of the Americas, New York, New York 10036

Made in the United States of America

Main entry under title:

Architectonics of the cerebral cortex.

   (Monograph series - International Brain Research Organization; v. 3)
   Includes bibliographical references and index.
   1. Cerebral cortex. 2. Cerebral cortex--Anatomy.
3. Electroencephalography. I. Brazier, Mary Agnes
Burniston, 1904–   II. Petsche, H. III. Series:
International Brain Research Organization. Monograph
series – International Brain Research Organization; v. 3.
[DNLM: 1. Cerebral cortex--Anatomy and histology.
2. Cerebral cortex--Physiology. W1 IN71s v. 3/W L307
A673]
QP383.A7   612'.825   77-83694
ISBN 0-89004-140-7

The IBRO Monograph Series

The International Brain Research Organization (IBRO) was founded in 1961 with the goal of fostering, in all countries, fundamental research leading to knowledge of the brain, both normal and abnormal. IBRO is represented by several hundred members drawn from 45 countries. Membership carries no dues and is focused essentially on the contribution that the individual is making to brain science.

Financial support comes from the dues and donations of 11 national committees for IBRO: Austria, Canada, Chile, Finland, Germany DDR, Hungary, India, Japan, Switzerland, the USA, and the USSR.

Eight categories of membership (the panels) subdivide the membership according to major interests, namely neuroanatomy, neurochemistry, neuroendocrinology, neuropharmacology, neurophysiology, behavioral sciences, neurocommunications and biophysics, and brain pathology.

In order to effect its major goal, IBRO, among its several activities, designs and runs educational workshops in brain science in less scientifically developed countries, sponsors fellowships, and, as evidenced by this volume, organizes major symposia, usually one a year on some special topic, to which members gather from many countries.

The first volume of the series was published in 1975 and contains the proceedings of a symposium held in New Delhi as a satellite to the XXVIth International Congress of Physiology: The subject was *Growth and Development of the Brain: Nutritional, Genetic, and Environmental Factors*.

The second volume, in October of 1975, was an invited symposium held in Toronto ancillary to the 1st International Congress of Child Neurology. The subject was *Brain Dysfunction in Infantile Febrile Convulsions* and forms the second in the IBRO Monograph Series, the third of which is this present volume.

Mary A. B. Brazier

Acknowledgments

Grateful appreciation is expressed to the following supporters of this symposium:

European Training Program in Brain and Behaviour Research (ETPBBR)
Akademie für Ärztliche Fortbildung
Der Bürgermeister der Stadt Wien, Herr Leopold Gratz
Die Herren Landeshauptleute für

    Niederösterreich (Senator h.c. Andreas Maurer)
    Oberösterreich (LA Dr. Erwin Wenzl)
    Tirol (ÖKR Eduard Wallnöfer)
    Burgenland (Theodor Kery)
    Kärnten (Leipold Wagner)
    Vorarlberg (Dr. Herbert Kessler)

Verband der Wissenschaftlichen Gesellschaftern Österreichs
Österreichischer Aero-Club
Comesa—Dr. Rolf Buchgeher KG, Wien
Fritz Schwarzer GmbH, München
Hewlett-Packard GmbH, Wien
Hoffmann-La Roche GmbH, Wien
Oesterreichische Nationalbank
Beckman Instruments GmbH, Wien
C. Reichert, Optische Werke AG, Wien
Siemens AG, Wien

Preface

This volume, the third in the Monograph Series of the International Brain Research Organization, is centered on the fine structure of the part of our brains that is responsible for our rational thought, our intelligence, our sensorimotor controls and the mechanisms by which these ends are achieved.

In the one-hundred years since the birth of the man, von Economo, who gave anatomy the atlas that became its major guideline for future research, great advances in technology have come to the aid of the scientist and these are reflected in this volume. Among them are such inventions as electron microscopy, computer analyses, and in neurochemistry, to mention only a few, the introduction of horseradish peroxidase for retrograde tracing in the live nervous system and the greatly improved staining techniques for use post-mortem.

IBRO owes the success of the symposium in Vienna, on which this volume is based, to the auspices of the Rector of the University of Vienna, Professor F. Seitelberger, and to the support received from several sources including the Austrian Academy of Sciences. This editor also wishes to express her appreciation to her editorial assistant, Gwen Garvin.

Mary A. B. Brazier

Contents

Contributors

O. S. Adrianov
Brain Research Institute
USSR Academy of Medical Sciences
Per. Obukha 5
Moscow 120, USSR

H. Braak
Anatomisches Institut der Universität
Kiel
Neue Universität, Haus 30
D-23 Kiel, Germany FDR

V. Braitenberg
Max Planck-Institut für Biologische
Kybernetik
Spemannstrasse 38
D-74 Tübingen, Germany FDR

M. A. B. Brazier
Brain Research Institute
University of California Medical Cen-
ter
Los Angeles, California 90024

Y. Burnod
Laboratoire de Physiologie
Pitié-Salpêtrière
91, Boulevard de l'Hôpital
F-75634 Paris, France

J. Calvet
Laboratoire de Recherches Neuro-
physiologiques de l'Association
Claude Bernard EPHE et INSERM
Hôpital de la Salpêtrière
75013 Paris, France

H. Caspers
Physiologisches Institut der Universi-
tät
Westphalian Wilhelm University
Westring 6
D-44 Münster, Germany FDR

O. D. Creutzfeldt
Abteilung für Neurobiologie
Max Planck-Institut für Biophysika-
lische Chemie
Postfach 968
D-34 Göttingen, Germany FDR

K. Detzer
Anatomisches Institut der Universität
Bonn
Nussallee 10
D-53 Bonn, Germany FDR

M. F. Diebler
Laboratoire de Neuropathologie
Hôpital St. Vincent-de-Paul
74, Avenue Denfert-Rochereau
Paris 14, France

F. Donate-Oliver
Departamento c. Morfologicas
C. U. Soria
Soria, Spain

E. Farkas-Bargeton
Laboratoire de Neuropathologie
Hôpital St. Vincent-de-Paul
74, Avenue Denfert-Rochereau
Paris 14, France

K. Fleischhauer
Anatomisches Institut der Universität
Bonn
Nussallee 10
D-53 Bonn, Germany FDR

L. J. Garey
Institut d'Anatomie
University of Lausanne
Rue du Bugnon 9
CH-1011 Lausanne, Switzerland

F. C. Hellweg
Max Planck-Institut für Biophysika-
lische Chemie
Postfach 968
D-34 Göttingen, Germany FDR

D. H. Ingvar
Department of Clinical Neurophysi-
ology
University Hospital
S-221 85
Lund 5, Sweden

R. W. C. Janzen
Physiologisches Institut der Univer-
sität
Westphalian Wilhelm University
Westring 6
D-44 Münster, Germany FDR

E. Lesky
Institut für Geschichte der Medizin
Währingerstrasse 25
A-1090 Wien, Austria

F. H. Lopes da Silva
Brain Research Department
Institute of Medical Physics TNO
Da Costakade 45
P. O. Box 5011
Utrecht, The Netherlands

I. B. Müller-Paschinger
Institut für Neurophysiologie der Uni-
versität Wien
Währingerstrasse 17
A-1090 Wien, Austria

K. O'Connor
MRC Clinical Psychiatry Unit
Graylingwell Hospital
Chichester, Sussex, PO 19 4PQ, Eng-
land

C. Ongley
MRC Clinical Psychiatry Unit
Graylingwell Hospital
Chichester, Sussex, PO 19 4PQ, Eng-
land

S. L. Palay
Department of Anatomy
Harvard Medical School
25 Shattuck Street
Boston, Massachusetts 02115

H. Petsche
Institut für Neurophysiologie der Uni-
versität Wien
Währingerstrasse 17
A-1090 Wien, Austria

H. Pockberger
Institut für Hirnforschung
Österreichische Akademie der Wissen-
schaften
Währingerstrasse 13A
A-1090 Wien, Austria

O. Prohaska
Institut für Hirnforschung
Österreichische Akademie der Wissen-
schaften
Währingerstrasse 13A
A-1090 Wien, Austria

P. Rappelsberger
Institut für Neurophysiologie der Uni-
versität Wien
Währingerstrasse 17
and
Institut für Hirnforschung
Österreichische Akademie der Wissen-
schaften
Währingerstrasse 13A
A-1090 Wien, Austria

D. Sanides
Max Planck-Institut für Biophysi-
kalische Chemie
Postfach 968
D-34 Göttingen, Germany FDR

*M. E. and A. B. Scheibel
Departments of Anatomy and Psychi-
atry
University of California Los Angeles
Los Angeles, California 90024

* Deceased

J. Scherrer
Laboratoire de Physiologie
Pitié-Salpêtrière
91, Boulevard de l'Hôpital
F-75634 Paris, France

A. Schüz
Max Planck-Institut für Biologische
Kybernetik
Spemannstrasse 38
D-74 Tübingen, Germany FDR

F. Seitelberger
Universität Wien
Wien, Austria

J. C. Shaw
MRC Clinical Psychiatry Unit
Graylingwell Hospital
Chichester, Sussex, PO 19 4PQ, England

E.-J. Speckmann
Physiologisches Institut der Universität
Westphalian Wilhelm University
Westring 6
D-44 Münster, Germany FDR

W. Storm van Leeuwen
Brain Research Department
Institute of Medical Physics TNO
Da Costakade 45
P.O. Box 5011
Utrecht, The Netherlands

J. Szentágothai
Department of Anatomy

Semmelweis University Medical
School
1450 Tüzoltó, Utea 58
Budapest 9, Hungary

T. Tömböl
Department of Anatomy
Semmelweis University Medical
School
1450 Tüzoltó, Utea 58
Budapest 9, Hungary

D. Volanschi
Academia Institutul de Neurologie e
Psihiatrie
Str. Povernei 42, Sect 1
71124 Bucharest, Romania

R. Vollmer
Institut für Neurophysiologie der Universität Wien
Währingerstrasse 17
A-1090 Wien, Austria

G. Werner
University of Pittsburgh
School of Medicine
Scaife Hall
3550 Terrace Street
Pittsburgh, Pennsylvania 15261

J. R. Wolff
Max Planck-Institut für Biophysikalische Chemie
Postfach 968
D-34 Göttingen, Germany FDR

Architectonics of the Cerebral Cortex,
edited by M. A. B. Brazier and H. Petsche.
Raven Press, New York © 1978.

Constantin von Economo (1876–1931): Life and Work

Erna Lesky

University of Vienna and Institute of the History of Medicine, A-1090 Vienna, Austria

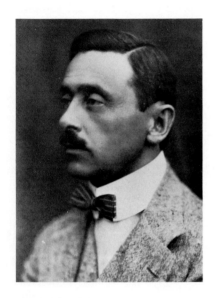

Constantin von Economo was born in Braila, Rumania, on August 21, 1876, the scion of a patrician family of Greek descent. The Vienna Institute of Neurology has seized the occasion of the recurrence of this date to devote this year's symposium to the memory of this scientist. We are proud to discharge a debt of honor that is legitimately ours. The question may be asked whether we have the right to claim a Greek, born in Rumania and raised in Trieste, as a representative of the Vienna School of Medicine. Answering this question at the same time spells recognition in Economo's life of the cultural radiance of the lost empire, the Hapsburg Monarchy.

The flourishing port city of the empire of many nations, Trieste — to become the home of the family in 1877 — gave the young Greek the chance to enter the precincts of German-speaking Austria through the Austrian schools of the city and adopt concurrently the values of the sensitive and broad-minded humanism which was to be characteristic of his future lifestyle. All things beautiful in nature and in the arts, ranging from Homer to Dante, Shakespeare and Goethe, stayed with him throughout his life and all things mysterious such as the Creator, remained the object of his adoration.

After having registered for the study of medicine at the University of Vienna in 1895, he penetrated even more deeply into the core of Austrian culture. We hail Constantin von Economo as one of our very own not only because he graduated from Vienna University (1901), became a docent (1913) and a "titular" full professor (1920), but because to his death he remained faithful to the Alma Mater Rudolphina despite flattering offers to

1

go abroad, and because he wrote in the preface to his principal work on cytoarchitectonics (5) about his University in Vienna and his chosen country, Austria: "The significance of Vienna University, of Vienna and all of German-speaking Austria as a European cultural center has never been truly comprehended and appreciated . . . , in the German language area . . . it has never been really understood that Austria, the foremost bastion of German civilization, has planted the outposts of its knowledge far to the East and has thus earned a special place of honor. . . ."

Around 1900 the Vienna medical faculty experienced its third period of reknown occasioned by mean like Billroth, Nothnagel, Meynert, and Krafft-Ebing, to name just a few. Economo never did meet his real scientific herald, Theodor Meynert (1833–1892); however, there were others who excelled in histological technique, such as the histologists Victor Ebner and Joseph Schaffer, the physiologist Siegmund Exner, and the neurologist Heinrich Obersteiner, world-famous founder of the Neurological Institute. Young Economo learned the subtle art of hardening, staining, and cutting microscopical preparations from these masters. In 1899 he had already advanced sufficiently in this difficult art to have his first work on the hypophysis of birds published by the supreme scientific forum of the country, the Academy of Science (1). The measure of certitude that had prompted Economo at this early age to decide on neurology as his chosen field and the inexorable diligence with which the young and rich baron continued to pursue this goal even though the splendor of the imperial city with its high society and the diversions of the belle époque were enticingly open to him, were indeed remarkable.

As early as 1902 he presented an experimental anatomical study on the central pathways of the masticating and swallowing processes (2). The thoroughness and accuracy displayed in this study are already typical of Economo's method and may serve as an example of his skill for combining animal experiments and microscopical anatomical techniques. However, the young researcher strove both to perfect his technique still further and to widen his horizons in neurology and psychiatry. The sovereign manner in which he approached his postgraduate training and the exactitude with which he adhered to his program are indeed impressive: 1 year in Paris with the disciples of Charcot; 6 months in Strasbourg with the master of neuroanatomy, Bethe; another 6 months in Munich with Kraepelin; followed by a few months in Berlin with the psychiatrist Ziehen and the neurologist Oppenheim. Thus, he knew everything that the European psychiatrists and neurologists of rank and distinction had to offer; in Munich he was thus able to enter into the then-pending dispute about the relationship between neurofibrils and ganglion cells and to clarify the role of the Golgi apparatus of the ganglion cells.

It redounds to the honor of both Julius von Wagner-Jauregg (1857–1940) and Economo that on the latter's return to Vienna he chose Wagner-Jauregg to be his principal teacher and master when he put himself at his disposal to work as volunteer assistant at his institute. Under the experienced guidance of Wagner-Jauregg, he became the clinician who, 11 years later, performed his clinical chef d'oeuvre, the discovery and description of encephalitis lethargica (4). However, before we go further into this major achievement, a few words must be said about Economo's career as a neuro-anatomist and neurophysiologist, which he pursued with great persistence and patience in addition to his clinical work during the period between 1906 and the outbreak of World War I.

His principal field of research remained the mesencephalon and the diencephalon; together with Paul Karplus he carried out experiments involving the severing of the cerebral peduncle in order to bring about experimental chorea. He wrote his habilitation thesis about pons tumors (1911) and published papers about the mesencephalon (1909) (3). Undoubtedly, these animal experiments and the histological work acquainted Economo so intimately with conditions in the brainstem that he was able to arrive at significant conclusions as to anatomical arrangement and localization.

This was important because during the winter of 1916–1917 there were several patients—a total of seven in April—who were admitted to the clinic of Wagner-Jauregg with various symptoms. The only feature common to almost all of them was a strange somnolence as well as an ocular muscle disturbance. It required a large measure of both a sense of combination and intuition to seize upon these few and by no means uniform cases and reduce them to the clinical and anatomical entity termed encephalitis lethargica.

When Economo announced the discovery of this new disease on April 17, 1917, to a gathering of the Psychiatric Association in Vienna with that particular quality of certitude so characteristic for his genius, he had already found out all the essentials: that this disease manifested a variety of symptoms, that it constituted an inflammation of the grey matter of the mesencephalon, that it was an infection[1] similar to poliomyelitis both in terms of the type of inflammation and its etiological aspects. Economo even sought to apply his own awareness of historical significance to the disease and assign it a place in medical history by recalling similar epidemics of an earlier day such as the so-called Nona in Northern Italy (1890) and the so-called Tübingen sleeping sickness of 1712 in Tübingen. When in 1920 encephalitis lethargica occurred pandemically and spread throughout the world, Economo had the satisfaction of having his original 1917 description of the disease confirmed. Additional observations concerned the

---

[1] Economo's disease, as encephalitis lethargica was later called after its discoverer, became known as encephalitis "A" to distinguish it from the insect-borne Japanese "B" encephalitis. The causative organism of Economo's disease, probably a virus, was never identified (see Walters in biographical and historical bibliography at the end of this chapter).

syndromes of postencephalitic complications, primarily the merciless Parkinson's disease.

Economo devoted 27 papers to the research on encephalitis lethargica and lectured on it in various countries, including the United States. Today, there is such a lively interest in this disease in the United States that in 1968 Economo's report of the disease in 1917 (4) was translated into English for the *Archives of Neurology* (9). In 1926 the epidemic subsided, and in 1929 Economo published a concluding treatise on it (6); by that time he had long since become a scientist of world renown.

If the discovery and description of encephalitis lethargica showed Economo to be an ingenious clinician, the conclusions as to the explanation of sleep he derived from the somnolent and ophthalmoplegic form of the disease proved him to be a biologist with the genius of universality. The frequent coincidence of ocular muscle disturbances and sleep disorders in encephalitis lethargica made him assume that in the immediate vicinity of the ocular muscle nuclei, i.e., in the grey matter of the aqueduct, a sleep control center (he himself coined this term) existed. The theory of sleep (7) that Economo based on this assumption is of particular interest because for the first time sleep is described as a complex biological condition, and differentiation is made between cerebral and bodily sleep.

It would be reasonable to presume that this research on encephalitis lethargica, on the physiology and pathology of sleep in addition to investigations about the hereditary aspects of mental disorders, would have exhausted the working capacity of a scientist carrying on all this research in the years from 1912 to 1925. Economo indeed performed an extraordinary feat by indefatigably devoting himself (with G. Koskinas) to his principal work, *The Cytoarchitectonics of the Human Cerebral Cortex* (5), published in 1925. "Everything about this work has monumental dimensions; the intellectual content, the amount of energy and time spent on it and, last but not least, the presentation. . . ." This was Wagner-Jauregg's judgment about the work of his disciple. Indeed, 107 areas of differing histological structure in the human cerebral cortex are described meticulously in a classic manner in 810 pages; measurements are detailed and shown in a separate atlas of illustrations. The latter consists of 112 40×40-cm photographic plates mounted on cardboard. Wagner-Jauregg described the infinite pains it must have taken to do thousands upon thousands of sections, to select the most characteristic ones, and to make 500 original large-scale photograms (not phototypes!). As a rule only the scientific and technological but not the financial aspects of this undertaking are properly esteemed. Economo, however, was not only the author of this work but also the generous patron. The printing of this work cost him a small fortune.

Economo dedicated this book to Theodor Meynert. He did so with the intention of erecting a monument to the founder of cytoarchitectonics (1867) in whose former laboratory he had worked while Meynert's picture looked down on him. Economo was privileged for two reasons to consider himself Meynert's heir: for one, he completed the work on cytoarchitectonics begun by Meynert and he also took up the latter's ideas about the correlations between the development of the cerebrum and that of mankind. Economo further expanded on it in his brilliant theory on progressive cerebration (8). In this endeavor, it proved to be most useful that the contemporary paleontologists, Abel and Osborn, had discovered the law about orthogenesis and rectigradation, which means that once an organ has acquired a certain direction of development, it continues to evolve in the same direction, the evolutionary process being irreversible (law of Dolo).

Economo understood progressive cerebration, i.e., the regional development characteristic for the human brain, to be a special case within the laws of orthogenesis and irreversibility as explained by Abel and Osborn and Dolo; in this connection he termed the frontal and parietal lobes as new acquisitions in the course of man-specific phylogenesis. Economo (similarly to Meynert) not only regarded the development of culture and civilization from the eoanthropus with his flintstone implements to modern man with his machines as a result of man's progressive cerebration, but, based on his optimism where evolution was concerned, he also thought that conclusions as to the future could be drawn. He believed that with the irreversible progressive development of his brain man would develop "new and yet unknown psychic capacities." He considered the development of music during recent centuries a case in point.

In the scientific field, the theory of progressive cerebration corresponded to Economo's faith in what is good, to his optimistic credo in man's potential. Only this faith can explain the ultimate devotion to his chosen task, which in 1928 prevented him from becoming the successor to his teacher Wagner-Jauregg and taking over this tradition-encrusted institution in Vienna. Only this faith can explain the tremendous workload that Economo carried during the final years of his life in order to complete his cerebral research. His work on elite brains, the brains of especially talented and one-sidedly gifted persons, illustrates the near-Faustian undertaking, searching for new and more perfect stages of progressive cerebration. Thus, he hoped to lift part of the veil covering the secrets of evolution, and to afford a glimpse into the future of homo sapiens.

For decades Economo carried out his technologically sophisticated research in Meynert's old microscopy room dating back to 1870, a premise which during Economo's time also had to serve as a general laboratory of a major clinic. Not until 1931 did Economo get his own department for cerebral research, which he inaugurated on May 7 with a brilliant lecture on the problems of cerebral research. Six months later everything came to a standstill: on October 21, 1931, Economo succumbed to the cardiac disease he had been suffering from for years.

Any description of Economo's personality would be incomplete if we were simply to talk about the daring researcher reaching out into time and to omit the equally daring aviator reaching for the skies. In a day when as yet there were no airplanes in Austria, he started in 1907 taking balloon trips, became one of the pioneers in aviation, president of the "Aeroklub" (1910), and the first reconnaissance pilot of the Austrian Army. The first Austrian airports in Wiener Neustadt and Aspern (near Vienna) owe their existence to his administrative skill. In 1931 Economo displayed his uncanny vision beyond the then current technological capacity when he stated: "Modern physics research indicates that we will have means available to utilize nuclear fission, and thus place at our disposal forces that will allow us to surmount gravity." Statements such as this once more manifest in a condensed version Economo's vision into utopia carried by a noble evolutionary idealism. The greatest boon that fate could bestow upon him was the fact that he did not live to see the reality of the atomic age. Even in the face of this reality there remains for us to pay due reverence to his idealism.

REFERENCES

1. Economo, C. von (1899): Zur Entwicklung der Volgelhypophyse. *Sber. Akad. Wiss. Wien,* Math.-nat. Cl., Abt. 3, 108:281–297.
2. Economo, C. von (1902): Die zentralen Bahnen des Kau – und Schluckaktes. *Pfluegers Arch. Physiol.,* 91:629–643.
3. Economo, C. von, and Karplus, J. P. (1909): Zur Physiologie und Anatomie des Mittelhirns. *Arch. Psychiat. Berlin,* 46:377–429.
4. Economo, C. von (1918): *Die Encephalitis lethargica.* Deuticke, Vienna.
5. Economo, C. von, and Koskinas, G. (1925): *Die Cytoarchitektonik der Hirnrinde des erwachsenen Menschen.* Springer, Berlin.
6. Economo, C. von (1929): *Die Encephalitis lethargica, ihre Nachkrankheiten und ihre Behandlung.* Urban & Schwarzenberg, Vienna.
7. Economo, C. von (1929): Schlaftheorie. *Ergebn. Physiol.,* 28/1:312–339.
8. Economo, C. von (1930): Cytoarchitectony and progressive cerebration. *Psychiatr. Q.,* 4:142–150.
9. Wilkins, R. H. (1968): Encephalitis lethargica. *Arch. Neurol.,* 18:324–328.

BIOGRAPHICAL AND HISTORICAL STUDIES

Economo, Caroline von, and Wagner-Jauregg, J. von (1932): *Constantin Freiherr von Economo.* Mayer, Vienna (English translation R. Spillman 1937, Burlington Free Press).
Huard, P., Théodorides, J., and Vetter, T. (1968): A propos du cinquantenaire de la découverte de l'encéphalite léthargique par C. von Economo (1917). *Histoire des Sciences Médicales,* 2:95–104.
Lesky, E. (1976): *The Vienna Medical School of the 19th Century.* The Johns Hopkins University Press, Baltimore.
Seitelberger, F. (1951): Nachruf für Constantin von Economo. *Wien. Med. Wochenschr.,* 101:907.
Seitelberger, F. (1966): Das wissenschaftliche Werk Constantin von Economos. *Wien. Med. Wochenschr.,* 78:729–731.
Spatz, H. (1931): Constantin v. Economo. *Münch. Med. Wochenschr.,* 78:2161–2163.
Stockert, F. G. von (1959): Theodor Meynert (1833–1892). In: *Grosse Nervenärzte, Vol. 2,* edited by K. Kolle, pp. 98–105. Georg Thieme, Stuttgart.
Sträussler, E. E. (1932): Constantin v. Economo. *Z. Gesamte Neurol. Psychiatry,* 139:649–657.

Stransky, E. (1931): Constantin Economo. *Med. Klin.*, 27:1611–1612.

Stransky, E. (1959): Constantin Economo (1876–1931). In: *Grosse Nervenärzte, Vol. 2*, edited by K. Kolle, pp. 180–185. Georg Thieme, Stuttgart.

Théodorides, J. (1964): Constantin von Economo (1876–1931) savant, humaniste, homme d'action. In: *Compte-Rendu du 19ᵉ Congrès International de l'Histoire de la Médecine*, pp. 624–636. Basel.

Wagner-Jauregg, J. (1931): Constantin Freiherr von Economo von San Serff. *Wien. Klin. Wochenschr.*, 81:1384–1386.

Walters, J. H. (1976): Constantin von Economo (1876–1931). *J. Operat. Psychiatry*, 7:75–79.

Architectonics of the Cerebral Cortex,
edited by M. A. B. Brazier and H. Petsche.
Raven Press, New York © 1978.

Architectonics of the Cerebral Cortex: Research in the 19th Century

Mary A. B. Brazier

*Brain Research Institute, University of California Los Angeles,
Los Angeles, California 90024*

Our knowledge of the architectonics of the cerebral cortex has developed part and parcel with those of the cerebellar cortex and the hippocampus, but in the space available this report will be restricted to those studies of the microstructure of the neocortex that anticipated the era of external mapping of the cortical surface, for this came to fruition in the following century.

Before the architectonics could be effectively explored, some identification of the individual components was imperative. This came rather late, since it had to wait for the development, not only of fixing and staining techniques, but for the invention of an adequate microscope.

Examination of cerebral tissue in aqueous solution made the quest hard for the early histologists. Alcohol, the first effective fixative to replace the weaker spirits of wine, was not employed before 1809, the year it was introduced by Reil. Malpighi (32), one of the first to give an account of what he observed about cerebral tissue through his primitive microscope, described and illustrated in 1685 some structures which he called "minute glands." In making his preparation, he had boiled the brains, removed the meninges, and then poured ink over the surface. Unfortunately, these structures were not nerve cells, although, just possibly, the strands were fibers (Fig. 1).

Perhaps at this time we might remind ourselves of some of the histological techniques being used by these early workers for these were crucial to the unravelling of architectonics. Formaldehyde did not come in to use as a fixative until 1893. In the 1850s von Gerlach (16) and his contemporaries were using a carmine dye for a stain. In the 1870s, workers like Bevan Lewis (30) were fixing the tissue with osmium tetroxide and staining it with aniline black, Cajal (44) was using silver reduction methods, while, in Italy, Golgi (17) was developing the use of potassium dichromate followed by silver nitrate, thus revealing the beautiful detail with which we are all familiar.

It was in 1873 that Golgi (17) first published the *reazione nera* (in the *Gazetta Medica Italiana*), giving, in the following year (18), a communication on "The Fine Anatomy of the Human Cerebellum" to the Istituto Lombardo, an Academy of Sciences and Letters. Later he was to improve

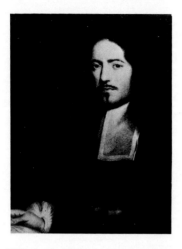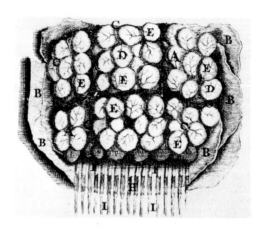

FIG. 1. M. Malpighi (1628–1694) and his illustrations of the "minute glands" which he saw through his primitive microscope when he examined brain tissue. (From De cerebri cortice. In: *De Viscerum Structure Exercitatio Anatomica.* Montinus, Bologna, 1666, pp. 50–70.)

the method by substituting osmic dichromate for the hardening process (19,20).

The innovative step of vital staining with methylene blue was made by Erlich in 1886 (9), a technique adopted by Cajal. Weigert's stains for myelin sheaths (58,59) had been in use since 1882, but it was not until just before the turn of the century that Nissl (39) discovered the "grummeaux basophiles" in the intracellular protoplasm and introduced aniline dyes for better staining of the nerve cell. This came at a time when attention was being paid to the neurofibrils inside the cell as revealed, for example, by Apáthy (1) using gold chloride and by Cajal with his silver reduction method.

A more serious problem at the beginning of the 19th century concerned the microscopes, which were inadequate to reveal the detail sought. Not only chromatic effects, but also spherical aberration, distorted the image, the latter being more difficult to correct.

But ingenuity was to come to the aid of the histologist from an inventor: Joseph Jackson Lister, who designed the first achromatic microscope that also had a correction for spherical aberration. Together with the physician Thomas Hodgkin, he published this in 1827 (26), a date which limits the exact exploration of neuronal detail to less than 150 years. A fuller account of this technical advance is found in the papers Lister left to his famous son, Lord Lister.

Those who have studied the development of microscopes will have noticed that all the historians rate this invention of Lister's as an outstanding breakthrough, and, indeed, for the field being discussed here, it was a crucial improvement. Lister's invention was to manufacture his object-glasses by joining together a planoconcave flint lens and a convex one by a transparent cement, such as Canada balsam, thus correcting for spherical aberration. Until that invention, some of the finest microscopes were those of the famous Giovanni Baptista Amici, a splendid collection that now can be seen in the Museum of Science in Florence.

With Lister's new arrangement of lenses, which avoided spherical distortion, Hodgkin examined brain tissue and described what he saw as follows (26):

> "If there is any organized animal substance which seems more likely than another to consist of globular particles, it is undoubtedly that of the brain. Our examination of it has yet been but slight; but we have noticed that when a portion of it, however fresh, is sufficiently extended to allow of its being viewed in the microscope, one sees instead of globules a multitude of very small particles, which are most irregular in shape and size, and are probably more dependent on the disintegration than on the organization of substance."

Within the next quarter century the two largest cells of the brain (though only their cell bodies) had been seen; Valentin in 1836 (54), 3 years before Schwann (49) enunciated his cell theory, described the cortical cell and depicted the cerebellar cell, later illustrated more accurately by Purkyně (42) who had acquired an achromatic microscope; and in 1849 Kölliker (29) sketched the pyramidal cell of the neocortex. It was Obersteiner, who as a medical student of 22, adopted the name of Purkyně for the cerebellar cell in his thesis written in 1869.

But cell bodies seen alone could give no hint of architectonics. The processes of neurons had been seen by Remak (45) and in more detail by Deiters (7), whose posthumous publication of 1865 gave us the first clear picture of dendrites, which he called "protoplasmic processes" (Fig. 2).

Remak, a pupil of Johannes Müller, had studied these processes intensely. He identified, in cells from the spinal cord, one process of considerable prolongation that we now know to be the axon. This he called the "organic fiber" (45).

> "The organic fibers" he wrote, "originate from the very substance of the nucleated globules, and this observation, although it is very difficult and requires great skill in preparation and observation, is nevertheless so clear that it cannot be doubted."

This was a point that had become very controversial, since, before this day, whether or not these so-called protoplasmic processes were indeed outgrowths from the parent nerve cell was still not settled, they being generally regarded as a plexus of fibers among which lay the independent nerve cells. That these processes of cells divided to form a net connecting many

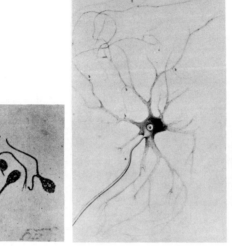
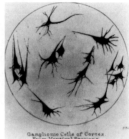

FIG. 2. Three pioneers in the identification of the processes of nerve cells. **R. Remak:** Nerve cells from the spinal cord of ox **(left).** (From *Observationes Anatomicae.* Reimer, Berlin, 1838.) **O. F. K. Deiters:** Anterior horn cell with axis cylinder and dendrites **(center).** (From *Untersuchungen über Gehirn und Rüchenmark.* Vieweg, Braunschweig.) **W. B. Lewis and H. Clarke:** The first illustration of pyramidal cells from the brain of man **(right).** (From *Proc. Roy. Soc., 27:38–49, 1878.*)

cells was outstandingly championed by Gerlach (16), who may be regarded as the father of the reticular theory.

Evidence against the network theory came early from two different workers with quite different approaches. The elder His (25), using human embryological material stained with hematoxylin, could find no evidence for network connections. Forel (12), also in Switzerland and employing retrograde degeneration, decided that nerve cells were in contact but never in continuity. But the controversy persisted.

Müller, in spite of his pupil's findings, accepted Valentin's strongly maintained postulate that nerve fibers surrounded the cell bodies but did not derive from them. Nevertheless, in spite of disagreeing with his student's position, Müller published it (46) in his journal together with Remak's description of a "primitive band" within the fiber (what later was to be known as the axis cylinder). Remak's "primitive band" was not immediately accepted and only later and after visiting Remak did Purkyně recognize (and name) the axis cylinder as a structure (42). In the days before photography, a direct demonstration proved more convincing than a sketch (Fig. 3).

This contribution of Remak's is really a turning point, since, by demonstrating more clearly than had Fontana, it ruled out once and for all the

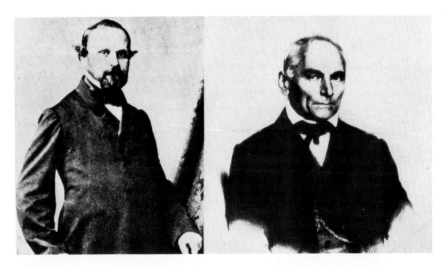

FIG. 3. Two early workers on the continuity of nerve cells and fiber: R. Remak **(left)** (1815–1865) and J. E. Purkyně **(right)** (1787–1869).

ancient Galenic concept of the core of the nerve fiber constituting a hollow channel for a nervous fluid. But the opposition was severe, especially from Valentin (54) and Henle (23), both of whom eventually relented, but not until the 1840s when the evidence became overwhelming. Valentin had undertaken the unusual course of founding a quarterly journal to publish solely his own work. This was called the *Reportorium für Anatomie und Physiologie* (55) and it is in volume 7, published in 1842, that we find his acceptance of Remak's axis cylinder.

In this museum, the locale of this symposium, surrounded by the magnificent wax models by Fontana, it is only appropriate to remind the audience of his classic work on the nerve fiber and its core, published as an appendix to the Florentine edition of his famous "Treatise on the Venim of the Viper" (11), to which Remak, at first skeptical, later gave recognition, although the interpretations of Fontana's findings were controversial and have remained so to this day.

The continuity of the fiber with the cell did not achieve universal acceptance until the time of Cajal, but it should be noted that the first confirmation of Remak's claim came from no less a scientist than Helmholtz in his doctoral thesis on invertebrate nerve, written in 1842 (22). The letters of Helmholtz to his father, in this period of his life, survive (28), and in them he tells how he was so certain of the origin of the fibers that he planned to offer his thesis in August of that year, but his teacher, Müller, being skeptical sent him back to examine a greater number of species. This he did, and finally obtained acceptance and his doctorate in November of 1842 (22).

Both Remak's work claiming this continuity and Helmholtz's confirmation were doctoral theses from the laboratory of Johannes Müller, who rejected the discovery, saying:

> "Concerning the direct connections of ganglionic globules with the grey fibers, I never was convinced of that in spite of the fact that Remak demonstrated to me often enough during his investigations the processes of the ganglionic globules" (37).

When Müller came to write his famous *Physiologie des Menschen* in 1844 (38), he gave considerable discussion to this problem (see p. 529).

The pioneer knowledge of the processes that emerge from nerve cells was largely gained from submammalian species or from the spinal cord. Only later do we find the groundwork for the study of architectonics in the brain.

For the cortex of man we have to wait until 1878 before we see pyramidal cells and these, described by their illustrators, Lewis and Clarke (31), as "ganglion cells," depict a number of processes emerging from the cell body. These workers found on the average seven such processes, and sometimes as many as 15 (Fig. 2). These are, of course, the giant pyramids that carry the name of Betz (6), professor at the University of Kiev who described them when making a special study of the motor region in dog, monkey, and man, publishing his results in 1874 and in 1881.

For the pioneers attempting to unravel the architectonics of the cortex there were two giant steps that had to be taken: first the unequivocal demonstration that the nerve fiber had its only origin in the nerve cell; and secondly, once that was accepted, that fibers deriving from different cell bodies did not form anastomoses. This second problem will be discussed later.

Throughout this search for the microstructure of the individual neuronal components lay the interest shown by all writers in the apparent lamination of the cerebral cortex, a feature observable by the naked eye, and therefore anticipating the work of the microscopists, which has just been discussed.

Our first description of this stratification comes to us just before the opening of the 19th century, from Gennari in 1782 (15), whose name is preserved as the eponym for the fine white line of myelinated fibers that runs parallel to the cortical surface. It is only fitting to add, here in Vienna, that it was Obersteiner (40,41) who named this white layer of the calcarine cortex "the line of Gennari" (Fig. 4).

Gennari described it as a "lineola albidior" and noted that, although he found it elsewhere in the brain, it was most conspicuous in "the internal part of the posterior lobe of the brain not far from the point in which it extends itself into the tentorium." Although he looked for it elsewhere in the horizontal strata of the brain and occasionally found what he called "a duplicate line," described as "subalbida," he notes that in no other place was it so evident as posteriorly.

At about this time, this "white line" was also described by Vicq d'Azyr (56,57) and by Soemmering (53), both being unaware of Gennari's descrip-

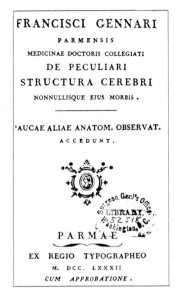

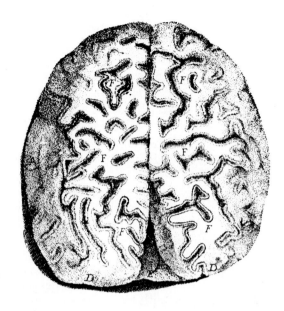

FIG. 4. The line of Gennari. Title page from F. Gennari (1752–1797) and his sketch of the brain (Parma, 1782).

tion. Vicq d'Azyr (in 1781), commenting that he found this only in the calcarine area, described it as follows:

"... la substance corticale y est interrompue suivant sa longeur, par un trait blanc linéaire qui suit tous les contours des convolutions, et qui donne à cette portion de la substance corticale, l'apparance d'un ruban rayé. ..."

The step taken, also by the naked eye, from detection of this prominent white stripe to the recognition of even other layerings in the cortex was contributed by a psychiatrist (or alienist as they were then called) at the asylum at Charenton near Paris. And this was Baillarger (3), who has also left an eponym to the cortex.

Baillarger, taking up earlier suggestions of Gall and of Nicholas Steno, approached the problem by regarding the grey substance of the cortex that he found in the convolutions as the prolongation of the fibers of the white matter, and therefore he may be regarded as the father of all the maps of the external surface of the brain that followed in such profusion at the turn of the century when localization of function became a major interest.

It was here in what he called "la substance grise extérieure du cerveau" that Baillarger hoped to find changes in brains from the insane as had, in fact, been reported by earlier French pathologists. To search for possible distortions he made it his goal to determine whether or not this grey substance was, in fact, made up of one or several layers. The great alienist, Pinel, had claimed that the three layers described by some earlier workers were abnormalities peculiar to the brains of manics and that the normal brain had one layer only.

Examination of 30 brains taken at random from patients who had died of various diseases convinced Baillarger that these layers were normal developments and not related to insanity. He also examined brains from calves, sheep, pigs, rabbits, cats, and dogs, and compared them with the less-laminated optic lobes of birds, reptiles, and fish. He was puzzled by the layers of fibers running parallel to the surface and thus crossing those ascending from the white matter and commented that they formed a "damier," a sort of checkerboard. He noted that they were less common in the brain of man than in those of lower animals.

Holding a thin slice of fresh cortex up to the light between two plates of glass [a technique used into this century by Elliot Smith (52)], Baillarger detected what he described as six layers and then published the famous picture which is familiar to all anatomists (Fig. 5). In this classic plate, published in 1840 (3), Baillarger gives great credit to Gennari, even reproducing two of his illustrations (Figs. 2 and 3, top center and top right). It is interesting that Baillarger with his naked eye perceived more detail in these thin slices of fresh tissue than Kölliker (29) with his microscope and fixed brains, who described (in 1854) just four layers. Remak, working with a magnifying glass, had, in 1844 (47), described and depicted six layers in the posterior lobe of the sheep.

For those of us who are electrophysiologists, it is interesting that Baillarger likened the stratification of the cortex to a voltaic pile, a suggestion made earlier by Rolando (48) for the cerebellum in which he had detected two layers. Rolando went even further, for he suggested that the alternate grey and white formed a "fluid" analogous to the galvanic "fluid," thought at that time to be the source of the electricity produced by the electric ray. To explain the unknown by analogy with electricity was, for years, very tempting. In a monograph entitled *Skull, Brain and Soul* by Emil Huscke (27), we find a section called "The Brain, an Electrical Apparatus," in which he views the two hemispheres as negative and positive, respectively, with their electrical connections running through the commissures. This model was strongly criticized by Meynert. It is in fact a surprise to find anyone speaking, as late as 1840, as Baillarger does, of a "fluide nerveux," since Remak had already demonstrated the axis cylinder filling the central core.

None of these investigators mentioned what the contribution of cell bodies might be to the appearance of these layers, i.e., their cytoarchitecture, although Remak made clear the role of fiber tracts and was aware that there were "ganglion" cells in the cortex. An idea of the cell content was first effectively contributed by Rudolf Berlin in 1858 (4) who, by using the carmine dye developed by Gerlach in the same year, was able to identify not only the layers but lying among them pyramidal cells, spindle cells, and granular cells.

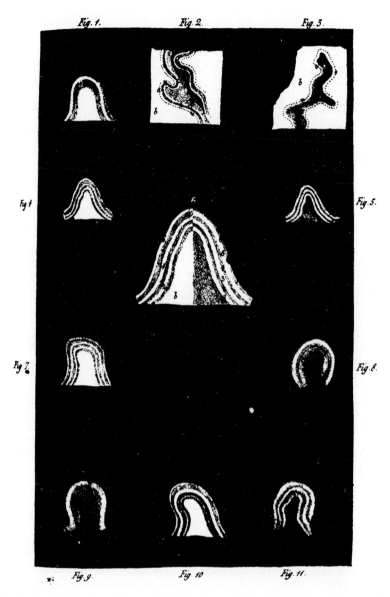

FIG. 5. Early depiction of the cortical layers and line of Gennari as drawn by Baillarger. His Figs. 2 and 3 are reproductions from Gennari. (From *Mem. Acad. R. Med.* (Paris), 8:149–183, 1840.)

But a major contribution was to come once again from a psychiatrist, and his motivation was essentially the same as Baillarger's before him: to link the functions of the mind with the intimate structure of the cortex — what he called the "organology of the cortical surface" (33). This was

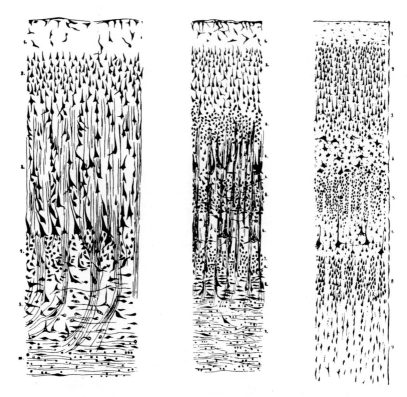

FIG. 6. Studies of cortical lamination. **Left and center:** Six-layered precentral cortex and eight-layered occipital cortex from Meynert. (From *Psychiatrie,* Braümuller 1884.) **Right:** Nine-layered calcarine cortex from Ramón y Cajal. (From *Histologie du Système Nerveux, Vol. 2,* 1911.)

Theodor Meynert, whose classic studies may be regarded as the starting point and basis of all modern histology of the cortex (34).

We find Meynert's depiction of the cortical layers in 1872 (35): Macroscopically, he said, one could discern three layers, but with his microscope he found five layers in the precentral cortex and eight layers in the occipital cortex. Figure 6 reproduces his specimen from the third frontal convolution of a human brain showing the extent of his third layer. This illustrates the point that was challenged later, namely that the large pyramids (the giant cells of Betz) are merged into the same layer as the angular cells above them.

Six years after the publication of Meynert's famous studies on the brains of mammals (35), Bevan Lewis, writing from the West Riding Asylum, that insane asylum that was also the workplace of David Ferrier, published in the inaugural volume of *Brain* in 1878 (30) and in the *Proceedings of the Royal Society* (31) in the same year, articles in which he described, for the first time in man, the giant pyramidal cells of the precentral gyrus (Fig. 2). He declared his belief that these cells had "motor significance," a conclusion that, in fact, Betz himself had reached from their counterparts in the lower animals.

In Bevan Lewis we meet our third psychiatrist in search of the architectonics of the cerebral cortex. He became director of the West Riding Lunatic Asylum and later Professor of Psychiatry at Leeds. Lewis and his colleague Clarke, working in the same institution as Ferrier, were undoubtedly influenced by the latter's extensive studies of motor function, for

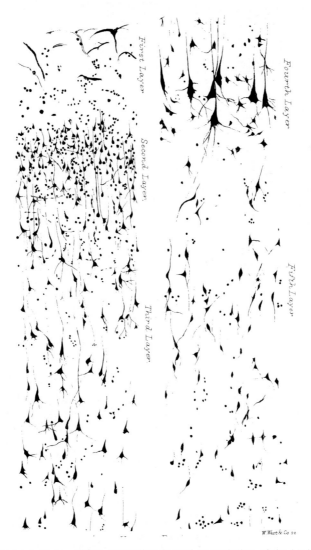

FIG. 7. Five-layered cortex of the ascending frontal convolution of the brain (Lewis and Clarke). (From *Proc. Roy. Soc.*, 27:38–49, 1878.)

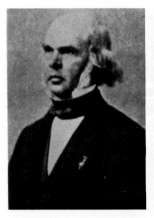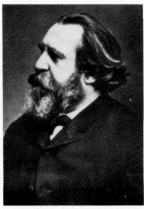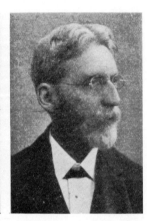

FIG. 8. Three psychiatrists who made major contributions to our knowledge of architectonics of the cortex: J. G. F. Baillarger **(left)** (1809–1890), T. Meynert **(center)** (1833–1892), and W. B. Lewis **(right)** (1847–1929).

we find their histological work focused on the precentral cortex. They were also working after Fritsch and Hitzig's demonstration (14) of the motor cortex by electrical stimulation, evidence not available to Meynert in his first writings.

After disagreeing on details with both Baillarger and Meynert, Lewis and Clarke proceeded to give detailed descriptions (and illustrations) of a five-layered human precentral cortex (Fig. 7). It is by their fourth layer that they challenged Meynert. Meynert had included in his third layer of the precentral cortex both the irregular angular cells and the large pyramids, giving the fourth layer to granule cells and numbering the spindle or fusiform cells as the fifth layer. Baillarger (who had named six layers) had put these irregular angular cells in the fourth layer and the spindle cells in the sixth (Fig. 8).

Lewis and Clarke's main emphasis (and remember that they were studying the precentral cortex) was on the very large pyramidal cells as shown in the layer they numbered as the fourth. They were immensely impressed by the size of these cells and differentiated them from the smaller angular cells. As a matter of fact, Meynert had indeed commented on their size, although he included them in his third layer together with the angular cells.

These giant cells are, as these workers pointed out, those described by Betz (6) and named by him "giant pyramids"—"die grossen Pyramidensellen"—and suggested by him as being motor in function. And Lewis and Clarke, using an ether-freezing microtome, by which they were able to get slices from different regions of the same human brain in rapid succession, were convinced that these cells predominated in the convolutions that Ferrier had demonstrated to be the motor area.

Because in other sections of the brain these cells of their fourth layer were not so large, they preferred to name them "ganglionic cells" rather than

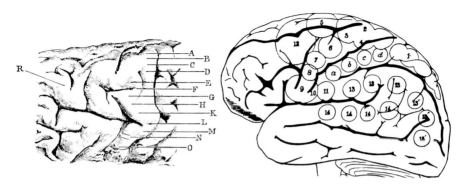

FIG. 9. Left: Location of motor cortex on the convolutions of the human brain. Lewis and Clarke's illustration in which they indicated area by A to D as analogous to numbers 2 and 4 on map **(right)**; published by D. Ferrier (1843–1928). (From *Proc. Roy Soc.,* 27: 38–49, 1878.) (Map from *Functions of the Brain,* Smith and Elder, London, 1876.)

"giant cells." The area of the precentral cortex in which they found the largest cells was labelled A to D in the sketch they published (Fig. 9). Correlating closely with Ferrier's work, they identified this zone of largest cells as that depicted by the numbers 2 and 4 in Ferrier's map (10). It should be remembered, however, that this map of Ferrier's is guesswork in which he transposed his findings in monkey to a map of the human convolutions. This method of transposition was also followed by Brodmann and by the Vogts.

In fact, most of the controversies between the earlier histologists concerning lamination lay in the fact that they were examining sections from different parts of the brain, a fact recognized by Meynert, who examined far more regions of the cortex than these workers. Meynert did not confine himself to the consideration of brain cells concerned only with motor function, for he was interested in sensory processes as they might be related to consciousness.

Figure 7 includes an illustration from Meynert of a sensory receiving area of cortex and is an example of his great contribution to the idea of receptor areas, the foundation of all the brain maps that were to follow in the first decades of the present century after Meynert's death in a period outside the scope of this review, and flowering in the classic work of von Economo and Koskinas (8). And when we come to the "sensations" evoked by sensory inflow we can perceive how much Munk was indebted to Meynert.

Meynert had started his work on the bat, work in which the goal was to follow the distribution and function of fiber tracts, a study which led him to introduce the terms now in use generally in their modern sense: namely, association and projection systems, a very great step forward in the understanding of the cortex. Meynert thus opened the field of exploration to the relationship of the cortex to other structures, such as the basal ganglia, (a term that had been introduced by Gall).

The science of architectonics then moved on from the detection of layers of nerve cells and fibers to the question of where these fibers went, where they came from, and what their function was. Far in the future, and unsuspected, lay the discoveries of laminar differences in chemical transmitters revealed by modern histochemistry in our own day.

From Meynert's work (33–35) we get the initial intense attack on the subject of the myelarchitectonics of the cortex: the arcuate fibers, the corpus callosum, the anterior commissure, the cerebellar peduncles, in other words, the destination and function of what he called the "conducting tracts" of his association and projection systems. He used the latter term for the fiber tracts running from the cortex to the thalamus and by connections via the brainstem to the spinal cord, as well as for connections from the retina to the occipital lobe. It is in an address given to the 9th International Congress of Medicine in Berlin (36) that we find Meynert's most philosophical analysis of the findings of interaction among brain regions.

Meynert should receive the credit for the sensory pathways to the cortex, including thalamocortical projections only guessed at by earlier workers. He called these tracts "Stiele" and distinguished four such: an anterior one to the frontal lobe, one from the anterior thalamus to what we now call the cingulate gyrus, and most clearly the connections between the occipital lobe and the pulvinar. This work foreshadowed that of the Swedish neurologist, Henschen (24), who at the end of the 19th century published his concepts, derived from autopsies, of the visual pathways to the calcarine cortex, ideas which were received with skepticism by Horsley, Hitzig, von Monokow, and other giants.

Early in this paper, reference was made to the second major problem facing the histologists of the cerebral cortex. Granted, eventually, that nerve fibers derived their origin from the nerve cell, there remained the question as to whether or not anastomoses formed between fibers from different nerve cells.

The idea of some degree of anastomosis died hard. Even Meynert, in his famous book on the brains of mammals (35), when announcing the postulate which he calls "the law of isolated conduction" states, he found "its morphological expression in the fact that the axes of the nerve cells appear to be elongated in the direction of the nerve fibre with which they are continuous." But, he makes some exceptions and states that: "Even in the grey masses, which doubtless constitute paths for transverse conduction by means of anastomoses, the law of isolated conduction holds good, though only conditionally."

He returns to this consideration of anastomoses when discussing the work of Arndt (2) and of Besser (5) who, he says, demonstrated them as occurring between the processes of cells in the cortex, and he later claims to have seen them.

"The fusiform body," Meynert wrote, "gives off laterally also from five to seven processes which, like the apical process, form demonstrable anastomoses." Later he writes: "On the occasion I distinctly saw the division of a medullary fibre in the cortex, or, in other words, the formation of such a fibre from the processes of two cells."

There was, at this time, some question as to whether or not a distinction had to be made between vertebrates (as studied by Meynert) and invertebrates. And one may take an example from the work of one of his pupils but one who made his career in a totally different field. In a paper written in 1882, Sigmund Freud (13) gives a camera lucida drawing of an apparent anastomosis of nerve fibers in tissue from fresh water crabs, the same animal used so much by Remak.

A variant of the problem of anastomoses reached into the present century in the form of a reticular theory of neurofibrils, but this lies beyond the period of this review.

But during and following the period under discussion, technical advances were to come once more to the aid of the histologist. In the last decades of the 19th century, these technical developments led to a tremendous expansion of work on the structure of the cortex and to the rise of the Spanish school spearheaded by Ramón y Cajal. His work is so well known to all that it will not be reviewed in detail.

Cajal's major publications in their original language are in Boletins, Gaceta, and Revista that were published in very few copies and remain rarities outside Spain. The greater number of them appeared in the last decade of the old century and the first of the new, including his magnum opus, the three volumes of which in their original language are dated 1894–1904. These, however, were not generally distributed until translated into French (as two volumes) in this century (44). Scientists all over the world are indebted to the many translators who have made these writings available in other languages.

After so much discussion of the mid-19th-century explorations of the laminar characteristics of the cortex, it is only fitting to look at those published toward the turn of the century by Cajal (Fig. 6). When describing the calcarine cortex, Cajal gives it nine layers as shown in this illustration of a Nissl preparation.

Cajal, as we know, added immensely to our knowledge of the intimate structure of the cerebral cortex. To mention just one example, we may take his analysis of the short-axoned cells of the first layers (43), the layer noted by Meynert to be so poor in cells and thought by Golgi to be solely occupied by neuroglia. Using several different staining procedures (including Erlich's methylene blue), Cajal produced beautiful pictures of the many short-axoned cells he found in this, first, plexiform layer—and not all were in immature cortex (Fig. 10). These studies of Cajal's mark the development of

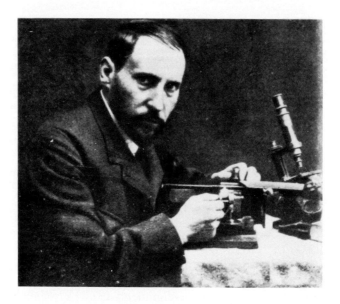

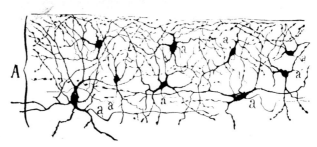

FIG. 10. S. Ramón y Cajal (1852–1934) and his illustration of short-axoned cells running parallel to the cortex. (From *Rev. Trim. Micrgr., 2*, 1897.)

interest moving from the solely vertically oriented distribution of neurons in the cortex to their horizontal interactions, and to the whole question of tangential spread of fibers, which was to interest a later generation.

Cajal had long been working with silver reduction methods but was jubilant when he first tried Golgi's technique of osmic dichromate fixation followed by silver. In French translation he exclaimed:

"Spectacle inattendu! Sur un fond jaune d'une translucidité parfaite, apparaissent, clairemés des filaments noirs, lisses et minces, ou épineux et épais, des corps noirs, triangulaires, étoilés, fusiformes! on dirait des dessins à l'encre de Chine sur un papier transparent du Japon."

It is most prominently in the work of Cajal and his contemporary, Golgi, that we find attention given to the mesh-work of the cortex, not only to the long projection pathways which were pioneered by Meynert and differentiated by Hammerberg in 1895 (21) into motor and sensory, but to the interplay between neurons in the form, for example, of collateral and recurrent collaterals (Fig. 11). We find beautiful illustrations of recurrent collaterals in Golgi's illustrations. Note here especially his Fig. 3 and the cell that bears his name in Fig. 6.

The period under review covers architectonics studied in two dimensions. Only later, a half century later to be exact, was an attack made on the three-dimensional architectonics of the cortex and was an attempt by Sholl (51) to quantify the neuronal arborizations found in his Golgi-Cox studies, thus opening up the whole field to a mathematical approach. For structure studied alone left open the question of function. How did these nerve cells intercommunicate?

The problem of function was a question not only for the anatomist but also for the physiologist. The premier English textbook of physiology in the 19th century, Michael Foster's *Textbook of Physiology,* had, by the 1890s, run to six editions. Foster planned as a seventh edition a volume devoted solely to the nervous system and asked a former pupil, Charles Sherrington, to write it (50). It is in this volume published in 1897 that we

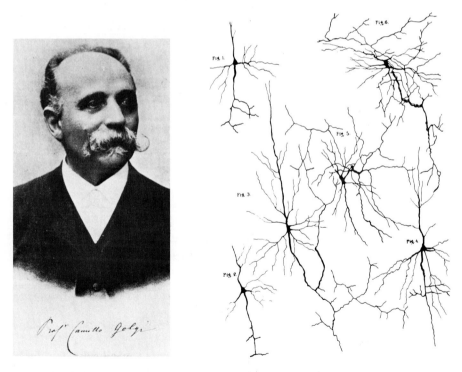

FIG. 11. C. Golgi (1843–1926) and one of his illustrations showing recurrent collaterals. (From *Untersuchungen über feineren Bau des centralen und peripherischen Nervensystems,* Jena, 1894.)

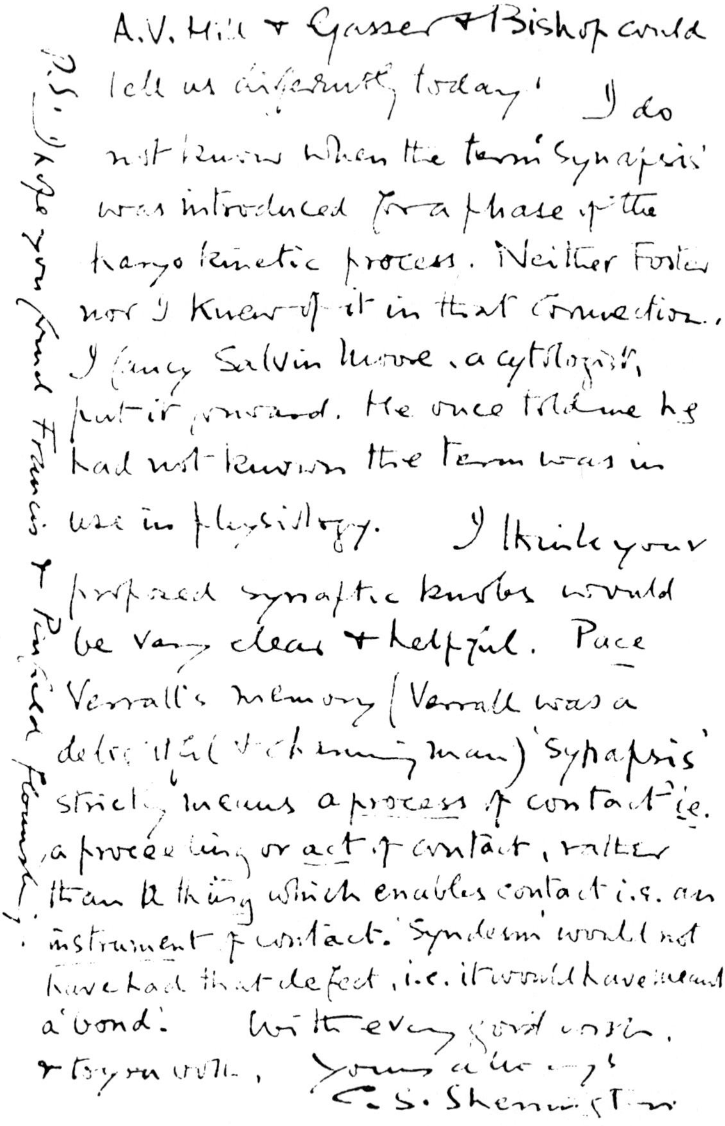
A.V. Hill & Gasser & Bishop could
tell us differently today! I do
not know when the term 'Synapsis'
was introduced for a phase of the
karyokinetic process. Neither Foster
nor I knew of it in that connection.
I fancy Salvin Moore, a cytologist,
put it forward. He once told me he
had not known the term was in
use in physiology. I think your
proposed synaptic knobs would
be very clear & helpful. Pace
Verrall's memory (Verrall was a
delightful & charming man) 'Synapsis'
strictly means a process of contact i.e.
a proceeding or act of contact, rather
than the thing which enables contact i.e. an
instrument of contact. 'Syndesm' would not
have had that defect, i.e. it would have meant
a 'bond'. With every good wish,
& to your work, Yours always,
C. S. Sherrington

P.S. I hope you & your friend Francis & Penfield flourish!

FIG. 12. Page of a letter from C. S. Sherrington (1857–1952) describing his choice of the word "synapse." (By courtesy of the Fulton Collection, Yale University Medical Library.)

find Sherrington's concern with how messages are carried between neurons and it is here that we find the first use of the word "synapse."

It is interesting that Cajal, who was naturally concerned with the interaction between cells since he rejected continuity and anastomoses, made no reference in his Nobel lecture to Sherrington or to his concepts of synapsis. Cajal stated there that, "Un ciment granuleux ou substance conductrice particulière servirait à relier très intimement les surfaces neuronales en contact." It was only much later, after the publication of the Silliman lectures, that we find Cajal acknowledging Sherrington's views on the synapse.

Decades later, when Sherrington was asked why he chose this word, he explained in a letter to Fulton (written in 1937) that when he had begun to write the part on the nervous system he had not got far with it before he felt "the need for some name to call the junction between nerve cell and nerve cell." He wrote Foster of his "wish to introduce a specific name" and suggested using "syndesm" from the Greek. He was talked out of this by Foster's friend Verrall who preferred "synapse" because it had an easier adjectival form (Fig. 12). Sherrington in the same letter expresses regret that he had been persuaded by Verrall to use "synapse."

As one reads from this original letter: "Synapsis," Sherrington says "strictly means a *process* of contact, i.e., a proceeding or *act* or contact, i.e., an *instrument* of contact. Syndesm would not have had that defect, i.e., it would have meant a bond."

But synapse it remained. This word, coming into the vocabulary of anatomists and physiologists at the end of the century under review, received worldwide adoption and has never been challenged. The synaptic organization of the cortex is the basis of all modern studies of the architectonics of the cerebral cortex.

REFERENCES

1. Apáthy, S. von (1897): Das leitende Element des Nervensystems und seine topographischen Beziehungen zu den Zellen. *Mitt. Zoo. Stat.,* 12:15–29.
2. Arndt, R. (1867): Studien über die Architectonik der Grosshirnrinde. *Schutze's Arch. Anat.,* 3 and 4: 441–476.
3. Baillarger, J.-G.-F. (1840): Recherches sur la structure de la couche corticale des circonvolutions du cerveau. *Mem. Acad. R. Med. Belg.,* 8:149–183.
4. Berlin, R. (1858): *Beitrag zur Strukturlehre der Grosshirnwindungen.* Junge, Erlangen.
5. Besser, L. (1866): Zur Histogenese der nervösen Elementartheile in den Centralorganen des neugebornen Menschen. *Arch. Pathol. Anat. Physiol. Klin. Med.,* 36:305–334.
6. Betz, V. (1874): Antomischer Nachweis zweier Gehirnzentra. *Zentralbl. Med. Wiss.,* 12:578–580; 595–599.
7. Deiters, O. F. K. (1865): *Untersuchungen über Gehirn und Ruchenmark des Menschen und der Säugethiere.* Vieweg, Braunschweig.
8. Economo, C. von, and Koskinas, G. N. (1925): *Die Cytoarchitektonik der Hirnrinde des erwachsenen Menschen.* Springer, Vienna.
9. Erlich, P. (1868): Über die Methyleneblaureaction der lebenden Nervensubstanz. *Dtsch. Med. Wochenschr.,* 12:49–52.
10. Ferrier, D. (1876): *The Functions of the Brain.* Smith Elder, London.
11. Fontana, F. (1781): *Traité sur le Vénin de la Vipère.* Florence (2 vols).
12. Forel, A.-H. (1887): Einige hirnanatomische Betrachtungen und Ergebnisse. *Arch Psychiatr. Nervenkr.,* 18:162–198.
13. Freud, S. (1882): Über den Bau der Nervenfasern und Nervenzellen beim Flusskrebs. *Sitz. Math-Natur. Akad. Wiss. Wien,* 85:9–46.
14. Fritsch, G. T., and Hitzig, E. (1870): Über die elektrische Erregbeit des Grosshirns. *Arch. Anat. Physiol. Wiss. Med.,* 37:300–332.
15. Gennari, F. (1782): *De Peculiari Structura Cerebri Nonnullisque Ejus Morbis.* Parma.

16. Gerlach, J. von (1872): Über die Structur der grauern Substanz des menschlichen Gros-shirns. *Zentralbl. Med. Wiss.*, 10:273–275.
17. Golgi, C. (1873): Sulla sostanza grigia del cervello. *Gazetta Med. Ital. Lombardia*, 6:244–246.
18. Golgi, C. (1874): Sulla sostanza grigia del cervello. Reale Istituto Lombardo. *Rep. II*, 7:69P.
19. Golgi, C. (1894): *Untersuchungen über den feineren Bau des centralen und peripherischen Nervensystems*. Fischer, Jena.
20. Golgi, C. (1900): Intorno alla struttura delle cellule nervose della corteccia cerebrale. *Verh. Anat. Ges.*, 14:164–176.
21. Hammerberg, C. (1895): Studien über Klinik und Pathologie der Idiote. *Druck der Akad.*, Bruchdruckerei, Uppsala.
22. Helmholtz, H. (1842): *De Fabrica Systematis nervosi evertebratorum*. Doctoral thesis, Nietahkianis, Berlin.
23. Henle, J. (1839): Anmerkung zum vorigen Aufsatz. *Müller's Arch. Anat. Physiol. Wiss.*, pp. 170–171.
24. Henschen, S. E. (1893): On the visual path and centre. *Brain*, 16:170–180.
25. His, W. (1888): Über die embryonale Entwickelung der Nervenbahnen. *Anat. Anz.*, 3: 499–506.
26. Hodgkin, T., and Lister, J. J. (1827): Notice of some microscopic observations of the blood and animal tissues. *Phil. Mag.*, 2:130–138.
27. Huscke, E. (1854): *Schädel, Hirn und Seele des Menschen und der Thiere nach Alter, Geschlecht und Race*. Mauke, Jena.
28. Koenigsberger, L. (1906): *Hermann von Helmholtz*. Clarendon Press, Oxford.
29. Kölliker, A. von (1850–1854): *Mikroskopische Anatomie, oder Gewebelehre des Menschen*. Englemann, Leipzig.
30. Lewis, W. B. (1878): On the comparative structure of the cortex cerebri. *Brain*, 1:79–86.
31. Lewis, W. B. and Clarke, H. (1878): The cortical lamination of the motor area of the brain. *Proc. Roy. Soc.*, 27:38–49.
32. Malpighi, M. (1666): De cerebre cortice. In: *Viscerum Structura Exercitatio Anatomica*, pp. 50–70. Montius, Bologna.
33. Meynert, T. (1884): *Psychiatrie: Klinik der Erkrankungen des Vordeshirns* (Erste Hälfe). Braumüller, Vienna.
34. Meynert, T. (1867–1868): Der Bau der Gross-Hirnrinde und seine örtichen Verschie-denheiten, nebst einem pathologisch-anatomischen Corollarium. *Viertejahrschr. Psychia-try*, 1867, 1:77–93 and 125–217; 1868, 1:381–403; and 1868, 2:88–113.
35. Meynert, T. (1869–1872): Vom Gehirne der Säugethiere. *Handbuch der Lehre von den Geweben des Menschen und der Thiere*, 2:694–808. Translated by the New Sydenham Society, 1870–1893 (edited by Stricker).
36. Meynert, T. (1891): *Über das Zussammenwirken der Gehirntheile. Tenth International Medical Congress*, Vol. 1, pp. 173–190. Hirschwald, Berlin.
37. Müller, J. (1839): Anastomosen oder Verästelungen der Fasern in den Ganglien wurden nie wahrgenommen. *Müllers Arch. Anat. Physiol. Wiss.*, p. 201.
38. Müller, J. (1844): *Handbuch der Physiologie des Menschen*. Hölscher, Coblenz.
39. Nissl, F. (1903): *Die Neuronlehre und ihre Arhänger*. Fischer, Jena.
40. Obersteiner, H. (1888): *Anleitung beim Studium des Baues der nervösen Centralorgane in gesunden und Kranken Zustande*. Deuticke, Wien.
41. Obersteiner, H. (1896): *Anleitung beim Studium des Baues der nervösen Centralorgane*. Deuticke, Wien, 572 pp.
42. Purkyně, J. E. (1838): Bericht über die Versammlung deutscher Naturforscher und Ärtze in Prag im September 1837. *Anat. Physiol. Verhandlungen*, 3 (Sect. 5) 177–180.
43. Ramón y Cajal, S. (1897): Las celulas de cilindro-eje corto de la capa molecular de cere-bro. *Rev. Trim. Microgr.*, 2:5–7.
44. Ramón y Cajal, S. (1911): *Histologie du Système Nerveux de l'Homme et des Verté-brés*. Maloine, Paris (2 vols).
45. Remak, R. (1838): *Observationes Anatomicae et Microscopicae de Systematis Nervosi Structura*. Reimer, Berlin, 41 pp.
46. Remak, R. (1841): Anatomische Beobachtungen über das Gehirn, das Ruckenmark und die Nervenwurzeln. *Müllers Arch. Anat. Physiol. Wiss.*, pp. 506–522.

47. Remak, R. (1844): Neurologische Erlauterungen Medicin. *Müllers Arch. Anat. Physiol. Wiss.,* pp. 463–472.
48. Rolando, L. (1809): *Saggio Sopra la Vera Struttura del Cervello dell'uomo e degl' Animali e Sopra le Funzioni del Sistema Nervoso.* Sassari, 98 pp.
49. Schwann, T. (1839): *Mikroskopische Untersuchungen über die Übereinstimmung in der Struktur und dem Wachsthum der Thiere und Pflanzen.* Reimer, Berlin.
50. Sherrington, C. S. (1897): In: Foster's *Textbook of Physiology,* 7th edition, Macmillan, New York.
51. Sholl, D. A. (1956): *The Organization of the Cerebral Cortex.* Methuen, London and Wiley, New York.
52. Smith, G. Elliot (1907): A new topographical survey of human cerebral cortex, being an account of the anatomically distinct cortical areas and their relationship to the cerebral sulci. *J. Anat. Physiol.,* 41:237–254.
53. Soemmering, S. T. (1788): *Vom Hirn und Ruckenmark.* Winkopp, Mainz.
54. Valentin, G. G. (1836): Über den Verlauf und die letzten Ende der Nerven. *Nova Acta Phys.-Med. Acad. Leopoldina, Breslau,* 18:51–240.
55. Valentin, G. G. (1842): *Report. Anat. Physiol.,* Vol. 7.
56. Vicq d'Azyr, F. (1781): Sur la structure du cerveau, du cervelet, de la moelle alongée, de la moelle épinière; et sur l'origine des nerfs de l'homme et des animaux. *Mem. Acad. R. Sci.,* pp. 495–622.
57. Vicq d'Azyr, F. (1786): *Traité d'Anatomie et de Physiologie.* Didot, Paris.
58. Weigert, C. (1882): Über eine neue Untersuchungsmethode des Zentralnervensystems. *Zentralbl. Med. Wiss.;* 20:753–757, 772–774.
59. Weigert, C. (1890): Bemerkungen über das Neurogliagerüst des menschlichen Central-nervensystems. *Anat. Anz.,* 5:543–551.

Architectonics of the Cerebral Cortex,
edited by M. A. B. Brazier and H. Petsche.
Raven Press, New York © 1978.

The Meynert Cell, an Unusual Cortical Pyramidal Cell

Sanford L. Palay

Department of Anatomy, Harvard Medical School, Boston, Massachusetts 02115

Although large nerve cells are not unknown in the mammalian central nervous system (spinal ganglion cells and ventral horn motor neurons are examples), certain large neurons in the human cerebral cortex have attracted an unusual amount of attention because they stand out in a field of generally small cells. The Betz cells in the precentral gyrus are probably the most famous examples of this group. These are gigantic pyramidal cells lying in lamina V, a layer heavily populated with large pyramidal cells, and they give rise to some of the nerve fibers in the corticospinal tract.

It is less well known that another group of giant pyramidal cells lies in the cortex lining the banks of the calcarine fissure and is especially numerous in the region where the macula of the retina is represented. Since these cells were first noticed in a description of the human visual cortex by Meynert (14) they have been given his name. Meynert's description of them was very brief: large, isolated, pyramidal cells with thick, heavy basal processes running horizontally within the laminae and particularly conspicuous in the deeper layers of the cortex. Ramón y Cajal (17) was more specific about their location, noting that they were arranged in a row in his seventh layer of the cortex, but he added nothing to their description. Le Gros Clark (8), however, in a study of Meynert cells in the monkey, placed them in lamina VI or at the boundary between laminae VI and V, according to the conventions that had been generally adopted by that time. He also carried out the first intensive study of them, measuring and counting them, describing their reactions to silver stains, and trying to trace their projections. Like the Betz cells, Meynert cells are difficult to distinguish from other pyramidal cells in the lower orders of mammals and it may even be doubted whether they exist as a separate entity in these animals. Shkol'nik-Yarros (18) reported that in the mouse, rabbit, and guinea pig the presumed Meynert cells are arranged in groups but are only slightly different from the other large pyramidal cells of lamina V. In carnivores and primates, however, Meynert cells are readily distinguishable from the other pyramids by their considerably greater size and their solitary disposition. In addition, they differ in various cytological features from ordinary pyramidal cells,

31

as will be described in the present paper. It is therefore inaccurate and perhaps misleading to regard them as merely large pyramidal cells (9,10).

MATERIALS AND METHODS

Meynert cells in 14 young adult *Macaca mulatta* were studied by means
of both light and electron microscopy according to methods previously
described (2). Golgi preparations were made from the brains of six of these
adult monkeys and also from two 6-week-old monkeys. The tissues of the
other eight adult monkeys were prepared for electron microscopy in the
usual manner (15). One to two micron sections from large blocks of cortex
were stained with toluidine blue. Thicker sections were treated with sodium
hydroxide in ethanol in order to remove the embedding resin and were then
stained with a modified Holmes silver stain. These two kinds of stained
preparations were used for counting and measuring Meynert cells and for
estimating intercellular distance.

CYTOLOGICAL FEATURES

In sections stained with toluidine blue, as in any Nissl preparation,
Meynert cells stand out by reason of their large size and their fleshy dendrites. According to the now generally used lamination scheme of Brodmann
(1), they lie in the lower half of the fifth cortical cell layer (2). The cell bodies
most often appear as irregular triangles, 20 to 30 μm wide at their base
and 40 to 50 μm high, with one or two thick and rapidly tapering dendrites
departing from one or more of their angles. Since none of the dendrites can
be followed very far in these thin sections, the cell bodies often appear
quite lopsided. The cytoplasm is generally voluminous and pale, with distinct, small and large Nissl bodies scattered about. At the base of each
dendrite the Nissl substance clears so that the dendrites appear as nearly
colorless channels cutting through the neuropil. The Meynert cell nucleus,
a large, round, vesicular body, is usually deeply creased on one side facing
the origin of a large basal dendrite. Nissl substance fills up the crease to
form a nuclear cap.

In electron micrographs the explanation for the usual pallor of the Meynert cell cytoplasm is evident. The cell body is laced with streams of parallel
microtubules and neurofilaments along with clusters of slender mitochondria. The granular endoplasmic reticulum is arrayed as a diffuse network
of predominantly small Nissl bodies, and the agranular reticulum is widely
dispersed as small Golgi complexes. All of these organelles also appear in
the stout dendrites, but longitudinally oriented neurofilaments and microtubules are the most prominent (Fig. 1). In fact neurofilaments are the most
conspicuous structures in the dendrites of Meynert cells. In this respect
the dendrites of Meynert cells differ from those of other pyramidal cells in

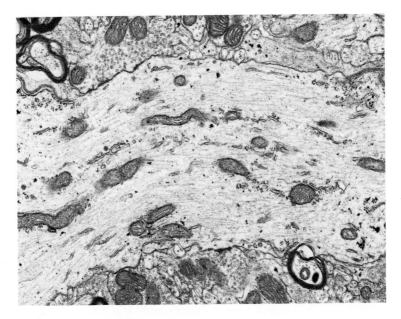

FIG. 1. Dendrite of a Meynert cell in longitudinal section. In addition to the usual organelles, the dendrite displays a large number of neurofilaments throughout. ×17,000. (From ref. 2.)

the visual cortex, which contain predominantly microtubules. The dendrites of certain other large neurons in mammals also display prominent neurofilaments, for example, the ventral horn cells of the spinal cord (23) and the Betz cells of the precentral cortex (7). In these dendrites, however, the neurofilaments travel in gently twisting cables confined to discrete longitudinal trajectories. In the dendrites of Meynert cells the neurofilaments also run in slender fascicles, but because they are so numerous they are dispersed throughout the cross section of the process. As a result of these characteristic features, the profiles of Meynert cell dendrites can be recognized even where they are separated from their perikaryon by the plane of section. The large number of neurofilaments may account for the dense staining of Meynert cells with silver methods.

Some of the Meynert cells in these animals contain crystalline mitochondrial inclusions enclosed within a membrane. One or several crystals may appear in a single mitochondrial profile, and they display a lattice structure comprised of plates 2 to 4 μm long and about 0.5 μm wide. Each plate contains repeating units about 20 nm in diameter. The nature of these crystals is unknown.

In each specimen a small number of pyknotic Meynert cells appear. These cells stain intensely with toluidine blue. In electron micrographs they are extremely dark and bear a highly irregular, ruffled surface. The nucleus is dense and the dark cytoplasm is full of mitochondria, membranes of the endoplasmic reticulum, and ribosomes. The Golgi apparatus is conspicuous because the lumina of its cisternae remain open. Apparently normal synaptic terminals are attached to the surface of such cells. The interstitial space is not enlarged and the adjacent neuropil as well as neighboring neuronal perikarya display no hint of disturbance.

GOLGI PREPARATIONS

The general form of Meynert cells is best displayed in Golgi preparations sectioned in a plane vertical to the pial surface so that the entire sweep of the dendritic tree is manifest. When several Meynert cells are impregnated in the same section, such preparations show that these giant cells belong to a relatively homogeneous class of cells with very similar morphological features (Fig. 2).

In addition to the broad pyramidal cell body, these cells have massive basal dendrites, which descend like stout roots from the basal angles of the perikarya into lamina VI and into the margin of the white matter. These basal dendrites spread out toward the horizontal plane and, without branching very much, occupy a cone-shaped territory in layers V and VI. The spreading basal dendrites overlap considerably, forming a mat of interwoven processes. The dendrites are richly supplied with long, slender spines, each fitted with a bulbous tip. The spines are usually 1 to 2 μm long, but occasionally one is as long as 3 or 4 μm, and they are spaced an average of 1.86 μm apart. Also originating from the basal side of the cell body or occasionally from one of the basal or apical dendrites is the axon, which springs from a low axon hillock and quickly narrows into a thin initial segment (Fig. 2). It then traverses lamina VI straight into the white matter, beyond which it could not be followed.

A single robust dendrite rises from the apex of the perikaryon and following a nearly straight trajectory passes through the successive overlying layers, until it subdivides at the beginning of lamina II into an umbellate terminal arbor that extends through laminae II and I and ends near the pial surface (Fig. 2). The terminal apical branchlets resemble the basal dendrites in occupying a cone-shaped territory and in being studded with spines, but the territories of neighboring Meynert cells overlap very little if at all and the spines are much farther apart. The apical dendrite itself is the most fascinating part of the Meynert cell (Fig. 3). It rises vertically from the apex of the perikaryon and for a distance of 30 to 60 μm it rapidly tapers to its definitive diameter. In this stretch its surface is smooth and it gives off two or three secondary branches which ramify weakly within lamina V. These collaterals are spiny like the basal dendrites, and since they are confined to lamina V, they probably should be regarded as filling out the territories of

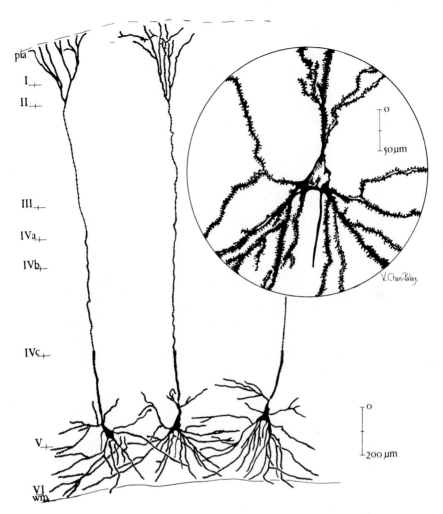

FIG. 2. Three neighboring Meynert cells in a Golgi preparation. The perikarya lie in the lower stratum of lamina V and their dendrites ascend to the pial surface. The cell in the center is shown in the inset at a higher magnification in order to display the differential spine density of the basal and apical dendrites. Rapid Golgi preparation, 600-g monkey, 90-μm section. (From ref. 2.)

the basal dendrites. For the next 250 to 300 μm of its path the apical dendrite traverses lamina V. On this stretch it exhibits a pubescent surface produced by closely set spines, 1 to 2 μm in length. At the margin of lamina V with lamina IV the density of spines suddenly diminishes and over the next 500 μm the spines become progressively farther apart. At the margin between laminae IVb and IVa (Fig. 3) the incidence of spines decreases again, so that there may be long stretches of dendrite without any append-

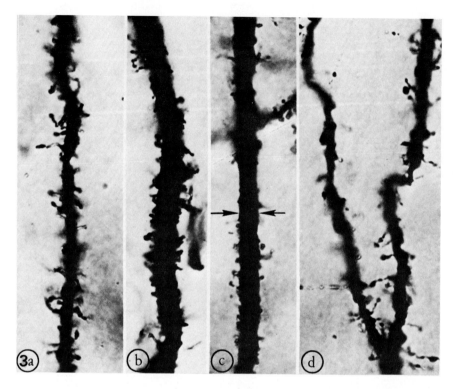

FIG. 3. Representative portions of the dendrites of a Meynert cell. **a:** Basal dendrite show-ing many slender, delicate spines with thin necks and bulbous tips. **b:** Apical dendrite in lamina V is covered with a fine pubescence produced by many close-set spines. **c:** The transition zone (arrows) at the boundary between laminae IVb and IVa, where the spines on the apical dendrite suddenly become markedly reduced. **d:** Terminal apical bouquet in lamina I and II with spines resembling those on the basal dendrites. Rapid Golgi prepara-tion, 90-μm section. ×3,750. (From ref. 2.)

ages at all, and those that do appear are only 1 to 1.5 μm long. This relatively smooth condition persists from the margin between laminae IVb and IVa to the terminal arborization in lamina II where spines reappear.

The counts of spines on a single representative Meynert cell are given in Table 1 (2). The total number of spines on a single cell is estimated in this way to be about 36,000. According to this single sample, over 77% of the spines of a Meynert cell are found on the basal dendrites, which account for only 66% of the total length of the dendritic arborization. It is interesting, however, that the short stretch of apical dendrite that crosses lamina V accounts for almost 10% of the total number of spines projecting from the whole dendritic tree. The rest of the apical dendrite before its terminal arborization possesses only 2.5% of the spines on the whole dendritic tree but 7.4% of the total length. The terminal arborization with about 23% of the total dendritic length has from 8 to 13% of the total number of spines.

TABLE 1. *Number of spines on the dendrites of a single Meynert cell (2)*

Segment	Visible spines (per 100 μm)	Total length of dendrites (μm)	Average diameter of dendrite (μm)	Circumference of dendrite (μm)	Distance between spines (μm)	Total spines
Basal dendrites	110	10,151[a]	2.94	9.24	.86	27,750
Apical dendrite and collaterals in layer V	127	622	4.4	13.80	.56	3,523
Apical dendrite in layers IVb and IVc	69	518	3.5	11.09	2.86	703
Apical dendrite in layers IVa and III	33	624	3.2	10.16	5.88	184
Terminal bouquet of apical dendrite in layers II and I	76	3,476[a]	2.96[b] 1.76[b]	9.24 5.53	2.63	4,636 2,774
Total for cell		15,391				35,865

[a] Total dendritic length calculated from the measured length of dendrites and branches within the section multiplied by the reciprocal of the volume fraction of the conical field occupied by the section. This fraction is given approximately by the ratio of the thickness of the section to the radius of cone of spread of the dendrites, i.e., 90 per 400 μm and 90 per 200 μm for the basal and apical dendritic cones, respectively.

[b] The two figures give the range of diameters of these tapering dendrites.

These figures, of course, are derived from only a single cell, but study of other Meynert cells indicated that the pattern of dendrites and spines is much the same in all. If it is recalled that each spine is the site of at least one synaptic junction with an afferent axon, then the typical Meynert cell can be assumed to receive at least 36,000 synapses. In fact, however, each cell must receive many more synapses, since each spine may have more than one junction and spine counts do not register the synaptic junctions on the shafts of the dendrites or on the soma. It would not be extravagant to propose that each Meynert cell may make as many as 100,000 synapses with afferent fibers. This number is comparable to Cragg's (4) estimate of 60,000 as the number of synapses made by an average pyramidal cell in the motor cortex of monkey.

The distribution of the spines, however, appears to differ from that shown by pyramidal cells elsewhere in the cortex. In a detailed examination of the distribution of spines along the apical dendrites of lamina V pyramidal cells in several mammals including man, Valverde (21) and Valverde and Ruiz-Marcos (22) showed that the number of spines first increases exponentially with distance from the perikaryon and then decreases again in the distal half of the dendrite. No indication was found of a relation between the distribution of spines and the cortical laminae through which the apical dendrite passes. Moreover, the pattern of spine distribution was found to be independent of the location of the pyramid in the cortex. However, only the vertically ascending part of the apical dendrite was considered, and the terminal arborization in laminae II and I was omitted. Marin-Padilla (12) and Marin-Padilla and Stibitz (13) reported very similar findings in human and hamster cortices, but included the entire trajectory of the apical dendrites of lamina V pyramids through the most superficial laminae. The latter authors, however, discerned sharp changes in the number of spines at the transition between laminae IV and III (an increase) and again in the upper portion of lamina III (a progressive decrease). They suggested that the distribution of the spines along the apical dendrite coincided with the distribution of different incoming cortical axons, which ramify specifically in different cortical layers. The apical dendrite of the Meynert cell displays a totally different pattern of spine distribution. After a smooth beginning it suddenly attains a high spine density which lasts for only 400 to 500 μm, during its traverse of lamina V. For the next 1,000 μm or so the spine density is quite low and steadily decreases until the terminal bouquet of branches is reached. These are modestly spiny again.

In comparing the results on ordinary pyramids with the distribution of spines on the Meynert cell, it becomes clear that the latter bears a strong relation to the lamination pattern of the cortex. According to the distribution of its dendritic spines the Meynert cell receives major inputs from laminae I and II and from laminae V and VI. These layers contain afferents from other cortical areas and axon collaterals of cells in the intermediate laminae of the same area. The small number of dendritic spines in laminae III and IV indicate that the Meynert cell receives relatively little input from the axonal plexus in these layers; consequently it appears to be little concerned with direct geniculocalcarine inputs and much more with the results of intracortical computations. This suggestion is in line with a recently discovered projection site for the axons of Meynert cells in the marmoset. In this animal, injections of horseradish peroxidase into the deeper layers of the middle temporal visual cortex resulted in labeling of Meynert cells in the ipsilateral visual cortex (20). Although it is not completely certain that such projections to another cortical area are the only or the primary target for Meynert cell axons, injections of peroxidase into the superior colliculus or the lateral geniculate body of macaques have failed to label Meynert cells in area 17 (11).

Measurements in Golgi, Nissl, and Holmes silver preparations permit one to estimate the overall size and shape of the territory occupied by a Meynert cell. As may be seen in Fig. 4, the cell body, the first part of the apical

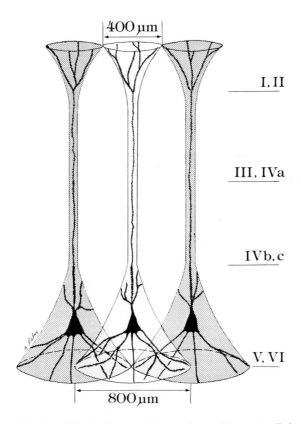

FIG. 4. Diagram of the dendritic territories of three adjacent Meynert cells in the perifoveal region of area 17. (From ref. 2.)

dendrite, and the basal dendritic arborization extend through a cone-shaped field about 800 μm across at its base in lamina VI and 650 μm tall. The apical dendrite connects this cone with another, smaller, and inverted cone, approximately 400 μm in diameter at the pial surface, which is occupied by the spreading terminal arborization in laminae I and II. The basal cones overlap extensively with their neighbors, since in the macular area of representation Meynert cells are spaced only 110 μm apart (center-to-center distance) and in the perifoveal area they are only 400 μm apart. The apical cones, however, barely touch in the perifoveal area and overlap extensively in the area of macular representation, which is the most crowded area.

Overlapping of the dendritic territories means, of course, an overlap in the synaptic input to neighboring cells from the axonal plexus of laminae V and VI especially and of laminae I and II to a lesser extent. Thus, neighboring cells may be in some respects redundant. The existence of a small number of dark or hyperchromic Meynert cells may be related to this redundancy. Le Gros Clark (8) estimated that in the monkey's macular area Meynert cells occurred at a density of 130 cells per cm^2 whereas our own data indicate a density of 8,000 per cm^2 in the same region (2). Our data came from animals that were all young (weighing 3 to 5 kg), but the age of the animals in Le Gros Clark's study is unknown. He refers to only one monkey of average size which weighed close to 4,000 g. He used the brain of this animal to measure the surface area of the visual cortex, but the size of the animals in which he made his cell counts is not specified. An intensive study of the numbers of Meynert cells in the visual cortex of members of the same species at different ages would be worthwhile, since it is possible that the number declines with increasing age. If Le Gros Clark's specimens came from older animals, a slow extinction of one Meynert cell after another could account for the discrepancy between his counts and ours. Overproduction followed by death of the excessive neurons is a well-known process in the developing nervous system. Although it is supposed that neuronal survival correlates with success in making the right connections with target cells (3,5,6), there is also evidence that at least some neurons undergo degeneration despite their success in reaching their targets (16). It is also well known that nerve fibers and nerve endings undergo apparently spontaneous degeneration in the brain of normal adult animals (see, for example, Sotelo and Palay, 19). Such phenomena may be regarded as part of a continuing renewal and modulatory process going on in the mature nervous system. Degeneration and elimination of cortical neuronal perikarya are also recognized as natural accompaniments of aging in the nervous system, but usually the dropout of neurons is considered to be random in distribution or related to local vascular insufficiencies. With respect to the dark Meynert cells, selective loss of a single cell type in an otherwise normal cortical area in young animals suggests that selective morphogenetic factors may be at work.

CONCLUSIONS

Meynert cells are a highly specialized and perhaps evanescent type of pyramidal neuron characteristic of the visual cortex in primates and carnivores. They are distinguished by their enormous size, thick basal dendrites, neurofilamentous cytoplasm, and peculiar distribution of dendritic spines. Variation in the numbers of such cells with advancing age deserves further study.

ACKNOWLEDGMENT

The original work on which this paper is based was supported by grants from the National Institute for Neurological and Communicative Disorders and Stroke, NS 10536, NS 03659, and NS 05591.

REFERENCES

1. Brodmann, K. (1905): Beiträge zur histologischen Lokalisation der Grosshirnrinde. Dritte Mittheilung. *J. Psychol. Neurol.,* 4:177–226.
2. Chan-Palay, V., Palay, S. L., and Billings-Gagliardi, S. M. (1974): Meynert cells in the primate visual cortex. *J. Neurocytol.,* 3:631–658.
3. Cowan, W. M. (1973): Neuronal death as a regulative mechanism in the control of cell number in the nervous system. In: *Development and Aging in the Nervous System,* edited by M. Rockstein, pp. 19–41. Academic Press, New York.
4. Cragg, B. G. (1967): The density of synapses and neurons in the motor and visual areas of the cerebral cortex. *J. Anat.,* 101:639–654.
5. Hamburger, V. (1975): Cell death in the development of the lateral motor column of the chick embryo. *J. Comp. Neurol.,* 160:535–546.
6. Hughes, A. (1968): Development of limb innervation. In: *Growth of the Nervous System,* edited by G. E. W. Wolstenholme, and M. O'Connor, pp. 110–117. Little, Brown, Boston.
7. Kaiserman-Abramof, I. R., and Peters, A. (1972): Some aspects of the morphology of Betz cells in the cerebral cortex of the cat. *Brain Res.,* 43:527–546.
8. Le Gros Clark, W. E. (1942): The cells of Meynert in the visual cortex of the monkey. *J. Anat.,* 76:369–376.
9. Lund, J. S. (1973): Organization of neurons in the visual cortex, area 17, of the monkey (*Macaca mulatta*). *J. Comp. Neurol.,* 147:455–496.
10. Lund, J. S., and Boothe, R. G. (1975): Interlaminar connections and pyramidal neuron organisation in the visual cortex, area 17, of the macaque monkey. *J. Comp. Neurol.,* 159: 305–334.
11. Lund, R. D., Lund, J. S., Bunt, A. H., Hendrickson, A. E., and Fuchs, A. F. (1974): Cells in area 17 of monkey (*Macaca mulatta*) which give rise to corticotectal and corticogeniculate pathways. *Soc. Neurosci. Abstracts,* page 319.
12. Marin-Padilla, M. (1967): Number and distribution of the apical dendritic spines of the layer V pyramidal cells in man. *J. Comp. Neurol.,* 131:475–490.
13. Marin-Padilla, M., and Stibitz, G. R. (1968): Distribution of the apical dendritic spines of the layer V pyramidal cells of the hamster neocortex. *Brain Res.,* 11:580–592.
14. Meynert, T. (1872): The brain of mammals. In: *Manual of Human and Comparative Histology, Vol. II,* edited by S. Stricker, translated by H. Power, p. 391. The New Sydenham Society, London.
15. Palay, S. L., and Chan-Palay, V. (1974): *Cerebellar Cortex, Cytology and Organization.* Springer-Verlag, New York, Heidelberg.

16. Prestige, M. C. (1976): Evidence that at least some of the motor nerve cells that die during development have first made peripheral connections. *J. Comp. Neurol.*, 170:123–134.
17. Ramón y Cajal, S. (1899): Estudios sobre la corteza cerebral humana. Corteza visual (1). *Revista Trimestral Micrográfica*, 4:1–63.
18. Sknol'nik-Yarros, E. G. (1974): *Neurons and Interneuronal Connections of the Central Visual System,* translated by B. Haigh, p. 109. Plenum Press, New York.
19. Sotelo, C., and Palay, S. L. (1971): Altered axons and axon terminals in the lateral vestibular nucleus of the rat. Possible example of axonal remodelling. *Lab. Invest.*, 25:653–671.
20. Spatz, W. B. (1975): An efferent connection of the solitary cells of Meynert. A study with horseradish peroxidase in the marmoset *Callithrix*. *Brain Res.*, 92:450–455.
21. Valverde, F. (1967): Apical dendritic spines of the visual cortex and light deprivation in the mouse. *Exp. Brain Res.*, 3:337–352.
22. Valverde, F., and Ruiz-Marcos, A. (1969): Dendritic spines in the visual cortex of the mouse: Introduction to a mathematical model. *Exp. Brain Res.*, 8:269–283.
23. Wuerker, R., and Palay, S. L. (1969): Neurofilaments and microtubules in anterior horn cells of the rat. *Tissue Cell,* 1:387–402.

Architectonics of the Cerebral Cortex,
edited by M. A. B. Brazier and H. Petsche.
Raven Press, New York © 1978.

The Dendritic Structure of the Human Betz Cell

*Madge E. Scheibel and Arnold B. Scheibel

*Departments of Anatomy and Psychiatry, University of California Los Angeles,
Los Angeles, California 90024*

Variety's the very spice of life
That gives it all its flavor.
— *Cowper*

Among the countless phalanxes of cortical pyramidal cells, the giant pyramids of Betz constitute a unique and highly individualized minority. The region of their distribution forms less than 2.8% of the surface of the human brain (17), and, in this prerolandic zone which forms their main setting, their total population of 30,000 to 40,000 cells (14) can scarcely make up more than 1 to 2% of all the pyramids present. Since their initial description by Vladimir Betz in 1874 (3), they have fascinated many observers including Campbell (6), Brodmann (5), Hammarberg (12), and Economo (7), whom we honor in this volume.

As striking as is their appearance in routine aniline or reduced silver stains, through phase contrast optics, or with the electron microscope, it is the Golgi methods which, alone, reveal the remarkable nature of these cells and their complex relationships to surrounding elements. As Cajal (21) indicated, it is their remarkable dendritic system, even more than their size, which sets them apart from all other pyramids, and which stimulates speculation about their almost certainly special functional role.

Limitations of available technology have made them rather difficult to analyze until recently. Walshe (31) critically reviewed information available at that time (1942), finally deciding that they did not make up a special structural and functional category and that they defied scientific description. Today, our position is more sanguine, and a group of studies relating their individual spike discharge patterns to events in the periphery are helping to provide hard facts which, with apologies to Walshe, have proven them highly amenable to scientific description. We are still early in this process, and much conjecture is still necessary, but the picture which has begun to emerge may provide a satisfactory first-order approximation.

---

* Deceased.

TECHNIQUE AND PURPOSE

The findings reported here are based on the study of approximately 150 well-impregnated Betz cells from the prerolandic cortices of four patients, aged 27 to 102. A number of partially impregnated giant pyramids plus comparative material from the motor areas of two rhesus macaques were also included in the study and provided background material. Thionine and reduced silver stains of human cortical material served as controls. Limited structural changes were noted in the oldest human material (aged 92 and 102) and will form the basis for a later report.

An introductory group of observations has been made with the electron microscope on several small blocks of tissue selected from the middle or deep portion of layer 5 precentral cortex near the vertex of the hemisphere. The tissue came from two patients aged 27 and 54. Choice of the location for electron microscope sections was based on examination of toluidine-blue-stained "thick sections" cut at 0.5 mμ from blocks already embedded in Epon and ready for final trimming before ultrasectioning. We selected cortical fields which were close and deep (100 to 300 mμ) to giant pyramids, and where there appeared to be satisfactory concentrations of dendritic profiles. Since these were usually sectioned transverse or oblique to their presumed long axes, we have only presumptive evidence that the constituent dendrites of any of these bundles may have come from a giant cell. The quality of the electron micrographs was unsatisfactory due to the usual problems of obtaining human autopsy material immediately after death. Although major membrane systems were intact and both axonal and dendritic profiles preserved, there was general blurring or loss of most of the smaller endocellular membrane-bound structures due to postmortem autolysis. For this reason the electron micrographs are not reproduced. Instead, we include tracings made from bundles that were seen on several of the plates and which were presumed to include shafts from giant pyramids.

Our present purpose is to describe basic patterns of dendritic architecture and relationships, the distribution of dendritic spines characteristic of Betz pyramids and dendrite bundle organization and to see how such findings may relate to the functional roles of these cells as presently understood.

DENDRITE STRUCTURE AND ORIENTATION

As already indicated, Betz cells are characterized by an enhanced number of primary dendrite shafts issuing from the cell body (Figs. 1 and 2). In the case of all other mature cortical pyramids, dendrite systems exclusive of the apical shaft leave the cell body almost entirely from the basal angles and are ordinarily limited to one to three shafts per basal angle as seen in the usual vertical section through the cortex. Thus, few large pyramids, even large fifth-layer elements, develop more than four to six primary basilar

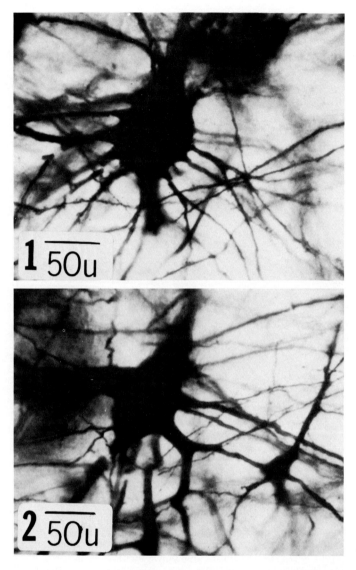

FIGS. 1 and 2. Betz cell bodies and dendrites from motor cortex of 27-year-old male. Note that dendrites issue from all portions of the circumference of the cell body rather than from the basal angles alone. In Fig. 1, a very large "tap root" shaft starts down toward deeper areas and is immediately lost to focus. In Fig. 2 a nongiant fifth-layer pyramid is shown for contrast. Rapid Golgi variant.

dendrites in the total basilar skirt system (Fig. 8). Betz cells do not seem to operate under the same structural constraints. Dendrites leave the cell body at almost any point around the circumference. This is reminiscent of immature cortical neurons where the basilar dendrite system also shows no

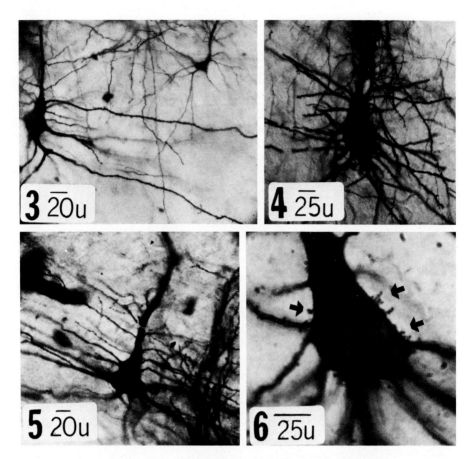

FIGS. 3, 4, 5, and 6. Details of dendritic and somal structure are shown. Figure 3 shows a Betz cell of smaller size with major dendrite shafts extending horizontally and in one general direction only. Figure 4 shows the number and density of dendrites that may issue from the circumference of a single Betz cell body. Twenty-two primary shafts were counted on this cell body. The characteristic appearance of Betz cells at the base of a sulcus is illustrated in Fig. 5. Many thin, essentially parallel dendrites issue from each side of the cell body and first portion of the apical shaft and extend for distances of 1 to 2 mm, approximately parallel to the cortical surface and grey–white interface. Figure 6 shows the presence of spines on the soma of a large Betz cell (arrows). The number and distribution of these are highly variable. Rapid Golgi variants. All material from 44-year-old male patient.

initial basilar preference (Fig. 4). In this regard it is worth remembering that the Betz cell primordia are among the first cortical immigrants, preceding by an appreciable interval those cells which will form the four outer layers (see Fleischhauer, *this volume*). While it would be unwarranted to assume that the Betz-cell dendrite distribution pattern marks it as a primitive cell, it might be noted that, in the late fetal and early newborn human cortex, the pattern of primary dendrite placement is already complete and maturation of these elements is limited to extension in length and the development of more elaborate secondary and tertiary branching (21, and Scheibel and Scheibel, unpublished data).

Three general groups of nonapical or circumferential dendrites (the term basilar does not seem appropriate) can be described; ascending oblique, horizontal, and descending oblique (Fig. 7), and the size and distribution of

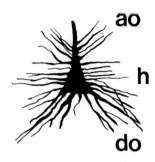

FIG. 7. Distribution of dendrites along the circumference of a typical Betz cell. They include varying numbers of ao, ascending obliques; h, horizontals; and do, descending obliques.

each group varies with the location of the individual Betz element. In general terms, the ascending oblique angles upward into the more superficial parts of layer 5 and occasionally into the area presumed to be layer 4, although this identification is always a difficult one in agranular cortex. The relative infrequency of invasion by these shafts into presumptive layer 4 is reinforced by Bonin's observation (4) that Betz-cell pyramids generally avoid the outer stripe of Baillarger, which is located in layer 4.

The horizontal contingent is limited to layer 5 and is especially prominent on those Betz elements located in the depths of the rolandic sulcus and on the lower portion of the anterior wall. In this type of cortical environment marked by somewhat thinner, concave laminae, multiple, horizontal shafts leave the cell body and maintain their relationship parallel to each other and to the cortical surface for 1 to 3 mm. Although these are not the largest Betz elements, they tend to be more numerous in these areas, and masses of long parallel dendrites, interwoven in bundle formation, form a veritable shelf which visually underlines the fifth layer (Fig. 5).

The descending oblique branches are similar to the basilar dendrites of non-Betz cells but are usually very much more numerous and extensive. It is from this contingent that the characteristic "tap root" dendrite (Fig. 11) usually arises. Such elements may run for enormous distances through layers 5 and 6 and occasionally into the underlying white matter.

Dendrite Length

The length of the Betz-cell dendrite may be very great, frequently exceeding 1 mm and sometimes extending more than 2 mm from the cell body. In some cases the length of one such shaft may exceed that of the apical

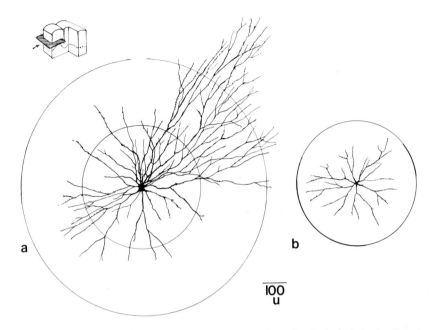

FIG. 8. The full extent of the dendrite system (exclusive of apical shafts) of a Betz-type pyramid **(a)** and a typical fifth-layer pyramid **(b).** Note the enormous number of Betz cell shafts emerging from the circumference of the body and the very great length of one sector of this dendrite envelope (>750 μm). The typical fifth-layer pyramid has a much smaller number of primary shafts, symmetrically arranged around the soma. Concentric circles measure 250-μm intervals from the center of Betz cell body. Section cut parallel to surface.

dendrite, which can extend through 2 to 3 mm of overlying cortex before generating its terminal arbor. However, the distribution of dendrites of this size are not symmetric. Indeed, the dendritic domains of these giant pyramids are hallmarked as much by their idiosyncratic geometry as by their size.

Domain Geometry

Some domains appear to be symmetrically arranged about the cell body. The best examples of these are found in those cells in the depth or along the anterior wall of the rolandic fissure where, as already noted, multiple horizontal branches generate broad skirts whose configuration, gently concave upward, parallels the cortical surface. Since Lassek (14) estimates that up to 82% of all Betz cells are located in the anterior wall, it seems clear that a majority of these giant pyramids are located in this environment and are configured so as to generate this type of domain. Due to their relative density, it follows that the association of such parallel arrays from adjacent Betz

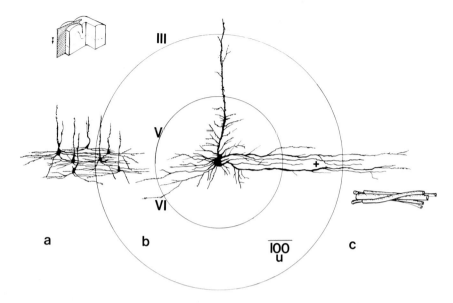

FIG. 9. Betz cell with major portion of dendritic domain developed on one side of cell body via several horizontal dendrite shafts. Part of the complement of fifth-layer pyramids which actually appear within this domain, +, are shown at **a.** Nature of the close apposition of Betz-cell shafts with basilar shafts of the fifth-layer pyramids are shown at **c.** Section cut perpendicular to surface.

cells to form dendrite bundles can be predicted and, in fact, appears with almost dramatic intensity in the deep cortical neuropil of sulcal cortex.

Betz cells are larger and somewhat more infrequent along the crown of the prerolandic gyrus and their dendritic domains tend to be dramatically asymetric. This type of configuration may express itself as (a) a cluster of horizontal dendrites extending in one direction only (as seen in vertical sections) with relatively short branches emerging from the rest of the cell body (Fig. 9); (b) a single long branch descending obliquely through layers 5 and 6 and sometimes projecting into the white matter (Fig. 11). A branch such as this usually generates numerous secondary radicles which leave the primary shaft at all angles, producing a cylindric domain often several hundred micra in diameter, which follows the parent shaft. Tap root dendrites may run vertically down through subjacent cortex and in this case, the Betz cell, by virtue of its ascending apical shaft, looks like a giant bipolar neuron whose major dendritic domain surrounds it like a long cylinder from white matter to cortical surface. (c) A variation of this configuration with a somewhat greater degree of symmetry is illustrated in Fig. 10 where a large number of dendrite shafts project directly downward both from the undersurface of the cell body and from the first one-third of the major horizontal dendrites. These vertical dendrites often remain unbranched, producing a short, thick cylindrical domain more or less centered on the vertical axis of the Betz cell

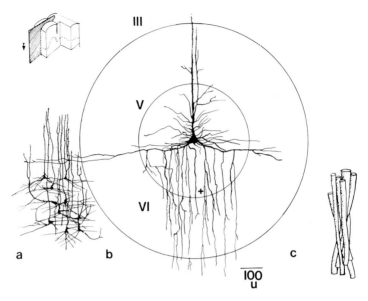

FIG. 10. Betz cell with major portion of dendritic domain developed over a presumably cylindrical area deep to the cell body in layers 5 and 6. The ensemble of fifth- and sixth-layer pyramids, shown at **a,** are actually located in the dendritic domain in **b,** centered on the +. Many of the apical dendrites of the pyramidal cell ensemble appear to form bundles **(c)** with the descending Betz-cell dendrites. Section cut perpendicular to surface.

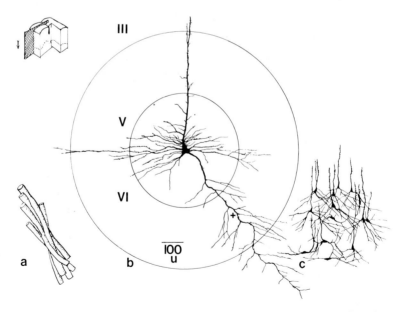

FIG. 11. Betz cell **(b)** with large oblique "tap root" type of dendrite angling downward into layers 5 and 6, among pyramidal cell ensembles shown in **c.** The Betz-cell shaft and branches form many close appositions and bundles with pyramidal cell basilar dendrites **(c).** Section cut perpendicular to surface.

and limited to the deep portion of layer 5 and, frequently, the superficial portion of layer 6.

Relatively greater degrees of symmetry are also seen in some Betz pyramids whose major domains appear generated by a veritable sunburst of dendrites, leaving the soma from every point on the circumference. The cell body shown in Fig. 4 generates at least 22 primary shafts (some may have been beyond our range of focus) and almost triple that number of secondary branches. Most of these elements extend for distances of 750 mμ or less and result in the generation of a spherical domain limited primarily to layer 5 and centered on the cell body.

Spine distribution along the surfaces of Betz pyramids remains a problem. Spines may — or may not — be present on the surfaces of the cell bodies (Fig. 6), apical shafts, and large primary dendrites of circumferential origin. We have traced several obliquely oriented tap root dendrites for over 1 mm without sign of a single spine. It is unlikely (although not impossible) that this is an artifact of fixation or staining, since surrounding dendrites of other cells frequently show normal complements of spines. In general, the more peripheral portions of large tap root and apical shafts are more likely to bear spines than the proximal segments; the finer branches more densely covered than the heavy branches. Since we have noticed the same peculiarities of distribution in perfused monkey cortex, we are inclined to believe that these patterns accurately reflect spine distribution on giant pyramids and indicate plastic plurifunctional roles for these shafts.

FORMATION OF DENDRITE BUNDLES

The preceding observations, while clearly introductory, emphasize certain features about the giant pyramidal cell of Betz, especially those seen in human cortex. Most obvious is their individuality, expressed in the pleomorphic nature of their dendrite domains, and the marked differences in sectors of surrounding cortical neuropil which their dendrite systems tap. The least variation in dendrite organization appears at the depths of sulcal cortex where the dendrite systems are predominantly horizontal and form powerful bundles which extend for many millimeters, approximately parallel to the cortical surfaces. Parenthetically, sulcal cortex is by far the thinnest portion of the sensorimotor complex. We have studied these bundle formations in cat motor cortex where they are generalized in distribution (22), suggesting more invariant structural-functional patterns in nonprimate forms.

In man, less than 25% of the Betz cells are apparently located on visible motor cortex, i.e., FA γ of Economo (7), but these are the largest cells and it is their dendrite systems which are the most highly individualized. Careful study of these dendrite systems indicates that the secondary and tertiary branches of the primary shafts enter close longitudinal associations with other dendrites, similar to the bundles of horizontal dendrites we have previously described in cat cortex (22) and in the deep sulcal regions of human prerolandic cortex. In these cases, however, the bundles are made up almost exclusively of the horizontal-oriented basal or circumferential dendrites of the giant pyramids themselves. In the case of the largest Betz cells on the crown of FA γ, bundles appear to be formed by apposition with dendrites of other types in many different locations throughout layers 5 and 6. Figures 9 to 11 show three configurations in which the domain of dendritic interaction is determined by the location and orientation of the major dendrites. In the case of the eccentric horizontal shafts (Fig. 9) bundles appear to be formed with horizontally oriented basilar shafts of fifth-layer pyramids. The long, oblique tap root dendrite in Fig. 11 forms large numbers of bundle relationships with the oblique basilar shafts of fifth- and sixth-layer pyramids. As far as we can determine, both the primary tap root shaft itself as well as its secondary branches are involved in bundle formation. The mass of downward-reaching, parallel shafts in Fig. 10 enter similar relationships with the apical shafts of appropriately placed pyramids deep to this Betz cell body in layers 5 and 6 (Fig. 10).

Bundles have now been described by several authors (10,16,20,25) and the details of their organization are fairly well known. Suffice it to say, they are made up of three to ten dendrite shafts whose cell bodies of origin may lie considerable distances apart. The constituent dendrite branches lie parallel to each other and may lie close enough to exclude formed intervening structures, even leaves of glia and individual synaptic terminals. In these cases, the plasma membranes are separated only by extraneuronal spaces 100 to 200 Å wide. So far, no evidence of synaptic specializations in the opposed membranes has been found. The constitution of the bundle, which may be traceable as an entity for some millimeters, constantly changes as individual shafts enter and leave the complex.

Electron microscopy of selected blocks of human precentral cortex, while not completely satisfactory from a technical point of view, has clearly shown clusters of dendritic profiles in the middle and deep portions of the fifth cortical layer where they have been identified in Golgi-stained material. Unlike the latter preparations, we are not able to trace the dendrites back to the cell bodies of origin and so, for the moment, the relation of any bundle dendrite shafts to giant cells must remain tentative. Nevertheless, many of the bundles appear to contain one or more large dendrite profiles (Fig. 12a) as well as a number of smaller ones, and lie in the vicinity of, and ventral to, giant pyramids identified in thick sections cut from the epon-embedded block. We therefore have at least the presumption that some of these represent bundles containing dendrites from both giant and nongiant pyramids, as identified in the Golgi-stained material. More satisfactory identification must await electron microscopy on individual Golgi-stained sections.

All examples from the tissue blocks sampled were sectioned in planes transverse or slightly oblique to the bundles. Each bundle contained three

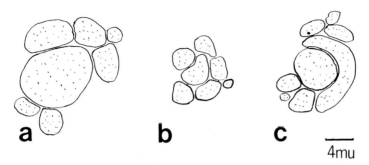

FIG. 12. Drawings of three dendrite bundles taken from electron micrographs of the fifth cortical layer of human precentral gyrus. In **a**, the very large dendrite profile is thought to come from a nearby giant cell of Betz, while at least some of the remaining dendrite sections undoubtedly come from adjacent nongiant cells. The bundle at **b** is made up of a more uniformly sized group of small dendrites. The bundle at **c** includes one dendrite section which appears deeply invaginated by another. We have not seen this type of structural relationship between dendrites of an individual bundle elsewhere in the nervous system. Original magnification of electron microphotograph, ×8,000.

to eight dendrite profiles with aggregate diameters for the entire bundle complex of 12 to 40 mμ. The apparent diameter of the individual constituent dendrites ranged from 3 to 14 mμ with about 90% of values below 8 mμ. Approximately one-half of the bundles visualized (n = 24) contained one of the larger dendrite profiles (> 8 mμ), and it is these larger elements which we assume may have their source in giant cells of Betz. Obviously, many of the smaller elements may also have been Betz-cell dendrite branches, but are not presently identifiable as such unless direct continuity can be demonstrated.

The structural organization of the bundles resembled what we have seen in other areas of the central nervous system (25–28) and appeared similar to descriptions by Matthews et al. (16), Fleischhauer et al. (10), Peters and Walsh (20), and others. Membranes of facing dendrite pairs and triads were often only tens of angstra apart, frequently with no visible intervening structures, and without obvious membrane specializations suggesting dendro-dendritic junctions, etc. (Fig. 12). One structural motif appeared unique to this system, however. In 7 out of 24 bundles studied, one dendrite profile, usually a large one, appeared deeply invaginated by one or two smaller elements (Fig. 12c). In one case, the smaller element appeared almost entirely encircled by the larger. We have no reason to suspect that these structural features are the result of postmortem change or laboratory processing. It is possible, therefore, that these apparently more intensive interrelationships between certain dendrite pairs within the bundle represent a specific feature of bundle organization unique — so far — to giant-cell-related bundles.

The functional role of dendrite bundles remains unknown, although several possible roles have been suggested including that of core substrate to cortical cell columns (20), electrotonic summation of events occurring in the associated elements (10), and as site for central programs controlling output patterns peculiar to the particular area (27). While the presently described associations between giant Betz cells and other pyramids do not provide specific functional information about these specialized dendritic relations, certain possibilities deserve mention. Antidromic studies by several investigators indicate a division of pyramidal tract cells into two major groups on the basis of conduction velocity (8,19,30). A small group of very rapidly conducting axons are phasically active during movement and generally precede EMG activity by 40 to 100 msec (9). The great remainder of more slowly conducting pyramidal elements tends to be tonically active with less dramatic change in firing rate, in either direction, no matter what is occurring at the level of motor output. The limited number of rapidly conducting elements are assumed to be the largest axons and are, undoubtedly from the Betz cells, whose axons are clearly the largest we have anatomically identified.

Differential counts by Lassek in man show that 75% of Betz cells are located in motor areas supplying the leg, 17.9% in the arm region, and only 6.6% in the head area, despite the dedication of much more extensive cortical areas to head and arm than to leg. These figures would appear to suggest a positive correlation between Betz elements and muscle mass or antigravity status, or both. The major antigravity operations of bipeds are localized in the lower extremities and back. It seems likely that the phasically programmed early output of Betz cells (8,9) is selectively directed toward extensor inhibition and flexor enhancement (15) as a necessary initial event in any patterned motor act superimposed on the background set of supportive, antigravity tone. The rapid burst of early activity (8) in the largest pyramidal cell axons probably initiates appropriate degrees of lysis in supportive activity across weight-bearing joints immediately before the development of definitive motor patterns initiated by the masses of surrounding pyramidal cells. The Betz element may accordingly be conceived as fulfilling an initial trigger function in motor activity by preparing the peripheral motor apparatus for the specific output program about to be implemented.

In our recent study of basilar dendrite bundle complexes in giant pyramids in the cat (22), we were interested in the possibility that the dendrite-to-dendrite relationships effected within bundle complexes might provide substrate for central programs which sequence and modulate the phasic discharge patterns of Betz-cell clusters. Such a role is, of course, speculative and is based on temporal correlations between development of dendrite bundles studied in spinal cord (25), brainstem (23), thalamus (26), and olfactory bulb (28) and the initial appearance of certain output patterns characteristic of these areas. In this regard, certain related assumptions were also made about the significance of the glycoprotein-sialic acid moieties along facing pairs of dendritic membrane and their interaction with extracellular divalent cations (27).

In the present situation, once again, it is difficult to conceive that the formation of dendrite bundle complexes between long horizontal or oblique Betz-cell shafts with dendrite systems of fifth- and sixth-layer pyramids is functionally irrelevant. At the moment there is no clear indication of the role these associations may play. However, we would like to propose that one function for these complexes may center upon the local electrical gradients which follow spike volleys generated by the Betz cell. Presently there are no data to support the possibility of spike generation in the dendrites of mature, healthy Betz pyramids. However, there is increasing appreciation of the potency of local graded processes and field effects in modulating threshold levels of polarization in adjacent neural elements. Studies by Grinnell (11) and Nelson (18) among others attest to the apparent range and strength of such coupling potentials in the motoneuronal pool of spinal cord where bundles are now known to constitute a significant part of the dendritic architecture (16,25). The remarkable sensitivity of neuronal membrane to low-level, imposed voltage gradients, as much as 10 orders of magnitude less than the potentials associated with spike-driven synaptic activity, has become clear through the studies of Adey (1) and co-workers. Even more recently, Kreutzberg (13) has provided evidence of intradendritic transport and secretion of peptides and glycoprotein precursor moieties, another putative means by which large Betz-cell dendrites may exert modulatory control over neural elements in the immediate surround. We are, therefore, suggesting that Betz pyramids exert considerable effects on their surround by means of local electrical and chemical gradients and that these "nonclassic" modes of operation may prove of importance in the processing of neural activity and in the interaction among neural ensembles (24,29).

Betz cells may serve two related functions: By virtue of their characteristic early phasic volleys projected upon the large antigravity muscle masses, they condition peripheral motor mechanisms for specific output sequences by introductory partial lysis of antigravity tone; and through their enormous dendritic apparatus, they generate field effects within their dendritic domains which effect large numbers of fourth-, fifth-, and sixth-layer pyramids. It is likely that both the local bioelectrical and biochemical mechanisms are time-locked to the axon spike volley, thereby conditioning large numbers of cortical pyramids about to be involved in the ensuing motor sequence.

The frequently noted asymmetry of the Betz-cell dendritic field and the presence of one or several unusually long dendrite shafts covering one sector of the surrounding neuropil fields may reflect the role of the pyramidal ensemble in this particular area in maintaining motor control over specific muscles, or over different aspects of the performance of one muscle (2) upon which the Betz cell in question exerts its initial effects.

A bipolar functional role of this sort need not be limited to Betz cells and may, in fact, serve as model for much neural activity. However, the structural characteristics of the giant cells of Betz are so boldly stated that they serve as an ideal paradigm for the cortical pyramid. In any case, they emphasize our increasing appreciation of the multimodal roles performed by dendrites and of the undoubted importance of nonclassic modes of information processing and neural control.

SUMMARY

The giant pyramidal cells of Betz are characterized not only by their great size but by the unusual length and idiosyncratic nature of their circumferential dendrites. Bundle complexes are formed with dendrites from great ensembles of non-Betz pyramids, especially in those neuropil sectors into which the Betz-cell dendrites project most powerfully. Betz cells are conceived as lead elements preparing the motor apparatus for the specific output sequences which follow, and the relevant sectors of cortical neuropil for appropriate control over those sequences.

Direct effects over peripheral musculature are probably limited to partial lysis of antigravity tone and are effected by the early phasic descending spike volley. Conditioning effects on elements of the surrounding neuropil may be produced in large part by nonclassic means such as graded bioelectrical fields and secretion and release of specific chemical substances.

ACKNOWLEDGMENT

These studies were supported by USPHS Grant NS 10567, NINDS. We thank Dr. Uwami Tomiyasu, Veterans Administration Hospital, Brentwood, for supplying most of the human cortical material upon which this study was based, and for help with the electron microscopy. We also thank Mr. Abe Green for his help in the preparation of the Golgi histologic material.

REFERENCES

1. Adey, W. R. (1975): Evidence for cooperative mechanisms in the susceptibility of cerebral tissue to environmental and intrinsic electric fields. In: *Functional Linkage in Biomolecular Systems,* edited by F. O. Schmitt, D. M. Schneider, and D. M. Crothers, pp. 325–342. Raven Press, New York.
2. Asanuma, H., and Rosen, I. (1972): Topographical organization of cortical efferent zones projecting to distant forelimb muscles in the monkey. *Exp. Brain Res.,* 14:243–256.
3. Betz, V. (1874): Anatomischer Nachweis zweiet Gehirncentra. *Centralblat Med. Wissensch.,* 12:578–595. Quoted in Lassek, A. (1954): *The Pyramidal Tract.* Charles C Thomas, Springfield, Ill.
4. Bonin, G. von (1950): *Essay on the Cerebral Cortex.* Charles C Thomas, Springfield, Ill.
5. Brodmann, K. (1909): *Vergleichende Lokalisationslehre der Grosshirnrinde in ihren Principien dargestellt auf Grund der Zellenbauer.* Barth, Liepzig (reprinted 1925).
6. Campbell, A. W. (1905): *Histological Studies on the Localization of Cerebral Function.* University Press, Cambridge, Mass.

7. Economo, C. von, and Koskinas, G. N. (1925): *Die Cytoarchitektonik der Hirnrinde des erwachsenen Menschen.* J. Springer, Vienna.
8. Evarts, E. V. (1965): Relation of discharge frequency to conduction velocity in pyramidal tract neurons. *J. Neurophysiol.,* 28:216–228.
9. Evarts, E. V. (1967): Representation of movements and muscles by pyramidal tract neurons of the precental motor cortex. In: *Neurophysiological Basis of Normal and Abnormal Motor Activities,* edited by M. D. Yahr and D. P. Purpura, pp. 215–253. Raven Press, New York.
10. Fleischauer, K., Petsche, H., and Wittkowski, W. (1972): Vertical bundles of dendrites in the neocortex. *Z. Anat. Etwickl. Gesch,,* 136:213–223.
11. Grinnell, A. D. (1966): A study of the interaction between motoneurons in the frog's spinal cord. *J. Physiol.,* 182:612–648.
12. Hammarberg, C. (1895): *Studien über Klinik und Pathologie der Idiote nebst Untersuchungen über die normale Anatomie der Hirnrinde.* Akad. Buchdrukerai, Upsala. Quoted in Lassek, A. (1954): *The Pyramidal Tract.* Charles C Thomas, Springfield, Ill.
13. Kreutzberg, G. W. (1976): Transneuronal transfer: Inter and extracellular pathways. In: Neuron-Target Cell Interactions, edited by B. H. Smith and G. W. Kreutzberg, pp. 275–293. Neurosciences Research Program, Boston.
14. Lassek, A. M. (1954): *The Pyramidal Tract.* Charles C Thomas, Springfield, Ill.
15. Lundberg, A., and Voorhoeve, P. (1962): Effects from the pyramidal tract on spinal reflex arcs. *Acta Physiol. Scand.,* 56:201–219.
16. Matthews, M. A., Willis, W. D., and Williams, V. (1971): Dendrite bundles in lamina IX of cat spinal cord: A possible source for electrical interaction between motoneurons. *Anat. Rec.,* 171:313–328.
17. Michails, J. J., and Davison, C. (1930): Measurements of cerebral and cerebellar surfaces. VIII. Measurements of the motor area in vertebrates and in man. *Arch. Neurol. Psychiatry,* 24:1212–1226.
18. Nelson, D. G. (1966): Interaction between spinal motoneurons of the cat. *J. Neurophysiol.,* 27:913–927.
19. Oshima, T. (1969): Studies of pyramidal tract cells. In: *Basic Mechanisms of the Epilepsies,* edited by H. Jasper, A. A. Ward, Jr., and A. Pope, pp. 253–261. Little, Brown, Boston.
20. Peters, A., and Walsh, T. M. (1972): A study of the organization of apical dendrites in the somatic sensory cortex of the rat. *J. Comp. Neurol.,* 144:253–268.
21. Ramon y Cajal, S. (1911): *Histologie du Système Nerveux de l'Homme et des Vertébrés, Vol. II.* Maloine, Paris.
22. Scheibel, M. E., Davies, T. L., Lindsay, R. D., and Scheibel, A. B. (1974): Basilar dendrite bundles of giant pyramidal cells. *Exp. Neurol.,* 42:307–319.
23. Scheibel, M. E., Davies, T. L., and Scheibel, A. B. (1973): Maturation of reticular dendrites: loss of spines and development of bundles. *Exp. Neurol.,* 38:301–310.
24. Scheibel, M. E., and Scheibel, A. B. (1955): The inferior olive. A Golgi study. *J. Comp. Neurol.,* 102:77–132.
25. Scheibel, M. E., and Scheibel, A. B. (1970): Organization of spinal motoneuron dendrites in bundles. *Exp. Neurol.,* 28:106–112.
26. Scheibel, M. E., and Scheibel, A. B. (1972): Specialized organizational patterns within the nucleus reticularis thalami of the cat. *Exp. Neurol.,* 43:316–322.
27. Scheibel, M. E., and Scheibel, A. B. (1973): Dendrite bundles as sites for central programs. An hypothesis. *Int. J. Neurosci.,* 6:195–202.
28. Scheibel, M. E., and Scheibel, A. B. (1975): Dendrite bundles, central programs, and the olfactory bulb. *Brain Res.,* 95:407–421.
29. Schmitt, F. O., Dev, P., and Smith, B. H. (1976): Electrotonic processing of information by brain cells. *Science,* 193:114–120.
30. Takahashi, K. (1965): Slow and fast groups of pyramidal tract cells and their respective membrane properties. *J. Neurophysiol.,* 28:908–924.
31. Walshe, F. M. R. (1942): The giant cells of Betz, the motor cortex, and the pyramidal tract: A critical review. *Brain,* 65:409–461.

Architectonics of the Cerebral Cortex,
edited by M. A. B. Brazier and H. Petsche.
Raven Press, New York © 1978.

Comparative Data on the Golgi Architecture of Interneurons of Different Cortical Areas in Cat and Rabbit

Teréz Tömböl

*First Department of Anatomy, Semmelweis University Medical School,
H-1450 Budapest, Hungary*

In the early years of this century, the entire cerebral cortex was first systematically studied and then divided into distinct areas on the basis of its cyto- and/or myeloarchitecture. These studies were carried out by Brodmann (1), Campbell (3), and Vogt and Vogt (37) in Nissl or myelin-stained material, and the details of the structure of different cortical areas were examined in various mammalian species. These first publications were confirmed, and cortical architectonics were considerably refined, leading to further areal subdivisions by Economo and Koskinas (6). From the beginning of the 1930s, a succession of experimental investigations started to test the validity of cytoarchitectural subdivisions by studying the connections between various cortical areas and subcortical nuclei (4, 5,7,8,10,15,16,23,24,26,27,38,39). Although the vertical organization of neuron chains was well recognized already by Lorente de Nó (18), it was only on the basis of recent physiological studies that the so-called columnar organization of the cortex (11–13,21,25) became firmly established.

The microphysiological approach to cortical organization substantiated the essential validity of the areal subdivision of the neocortex into fields of differing connections and functions, and revived the interest for a more detailed Golgi architecture which would help us to understand neuronal architecture as the structural basis of intracortical functions.

An elementary knowledge of neuronal architecture and basic concepts about functional connectivity was established already by Ramón y Cajal (2). This outstanding work was continued and extended by Lorente de Nó (17,18) and more recently by the resurging interest in Golgi studies (5,14, 19,22,26,29,30,31,35,36).

After the first attempts by Sholl (28) to introduce the quantitative aspect into cortical connectivity, speculations about neuron connectivity models were resumed by Globus and Scheibel (9) and Szentágothai (29). This latter model was subsequently developed (32–34) into a more complex neuronal circuit concept which includes most of the presently known neuron types.

59

This Golgi study deals with the interneurons found in different cortical areas of the cat and rabbit, and an attempt is made to emphasize both similarities in the organization and differences in detail.

There is a great variety in the cortex of neurons that in analogy to subcortical structures might be called "interneurons." However, the term interneuron was prompted by functional considerations, and it is now difficult to arrive at a satisfactory general anatomical definition because of the great variety of shapes and positions of local neurons in the continuity of the neuron chains. The term "nonpyramidal" is now widely used by morphologists; however, the anatomical description of interneurons reveals that interneurons have been found that are pyramidal in shape. The term "short axon cells" also seems not to be quite adequate due to the fact that there are interneurons in the cortex with relatively long axons transgressing more often all the cortical layers but without leaving the cortex. Conversely, there are the small stellate cells, mainly in layer IV, that in spite of their short axons cannot be really labeled interneurons, since they are an essential link in the main neuron chain. Let us for the time being, and the sake of expediency, distinguish two main groups: (a) interneurons with short-, and (b) interneurons with medium-range axons. The short axon cells are morphologically various kinds of Golgi type II neurons; axonal arborizations do not significantly extend beyond the reach of the dendritic tree and are located mostly in one layer.

The interneurons with medium-range axon are of three kinds according to their axonal extensions, which may be arranged either in horizontal, vertical, or both directions.

The "short axon cells" found in layers II, V, and VI belong to the first group of interneurons both in the cat and the rabbit, and occur in different cortical areas (Figs. 1–4). They are characterized by poorly arborizing dendrites which are radially oriented and a few spines can be observed on their surface. These cells roughly correspond in size and shape and dendritic arborization, as well as surface characteristics to the stellate neurons of lamina IV, which have been recognized recently as the direct monosynaptic targets of the specific sensory afferents. The terminal portions of the axon arborizations of these layer II, V, and VI "short axon cells" are oriented predominantly horizontally and descending, so that they could well establish synapses primarily with either basal dendrites of the deeper pyramidal cells or with horizontally and obliquely oriented dendrites of other efferent neurons in the deeper strata.

It was established recently that thalamic afferents terminate predominantly on the spiny stellate neurons. In the Golgi picture, the contacts between the terminals, for example, of optic radiation fibers and the dendrites both with spines and dendritic shafts of small and medium-size stellate neurons are conspicuous.

The described type of spiny "short axon interneurons" in layers VI, V, and II are most likely to be contacted mainly by thalamic afferents;

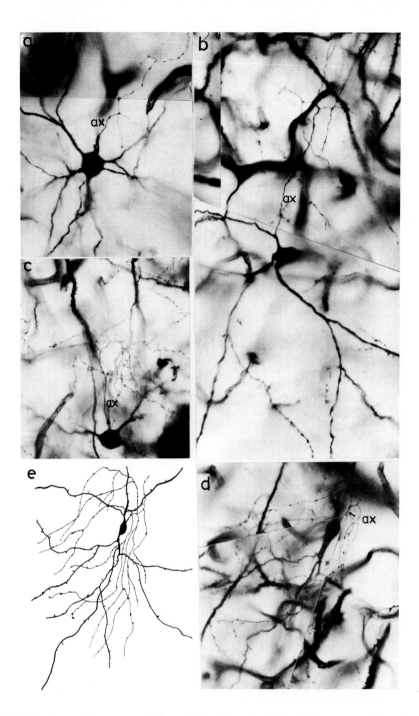

FIG. 1. Short axon interneurons in layer V of cat visual cortex. **a:** Interneuron with varicose dendrites and with ascending, sparsely arborizing axon **(ax). b:** Interneuron with few, long dendrites. Spines are rarely arranged on the dendrites; the axon **(ax)** ascends and branches into ascending and descending rami. **c, d:** Interneurons with spiny dendrites. Their ascending axon **(ax)** ramifies into descending branches. **e:** Drawing on the interneuron in **d.**

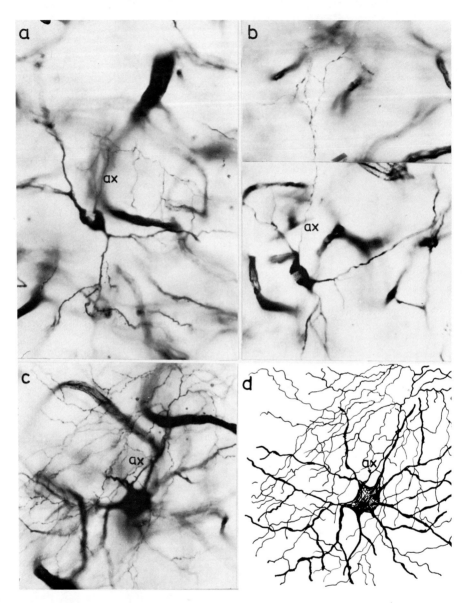

FIG. 2. a, b: Short axon interneurons with ascending axon **(ax)** in layer V of rabbit visual cortex. Interneuron with spiny **(a)** and with varicose **(b)** dendrites. **c:** Neurogliform neuron in rabbit somatosensory cortex. The origin and dense ramification of axon **(ax)** is well seen. **d:** Drawing of the neurogliform neuron.

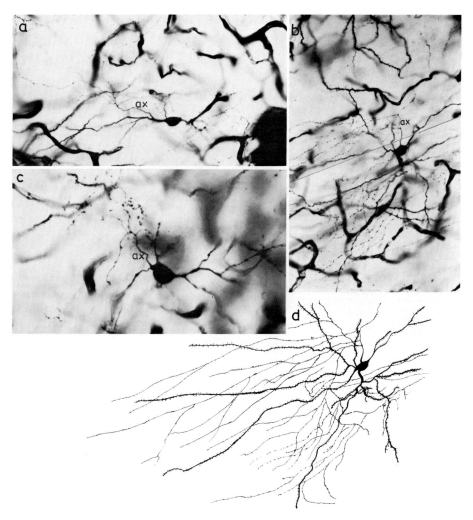

FIG. 3. Short axon interneuron in layer VI of cat visual cortex. Interneuron with spiny **(a)** and with varicose **(c)** dendrites. **b, d:** Interneuron with parallel and obliquely arranged axonal arborization **(ax).** The dendrites are spiny.

however, since they occur also in nonprimary sensory areas, these afferents may be of nonsensory thalamic nature. This tentative suggestion has, of course, to be substantiated by electron microscopy level degeneration or axonal flow-labeling studies.

In layers V and VI, "short axon cells" characterized by varicose dendritic branches and completely lacking spines were also found. Their very short axonal branches of similarly beaded appearance are ascending and arborizing poorly in their parent or in the adjacent layer.

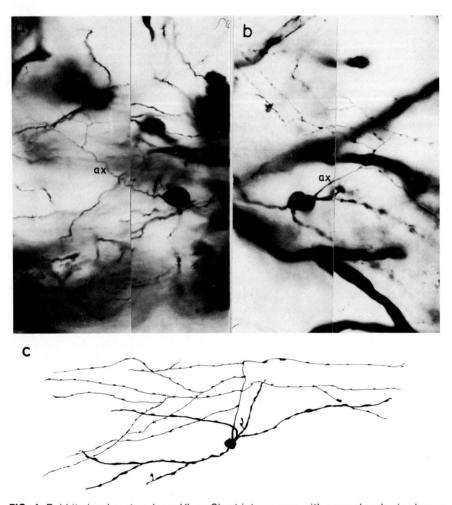

FIG. 4. Rabbit visual cortex, layer VI. **a:** Short interneuron with sparsely arborized axon **(ax). b, c:** Interneuron with parallelly and obliquely arranged axonal arborization **(ax).**

A third Golgi type II cell or "short axon interneuron" belonging to the first group, are the "neurogliform" neurons found in all layers except the first in different cortical areas both in cat and rabbit. This type of interneuron corresponds to type 5 described by Jones (14). Their cell body is of medium size, 18 to 22 μm in diameter. The pattern of their dendritic and axonal arborization is strikingly characteristic. The dendritic arbor is extremely dense, with sinous dendrites, which after repeated divisions become as thin as the axon branches. Neither protrusions nor spines can be observed on the dendrites. The axon arises usually from a dendritic shaft near the cell body and after a short course issues countless branches, which by further ramifications develop a very compact network consisting of very delicate beaded branches. The axonal arborization is usually a sphere of a diameter of about 300 μm. The axonal arbor corresponds to a slightly larger sphere than that of the dendrites and is often somewhat shifted against the latter. No specific orientation of either the dendritic or axonal branches is discernible. Consequently, the dendritic tree can receive different axon terminals and the extremely delicate terminal axonal lacework may contact similarly, very probably, dendrites and dendritic spines of numerous neurons located within the axonal arborization sphere. The extreme delicacy of the axonal branches and terminals, and the fact that the synaptic vesicles in such small terminals are usually of the spheric shape, might suggest that these neurons are more likely to be excitatory.

A second group of interneurons with medium-range axons (Figs. 5 and 6) and with horizontal arborizations have been described in layers I and VI. In the first layer, the horizontal cells of Ramón y Cajal (2) emit their axons horizontally and they remain confined to this layer. Such axons could be traced in our material for distances up to 500 to 800 μm. The horizontal cells of layer VI are also characteristic. The cell body is fusiform and oriented in the horizontal direction. The dendrites are few and are branching sparsely. However, the main dendrites are very long (about 700 μm) extending in both directions horizontally within the layer, and are densely covered with spines. The axon breaks up into delicate branches that spread almost horizontally over layer VI. The axon branches bear thorn-like terminal appendages. These neurons very probably establish contact with the efferent neurons in layer VI. Both horizontal cells are present in the cat and the rabbit in various cortical areas.

The vertically arranged neurons in the cortex are the Martinotti cells of layer VI, the double bouquet cells (2,14,29–31) in layers II and III, and the multiangular cells in layer I (35). These cells have been found both in cat and rabbit cortex and are present in different cortical areas. The Martinotti cells of layer VI and the multiangular neurons of layer I establish mutual connections between the two marginal layers (Figs. 5 and 6).

A great many studies have been dealing, especially recently, with the basket cells of the cortex (2,14,20,29–34). Both small and large basket cells can be found in various cortical areas of the cat and the rabbit (Figs. 7 and 8). Their axon arborizations extend both in horizontal and in vertical directions; hence, they belong to the third group of cortical interneurons with medium-range axons. The small basket cells in layer II send their main axon in the vertical direction, generally with an arciform turn. The axon stem gives off several vertical and horizontal varicose side branches. The axon branches invade the outer three layers establishing axosomatic contacts in a field of about 150 to 200 μm width (Fig. 7).

The large basket cells [type 1 according to Jones (14)] are found mainly in layers III, IV, and V. Their huge dendritic trees extend across several layers, as do their axonal arborizations. The dendrites are thick and varicose,

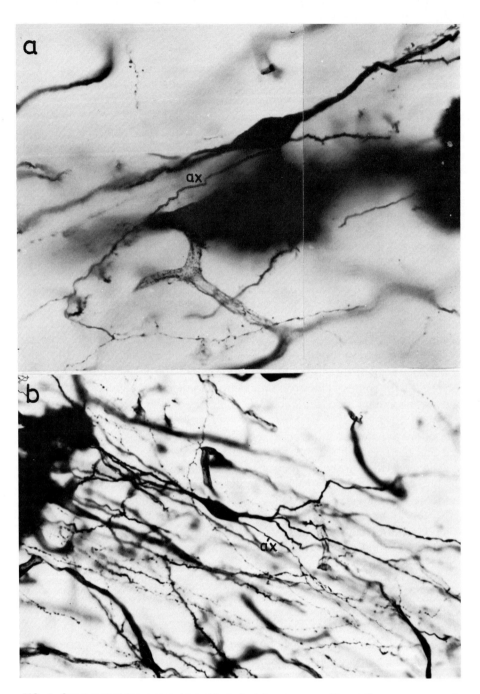

FIG. 5. Cat suprasylvian gyrus, layer VI. **a, b:** Interneurons with medium-range axonal arborization **(ax).** Fusiform neurons with long, polarly arranged dendrites, which are densely packed with spines. The axon branches are arranged horizontally. Some spine-like terminal side branches are on the axon branches.

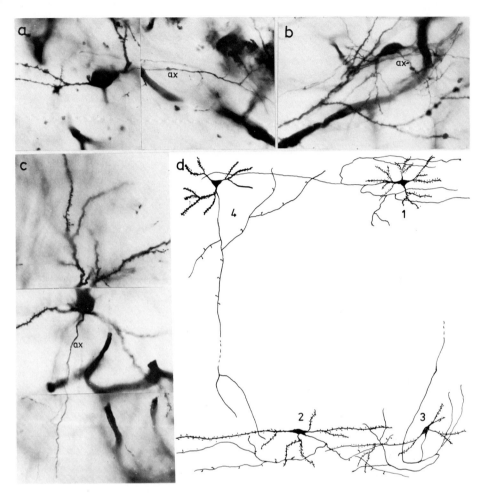

FIG. 6. Interneurons with medium-range axonal arborization in rabbit visual and somato-sensory cortex (**ax** = axon). **a:** Fusiform neuron in layer VI of visual cortical area. **b:** Horizontal cell of Cajal in layer I of somatosensory cortex. **c:** Multiangular neuron in layer I of visual cortex. **d:** Schematic drawing of the vertically and horizontally arranged inter-neurons. **1:** Horizontal cell of Cajal. **2:** Fusiform neuron in layer VI. **3:** Martinotti cell in layer VI. **4:** Multiangular neuron in layer I.

and spine-like protrusions can usually be observed on their surface. The usually arciform stem axon gives off vertical branches. The vertical axon branches, in addition to some preterminals, emit horizontally oriented collaterals at regular intervals generally in anteroposterior direction. These collaterals could be traced for distances up to 500 to 1,000 μm. Fine pre-terminal branches originate from these horizontal, long collaterals and after a short vertical course ramify into two or more beaded terminals that surround and contact the pyramid cell somata. Both the small and

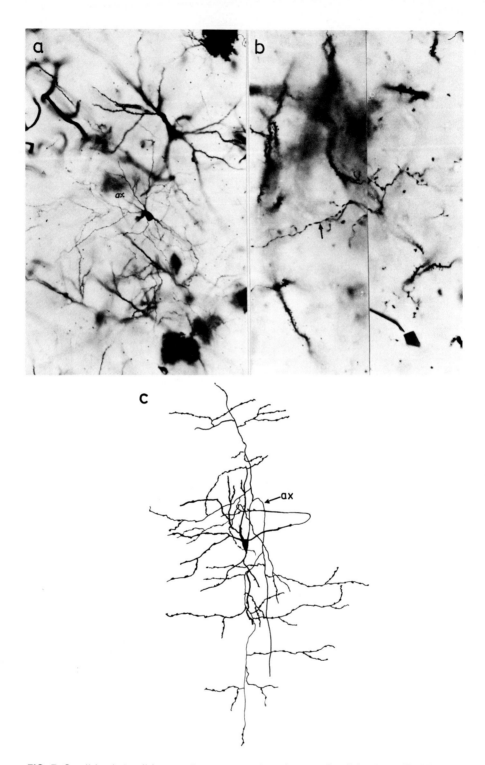

FIG. 7. Small basket cell in somatosensory cortex of cat. **a:** Small basket cell with axon (**ax**) in layer II. **b:** A horizontal axon branch with small varicose side branches of the small basket neuron. **c:** Drawing of the same small basket neuron.

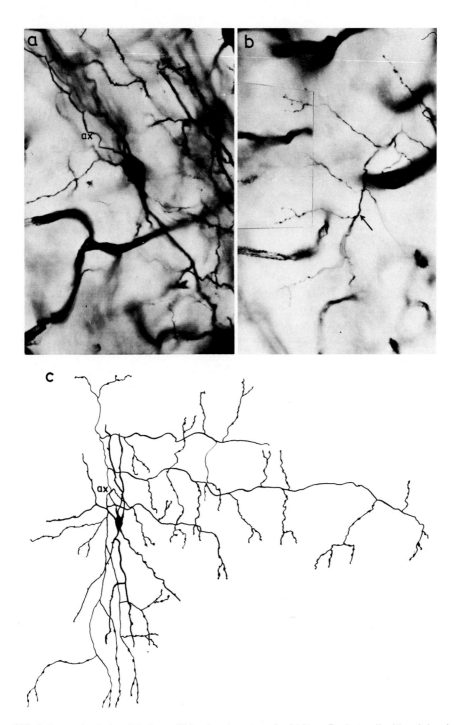

FIG. 8. Large basket cell in layer IV in visual cortex of rabbit. **a:** Basket cell with origin of axon **(ax). b:** A horizontal axon branch with several preterminal side branches ramifying into some varicose terminals. **c:** Drawing of the large basket cell in **a.**

the large basket cells have been widely discussed as inhibitory interneurons (31,32,34) (Fig. 8).

A separate cell type of this group deserves a somewhat more detailed discussion. This is a cell corresponding to the "chandelier" cell of Szentágothai (33,34), found in the upper layers, or the type 4 interneuron of Jones (14) described in all layers of the somatosensory cortex, respectively. In the cat visual, somatosensory, and other cortical areas the chandelier cells occur—in our material—in all layers, except the first (Figs. 9–11). No chandelier cells have been found so far in the rabbit cortex; however, a negative result in Golgi material is of little value. Their cell body is of medium size, fusiform with vertically oriented long axis. The long dendrites, which bear no spines, are similarly vertically arranged. The distinctive feature of these chandelier neurons is their axonal arborizations. After a variable vertical course, the axon turns into horizontal direction and gives off several vertical, ascending or descending, and repeatedly ramifying branches. The secondary or tertiary axonal branches are often thicker than the axon at its origin. Most characteristic of these cells are the candlestick terminal portions forming a strictly vertical bunch either in straight continuation of the preterminal fiber or curving back into the opposite direction. These vertically oriented terminal portions are found virtually in all layers but the first. From this orientation and also from electron microscopic observations (34), it seems evident that the axons contact selectively apical dendrites of pyramidal cells. The axonal arborization in layers V and VI slightly differ from those found in the outer layers. The vertical expansion of the axon arborization is not as large as in lamina IV. The courses of the terminal portions correspond to the less regular vertical courses of the apical dendrites in the deeper layers of the cortex (Fig. 11).

A comparison of the axonal arborizations of the chandelier neurons in layers IV and above show a difference between their dimensions. In the horizontal direction their spread is about the same, about 250 to 300 μm. Their vertical diameter is largest in layer IV where terminal portions of the same may also invade layers III and V. The axonal arborization can be found in three successive sections in both cases. Correspondingly, one might suppose that the chandelier neurons occupy well-circumscribed columns of 120 to 150 μm radius of the cortical tissue.

The number of "candlestick" terminal portions of one axonal arborization varies between 150 and 250. The length of one terminal portion is about 20 to 50 μm containing 8 to 10 boutons of 2 μm diameter each (Fig. 11).

These numerical data of the chandelier neurons suggest a massive and compactly organized structure that can establish a cuff of concentrated contacts on the apical dendrites of numerous pyramidal neurons or possibly on more or less vertically oriented main dendrites of other projective neurons in layer VI. On the basis of recent electron microscopic observations (34), this type of cell is very likely to be inhibitory in nature.

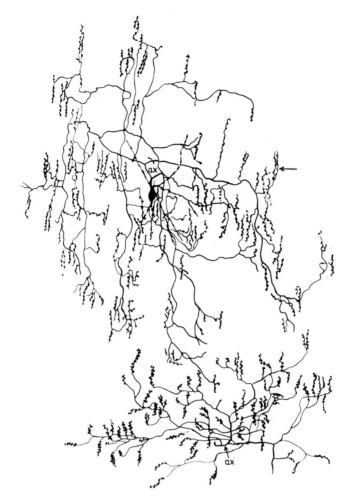

FIG. 9. Drawing of a chandelier neuron in cat visual cortex, layer IV. The axon **(ax)** arborization with numerous terminal portions is well seen.

What is most striking in the comparison between the Golgi architectonics of the neocortex of the cat and the rabbit is the essential similarity in principal organization reflected even in minute details of shape and arborization pattern of various interneurons (Fig. 12). The lack of the so-called "chandelier" cell in the rabbit cannot be taken too seriously; this very characteristic cell type has not been found in so many studies up to very recently. Golgi architectonics—in spite of its fundamental value—seem to bear little relevance for areal distinction. Apparently, the same cell types occur in very different relative numbers, as clearly reflected in the Nissl cytoarchitectonics, but this is just what would escape totally in the Golgi picture. Additionally, it obviously is the input and output in which

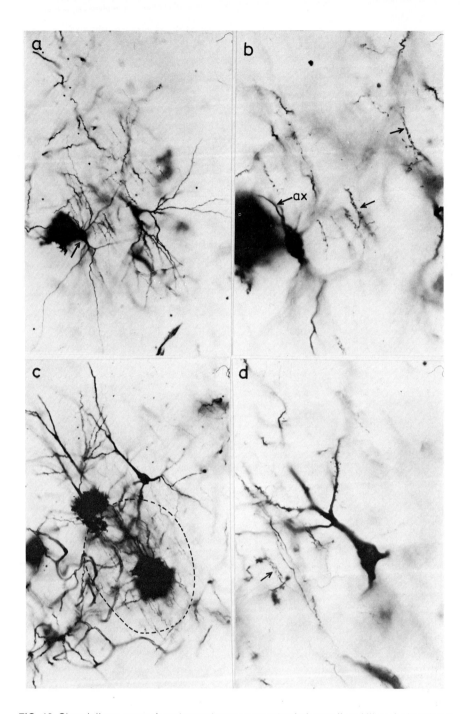

FIG. 10. Chandelier neurons in cat somatosensory cortex in layers II and III. **a:** A chandelier neuron with axonarborization. **b:** The same neuron with higher magnification. Arrows point to the terminal portions. **c:** The arborization field of a chandelier neuron is circumscribed with dotted line. **d:** Arrows point to the terminal portions of chandelier neuron.

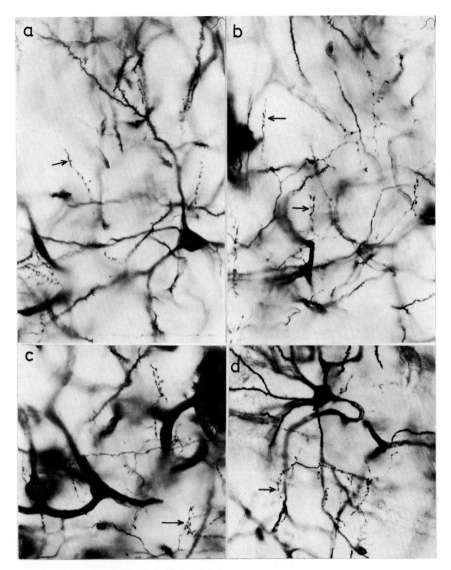

FIG. 11. Terminal portions **(arrows)** of axon arborization of chandelier neurons in layers V **(a, b, and c)** and VI **(d)**.

the fundamental areal differences are invested. Typology of nerve cells in itself would tend to overemphasize similarities both between different species and different areas of the same species. This is to caution us against overrating the significance of cell typology and a challenge to concentrate on other more distinctive features of different cortical regions.

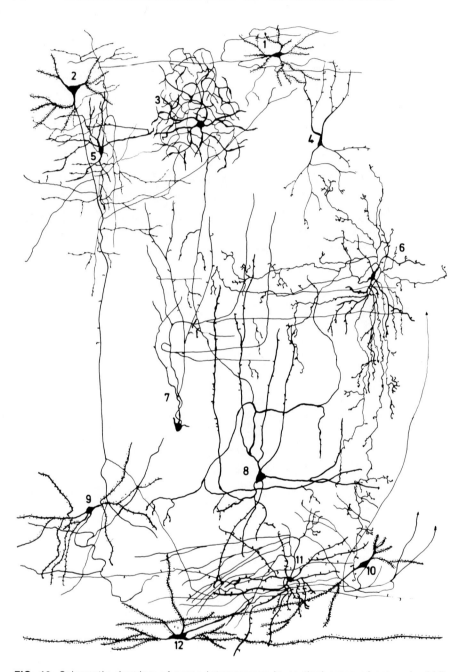

FIG. 12. Schematic drawing of some interneurons in cortical areas of cat and rabbit. **1:** Horizontal cell of Cajal. **2:** Multiangular cell of layer I. **3:** Neurogliform neuron. **4:** Golgi type II interneuron. **5:** Small basket cell in layers II and III. **6:** Interneuron with medium-range axonal arborization extending both in vertical and horizontal directions. **7, 8:** Large basket cells. **9:** Golgi type II interneuron in layer V. **10:** Martinotti cell. **11:** Golgi type II interneuron in layer VI. **12:** Horizontal fusiform neuron in layer VI.

REFERENCES

1. Brodmann, K. (1903): Beiträge zur histologischen Localisation der Grosshirnrinde. Erste Mitteilung. Die Regio Rolandica. *J. Psychol. Neurol.*, 2:79–132.
2. Ramon y Cajal, S. (1911): *Histologie du Système Nerveux de l'Homme et des Vertébrés, Vol. 2.* Maloine, Paris.
3. Campbell, A. W. (1903): Histological studies on cerebral localisation. *Proc. R. Soc.*, 72:488–492.
4. Clark, W. E. Le Gros, and Boggon, R. H. (1935): The thalamic connections of the parietal and frontal lobes of the brain in the monkey. *Philos. Trans. R. Soc. Lond.* [*Biol.*], 224:313–359.
5. Colonnier, M. (1966): The structural design of the neocortex. In: *Brain and Conscious Experience,* edited by J. C. Eccles, pp. 1–23. Springer Verlag, New York.
6. Economo, C. von, and Koskinas, G. N. (1925): *Die Cytoarchitektonik der Hirnrinde des erwachsenen Menschen.* Springer, Wien.
7. Garey, L. J., and Powell, T. P. S. (1967): The projection of the lateral geniculate nucleus upon the cortex in the cat. *Proc. R. Soc. Lond.* [*Biol.*], 169:107–126.
8. Garey, L. A., and Powell, T. P. S. (1971): An experimental study of the termination of the lateral geniculo-cortical pathway in the cat and monkey. *Proc. R. Soc. Lond.* [*Biol.*], 179:41–63.
9. Globus, A., and Scheibel, A. B. (1967): Pattern and field in cortical structure: the rabbit. *J. Comp. Neurol.*, 131:155–172.
10. Guillery, R. W. (1966): A study of Golgi preparations from the dorsal lateral geniculate nucleus of the adult cat. *J. Comp. Neurol.*, 128:21–69.
11. Hubel, D. H., and Wiesel, T. N. (1963): Shape and arrangement of columns in cat's striate cortex. *J. Physiol. (Lond.)*, 165:559–568.
12. Hubel, D. H., and Wiesel, T. N. (1965): Receptive fields and functional architecture in the cat's visual cortex. *J. Physiol. (Lond.)*, 160:106–154.
13. Hubel, D. H., and Wiesel, T. N. (1969): Anatomical demonstration of columns in the monkey striate cortex. *Nature,* 221:747–750.
14. Jones, E. G. (1975): Varieties and distribution of nonpyramidal cells in the somatic sensory cortex of the squirrel monkey. *J. Comp. Neurol.*, 160:205–268.
15. Jones, E. G., and Powell, T. P. S. (1969): An electron microscopic study of the mode of termination of cortico-thalamic fibers in the thalamic relay nuclei of the cat. *Proc. R. Soc. Lond.* [*Biol.*], 172:173–185.
16. Jones, E. G., and Powell, T. P. S. (1970): Electron microscopy of the somatic sensory cortex of the cat. I. Cell types and synaptic organization. *Philos. Trans. R. Soc. Lond.* [*Biol.*], 257:1–11.
17. Lorente de Nó, R. (1922): La corteza cerebral del raton. (Primera contribucion. La corteza acustica). *Trab. Lab. Invest. Biol. Madrid,* 20:41–78.
18. Lorente de Nó, R. (1938): Cerebral cortex: architecture, intracortical connections, motor projections. In: *Physiology of the Nervous System,* 1st edition, edited by J. F. Fulton. Oxford University Press, London.
19. Lund, J. S. (1973): Organization of neurons in the visual cortex area 17, of the monkey (*Macaca mulatta*). *J. Comp. Neurol.*, 147:455–496.
20. Marin-Padilla, M. (1969): Origin of the pericellular baskets of the pyramidal cells of the human motor cortex: A Golgi study. *Brain Res.*, 14:633–646.
21. Mountcastle, V. B. (1957): Modality and topographic properties of single neurons of cat's somatic sensory cortex. *J. Neurophysiol.*, 20:408–434.
22. O'Leary, J. L. (1941): Structure of the area striata of the cat. *J. Comp. Neurol.*, 75:131–164.
23. Otsuka, R., and Hassler, R. (1962): Über Aufbau und Gliederung der corticalen Sehsphäre bei der Katze. *Arch. Psychiatr. Z. Ges. Neurol.*, 203:212–234.
24. Polyak, S. (1932): *The Main Afferent Fiber Systems of the Cerebral Cortex in Primates.* University of California Press, Berkeley, California.
25. Powell, T. P. S., and Mountcastle, V. B. (1959): Some aspects of the functional organization of the cortex of the postcentral gyrus of the monkey: A correlation of findings obtained in a single unit analysis with cytoarchitecture. *Bull. Johns Hopkins Hosp.*, 105:133–162.
26. Rose, J. E., and Woolsey, C. N. (1948): Structure and relations of limbic cortex and anterior thalamic nuclei in rabbit and cat. *J. Comp. Neurol.*, 89:279–348.

27. Rose, J. E., and Woolsey, C. N. (1948): The orbitofrontal cortex and its connections with the medio-dorsal nucleus in the rabbit, sheep and cat. *Assoc. Res. Nerv. Ment. Dis.*, 27:210–232.
28. Sholl, D. A. (1963): Dendritic organization in the neurons of the visual and motor cortices of the cat. *J. Anat.*, 87:387–406.
29. Szentágothai, J. (1967): The anatomy of complex integrative units in the nervous system. In: *Recent Development in Neurobiology in Hungary, Vol. 1.*, edited by K. Lissák, pp. 9–45. Akadémiai Kiadó, Budapest.
30. Szentágothai, J. (1969): Architecture of the cerebral cortex. In: *Basic Mechanisms of the Epilepsies*, edited by H. H. Jasper, A. A. Ward, and A. Pope. Little, Brown, Boston.
31. Szentágothai, J. (1970): Les circuits neuronaux de l'écorce cérébrale. *Bull. Acad. R. Méd. Belg.*, 10:475–492.
32. Szentágothai, J. (1973): Synaptology of the visual cortex. In: *Handbook of Sensory Physiology, Vol. 713: Visual Centers in the Brain*, edited by R. Jung. Springer-Verlag, Berlin.
33. Szentágothai, J., and Arbib, M. A. (1974): Conceptual models of neural organization. *Neurosci. Res. Program Bull.*, 12:313–510.
34. Szentágothai, J. (1975): The "module-concept" in cerebral cortex architecture. *Brain Res.*, 95:475–496.
35. Tömböl, T. (1972): A Golgi analysis of the sensory-motor cortex in the rabbit. In: *Synchronization of EEG Activity in Epilepsies*, edited by H. Petsche and M. A. B. Brazier, pp. 25–36. Springer Verlag, Vienna.
36. Valverde, F. (1971): Short axon neuronal subsystems in the visual cortex of the monkey. *Int. J. Neurosci.*, 1:181–197.
37. Vogt, O., and Vogt, C. (1963): Zur anatomischen Gliederung des Cortex cerebri. *J. Psychol. Neurol.*, 2:160–180.
38. Walker, A. E. (1938): *The Primate Thalamus*. Chicago University Press, Chicago.
39. Walker, A. E. (1940): A cytoarchitectural study of the prefrontal area of the macaque monkey. *J. Comp. Neurol.*, 73:59–86.

Architectonics of the Cerebral Cortex,
edited by M. A. B. Brazier and H. Petsche.
Raven Press, New York © 1978.

Specificity Versus (Quasi-) Randomness in Cortical Connectivity

J. Szentágothai

*First Department of Anatomy, Semmelweis University Medical School, H-1450,
Budapest, Hungary*

Whenever he is looking at any piece of neural tissue, the investigator becomes immediately confronted with the choice between two conflicting issues: the question of how much of the intricate wiring of the neuropil is strictly predetermined by some genetically prescribed blueprint, and how much freedom is left to chance within some framework of statistical probabilities or some secondary mechanisms of trial and error, or selecting connections according to necessities or the individual history of the animal. Even on brief reflection one has to arrive at the conclusion that the case may not rest on either extreme. I shall not enter into a discussion of the ultimate consequences of either stand; this has been done repeatedly by various authors, and the difficulties encountered on both ends are insurmountable. The fundamental question is phrased usually more carefully as "specificity versus plasticity," and with good reason. Plasticity of neural connexions is a legitimate concept with a good deal of experimental proof, especially in the recent literature, whereas "randomness" is some kind of anathema. In spite of this I should like to keep away from the issue of plasticity—with which I have been concerned in earlier times (27,35), well before the recent elegant experimental models (8,9,14,21–23) became available—mainly because of my skepticism against the use of the crude growth mechanisms involved as models for memory and learning. What I intend to do instead is to take a look at cortical connectivity with the mental strategy of trying to understand how much of it could be explained as being determined by the principles that we know to be operative during neural tissue development and, conversely, how much would have to be left to chance within a certain deterministic framework.

There cannot be much doubt today that afferent input to cortex or cortex-like-layered neural structures is geometrically highly ordered, excellent examples being available in the optic tectum, the cerebellar cortex (11,36), and the visual cortex (6). The basic principle of order appears in many cases to be simply some parallel lamination of fibers of common origin or some other feature that they have in common. In other cases the ordering principle is more complex and may be the preservation of an almost complete isomorphism in the cortical representation of the periphery, as exemplified by the so-called "cortical barrels" (37). It is certainly remarkable that the tangential spread within the layered structure of the specific afferents is within the size or often somewhat less than the spacing of the lamination of the input. In the cerebellum there is some indication that the organization of input is even more delicate, possibly a fraction of the 1-mm-wide strips seen anatomically. However, when translated into connectivity on the cellular level, the situation becomes more intricate. We believe we know now the main direct target cells of the sensory afferents: the spiny stellates of lamina IV. But what is the divergence and what the convergence? The situation becomes even more difficult with the other systems like the corticocortical afferents. Although they have a largely columnar organization (3), they reach layers I and II chiefly, where it is less likely that massive contacts between any given afferent and any single cortical cell could exist.

Using considerably improved degeneration techniques and taking advantage of the possibility of fine adjustment of contrasts in dark-field microscopy Záborszky et al. (38) could show that even regions of apparently massive degeneration of callosal fibers in the upper cortical layers can be resolved into distinct groups of degeneration fragments of about 300 μm diameters (in the tangential direction). This means that the basic units of corticocortical input are vertically oriented cylindrical—or more correctly speaking hourglass (= rotation hyperboloid) shape—columns of cortical tissue penetrating through the entire depth of the cortex. Consequently, even in the tangentially oriented neuropil of lamina I, contacts of any given corticocortical afferent would be limited to the space of a relatively flat disc of 300 μm diameter and, apart from the few nonpyramidal cells, virtually to the branchings of the apical dendrites of the pyramidal cells situated in this column and to some entering branches from pyramidal cell apical dendrites of the neighbouring columns. Extrapolating this system of 300-μm-wide vertical cylinders as the basic unit of corticocortical connectivity—in one direction, i.e., from looking at what comes into a certain locus of cortex from other cortical regions—we have to arrive at the conclusion that the spatial specificity of corticocortical connexions is much more complex than one could have expected.

Unfortunately, the spatial resolving power of our present anatomical methods for tracing neurons in the reverse sense i.e., for asking the question, "From what other cortical loci do afferents impinge upon a certain cortical locus?," is not yet refined enough to detect such delicate "point-to-point" relations. From the vast material now quickly accumulating from the use of the horseradish peroxidase method for tracing corticocortical connexions in backward direction, there are at least indications that specific connectivity in the sense of the specificity of the sources of corticocortical afferents directed to a given locus is as refined (although probably in a different sense) as that of the convergence at specific cortical loci of fibers arising from a wider field of cortical sources.

The question of the spatial specificity of the relatively long-range connexions of the cerebral cortex, however, is of relatively little concern for
the basic problem that I want to discuss. We, therefore, may leave this issue
with the preliminary conclusion that, although there is virtually no possibility, anatomically, for anything like a "point-to-point" connectivity on the
level of single cells in long- or medium-range connexions, such a predetermined specificity can be realistically assumed for relatively small pieces
(columns) of cortex with cell numbers within the order of magnitude of 100.

The central problem of these considerations is the internal — or in other
words local — connectivity, because it might be in this field that, at the present stage of our understanding of the cerebral cortex, the most important
questions can be raised. As we have just seen, we have all the specific wiring
in long- and medium-range connexions that one might wish for, but how
about the local neuronal apparatus? What kind of specific wiring and connectivity can be expected from cells that have dendrites (i.e., receiving processes) that extend for hundreds of microns, and axon arborizations that
might look as diffuse brushes of branches without any apparent spatial
orientation or specific targets? I have been trying, for over 10 years, first
on the basis of the very scanty material available on local connectivity
(24,25) and first in a somewhat simplistic manner (26,28) to develop a coherent concept of internal neuron circuitry. Aided by the quick accumulation
of new Golgi data (5,7,10), I was able to give shape to the concept in a sequence of iterative attempts (29–31,34) until it reached the level reflected
in a paper written for the Brodal Festschrift (32).

A relatively high degree of specificity appears to prevail in local neuron
circuits in two major respects: (a) a number of specific interneurons are
highly selective not only concerning the kind of other neurons with which
they establish synapses, but also concerning what part of these neurons they
contact; (b) there is a relatively strict geometric order in the distribution
of local interneuron axons, i.e., each axon appears to have available for its
arborization a space unit of cortical tissue having a well-defined size, shape,
orientation, and localization.

In other words, the synapses established by the axon of an interneuron
are distributed and, hence, their action is exercised within a well-defined
space module of the cortex. In some cases these synapses are so densely
distributed that virtually all neurons — of course, those that are the specific
targets of that interneuron — of this space module receive a synapse from the
axon belonging to the module. This is particularly apparent in some of the
putative inhibitory interneurons that have thus far been identified on the
basis of structural criteria of their synapses (32,33). The large basket cells,
for example, appear to establish synapses with the somata of all pyramidal
cells situated within their narrow vertically oriented trench-like spaces that
cut through a large part of laminae III, IV, and V (10,29). This does not
mean, of course, that there is no convergence under such circumstances. On
the contrary, the relatively small number of boutons — at least in the large

basket cells (31) — given to a pyramid cell body by a single preterminal axon (in the order of 10) in contrast to the large number of axosomatic synaptic contacts of the assumed inhibitory type (so-called SF boutons, standing for *symmetrical* membrane contact and *flattened* synaptic vesicles) would strongly suggest a major convergence from several basket cells to any given pyramid cell. This would be a case somewhat similar to the basket cells of the cerebellar cortex, where the convergence upon any given basket surrounding a Purkinje cell would be, according to the calculation of Palkovits et al. (12), about 50:1. This is not necessarily so, however, because the so-called "chandelier" cell (32), (see also illustrations by Tömböl, *this volume*) yields so many groups of terminals densely arranged around a certain short stretch of pyramid-cell dendritic shafts, that no more boutons of the same SF type could be accommodated on the same portion of the shaft. Obviously, this would not exclude the possibility that groups of axon terminals of several "chandelier" cells are arranged sequentially at different portions of a dendritic shaft, but there is neither any Golgi nor electron microscopic evidence so far that would support such an assumption.

The geometric and modular specificity is less clearly demonstrable in putative local excitatory connexions, but there are some good reasons to assume that the situation is similar. There is considerable evidence now for the assumption that a specific kind of spiny stellate cell (5,7) of lamina IV is the main target in the primary sensory regions of the cortex for the specific afferents. The axonal arborization of these cells is mainly vertically ascending, therefore, in dense vertical strands of thin terminal fibers that appear to establish synapses mainly with the spines of the apical dendrites of the pyramid cells (28,31). Another prime target for specific afferents may be small neurogliform cells with vertically descending axons also arborizing in strands of delicate terminal fibers mainly of vertical orientation (30,32). This would mean that specific sensory impulse patterns arriving in lamina IV and bringing a quasi-two-dimensional spatiotemporal pattern of excitation (neglecting for the sake of simplicity any interference by simultaneously excited inhibitory interneurons), would be translated into a vertical projection of this pattern ascending toward the upper and descending toward the lower layers of the cortex. Since there would be, obviously, some interference by inhibitory mechanisms and some lateral interaction between the projections from neighbouring regions of lamina IV, this might easily account for the fact that while, for example in the visual cortex, the cells of the receiving layer are mainly monocularly driven, the cells vertically above and below are already binocularly driven and show in addition various specific receptive field properties (orientation, movement, sensitivity, etc.).

The basic functional organization of the cerebral cortex would thus vaguely resemble that of the cerebellar cortex with two important differences: (a) the input patterns are delivered in both cases in quasi-two-dimensional sheets, in the cerebellar cortex in sagittally oriented, very thin discs of the granular layer (in the case of the mossy afferents) and in the cerebral cortex to sublaminae of lamina IV; (b) from here the pattern is bidirectionally projected, in the case of the cerebellar cortex in the transverse direction (i.e., parallel to the surface and the axes of the folia) by the T-shaped branches of the granule cell axons (= the parallel fibers in the molecular layer). Conversely in the cerebral cortex the input pattern is projected in the vertical direction upward toward the superficial and downward toward the deeper laminae. This very vague similarity in basic organization does not, of course, suggest any similarity in the details; on the contrary, it is more suited to emphasize the overwhelming differences in the complexity of the two neural structures.

The picture emerging from such considerations is one of a very high degree of specific wiring both in distant and in local connexions of the cerebral cortex. We have to be aware of the fact that anatomical techniques can indicate only the maximal "grain" size of the spatial resolution (for example, 300-μm-wide strips or columns), and that the true resolution in connectivity may in fact be one order of magnitude finer. The specificity in connexions is aided by two further mechanisms (one might venture to use the expression "operators"): one being the specificity of certain axons to establish synaptic contacts only with certain loci of certain types of neurons, the other the aforementioned "modular principle" of axonal arborizations. This latter can, on the basis of a given density (i.e., determined spacing of certain neuron types), simply bring about a very high degree of specific connectivity, without having recourse to the assumption of an unreasonable degree of inbuilt almost individual specificities in the selection of connexions.

However, all this is only one side of the matter. A single look at one of the classic illustrations of Golgi-stained pyramidal cells or at the impressive drawing of three neighbouring pyramids by M. E. and A. B. Scheibel (19, Fig. 7) may convince anybody that the uniquely rich initial collateral system of the pyramid cells contributes to a type of connectivity that is highly different from that which has been discussed in the preceding paragraphs. Most important, the distances covered by these collaterals are much larger — 1 to 1.5 mm — than those of the "columnar" systems established by various types of cortical afferents. This is also supported by direct degenerative evidence in the case of small intracortical lesions in chronically isolated pieces of cortex (2). The highly systematic mode of orientation and distribution of these collaterals — the first (most proximal) collaterals almost invariably ascend nearly vertically, while the next have an increasingly oblique ascending, horizontal, and eventually an oblique descending course (32, Fig. 1) — leaving little room for any specific "addressing" of the collaterals to other neurons of any specific locations.

Earlier Golgi studies in chronically isolated cortical slabs (24) have shown that these collaterals appear to contact any neuronal element that they come across, mainly spines of other pyramid cells. Figures 1 and 2 show drawings

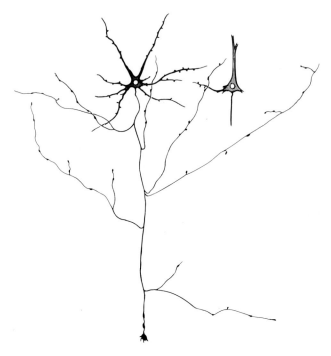

FIG. 1. Upper lamina II pyramid cell and its collateral system from chronically isolated cortical slab in rapid Golgi stain. The cut runs through the middle of lamina III, where the transected axon shows abortive growth cones. One collateral appears to establish contact with basal dendrite of neighbouring pyramid cell. Adult cat visual cortex.

of such pyramid cells and their collaterals in isolated cortices. The Golgi pictures are, of course, little suited for extracting exact information about synapses, apart from axon–spine synapses that can be recognized relatively easily, and from the negative statement that even the most terminal branches of the pyramid collaterals do not attach themselves in specific ways (for example, by forming baskets or surrounding apical dendrites) to specific parts of other nerve cells. There is, hence, little possibility for any kind of specific connectivity established by the pyramid collaterals; on the contrary, it looks as though an extremely diffuse, almost random connectivity would be established by any pyramid cell in a surround of 3-mm diameter (we do not know as yet whether this surround is indeed circular, i.e., a cylinder, or whether the cylinder might be elliptic with the longer axis in some specific direction). Additionally the number of synapses given by any collateral to any given other neuron has to be small, apart from the vertically ascending first collaterals that might give repeated contacts to the spines of a neighbouring apical dendrite.

Figure 3 tries to give an impression of the quantitative relations by viewing from above the collateral system of a single pyramidal cell, placed into

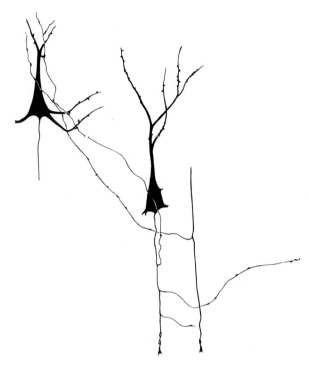

FIG. 2. Same as Fig. 1 showing two pyramid cells and the axon of a third with part of their collateral system and some axon–spine synapses established with dendrites of pyramid cell at left.

the center of the drawing. The number and arborization pattern of this cell corresponds to that of the already mentioned drawing by Scheibel and Scheibel (19, Fig. 7) and to that observed in isolated cortical slabs (Figs. 1 and 2). The maximal spread of the collaterals is indicated by a circle having the diameter of 3 mm. All cells situated within this circle—and additionally some whose dendrites invade the corresponding cylinder—are potential recipients of synapses from the central cell. An approximate idea of the number of pyramidal cells located within this cylinder is indicated by the group of small circles right below the central cell, corresponding to the bundles of apical dendrites as described by Peters and Walsh (13). Such a "cluster" of pyramidal cells corresponds to about 20 to 30 pyramidal cells arranged in the entire depth of the cortex, and contributing their apical dendrites to bundles of around 100 μm diameter (in lamina II), where the bundling disappears partly by merging of the neighbouring bundles and partly by the arborization of the dendritic shafts.

It is easy to calculate that roughly 700 of such bundles, i.e., 20 to 30 times as many pyramidal cells are within such a 3-mm-wide cylinder, and the

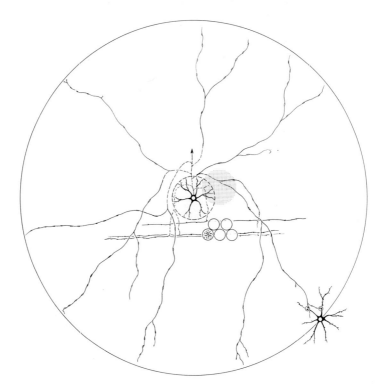

FIG. 3. Collateral system of a pyramid cell **(center)** as it would appear in the view from the surface (semidiagrammatic reconstruction). The large circle having a diameter of 3 mm indicates the potential territory reached by the collaterals. The pyramid cell below right on the perimeter would be a potential recipient of synaptic contacts from the central cell. The small circles (100 μm diameter) correspond to the apical dendrite bundles (ref. 13) containing 20 to 30 apical dendrites of a pyramid-cell cluster. The round stippled area at right of central pyramid cell (± 300 μm diameter) indicates width of an "arborization-column" of corticocortical afferents. See text for further explanation.

density of collaterals from the same cluster is obtained by multiplying the illustrated collateral arborization 20 to 30 times. The total density of this collateral system at any point of the circle would correspond then to the spatial interpenetration of 700 cluster arborizations, i.e., 700×20 to 30 of the density shown in Fig. 3. For the sake of comparison the minimal size (300 μm) of a corticocortical connectivity column (see earlier in this chapter) is indicated by the hatched area.

Although each pyramidal cell has apparently only very few contacts with any other cell within reach of its collateral system, one should think that the simultaneous activity of neighbouring pyramidal cells (for example, within a column of cells having the same receptive field properties) ought to exercise a significant action on a large field of cortical tissue. Considering that pyramidal cells can be assumed to be excitatory in character [also supported by the anatomical information, on the mode of termination of corticocortical fiber systems by AR-type—standing for *asymmetrical* membrane contact and *round* synaptic vesicles—axon–spine synapses (31) and of corticothalamic fiber systems by the same type of AR synapses] and that many of the synapses given by the pyramidal cell collaterals appear to contact other pyramidal cells (Figs. 1 and 2), one should expect a strong positive (excitatory) feedback action between pyramidal cells. Curiously enough, little of this is experienced in physiological studies (2,4); if anything, the local corticocortical influence appears to be rather inhibitory. This calls for an inquiry into the local synaptic connectivity on the electron microscopic level with special attention to the synapses of the pyramid-cell collaterals.

In such a study it is best to take advantage of the cortical isolation technique, in order to get rid of the afferent pathways. Considering the possibility of sprouting, or other types of rearrangement, relatively short survival periods have been chosen (3 to 4 days). This is permissible in view of the relative rapidity of secondary degeneration in the cortex. In isolated cortical slabs containing all the six layers, the changes of synaptic structure are not very dramatic. As could be expected from earlier studies (1,25,32) the axosomatic synapses persisting on pyramidal cells are exclusively of the SF type (obviously basket-cell terminals) (Fig. 4). In the neuropil the typical AR–dendritic spine synapses (Figs. 4–6) are the most prominent persisting elements. They correspond in all fine cytological characteristics to the terminals of corticothalamic (geniculate) pathways that have been identified in scores of studies, and which originate mainly from pyramidal cells of the deeper layers (V and VI), so that one would have no difficulty to identify them as the synapses of pyramid-cell collaterals.

The persisting SF-type synapses on the apical dendrites (Fig. 5) could be identified without difficulty with the "chandelier-cell" synapses (32). It is, however, already apparent in such isolated slabs of entire cortex that numerous other types of synapses persist either with clearly round, or often with somewhat pleomorphic, vesicles (Fig. 6) that are neither of the usual "inhibitory" SF-type synapses, nor the AR-type spine synapses that are such good candidates for the terminals of the pyramid collaterals. But this is not astonishing if one thinks of the very large number of different types of neurons that obviously persist in such isolated slabs.

In order to reduce the number and diversity of surviving neuron types, isolated cortical slabs were prepared containing only $2\frac{1}{2}$ layers, i.e., they were undercut through the midportions of lamina III. (Most of these undercut slabs were virtually isolated from the remaining cortex; they were small, lense-shaped fragments of cortical tissue with their blood supply from the pial vessels.) The difference from isolated slabs of the entire cortex is remarkable. This is due partially to a massive degeneration of dendrites, which is to be expected especially for the apical dendrites of pyramidal cells located below the cut. Unfortunately, the shape of the synaptic vesi-

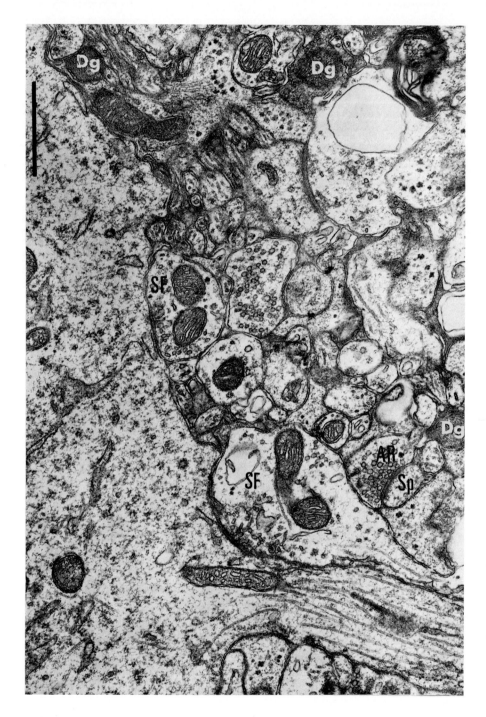

FIG. 4. Electron micrograph from isolated total cortical slab (visual cortex, cat) with part of pyramid cell body (in lamina III). Besides several axonal profiles in degeneration **(Dg)** two SF-type contacts (symmetrical membrane contact, flattened vesicles) one typical AR-type (asymmetrical membrane contact, round synaptic vesicles) axon–spine **(Sp)** contact remained intact. Scale 1 μm, 3 days after isolation.

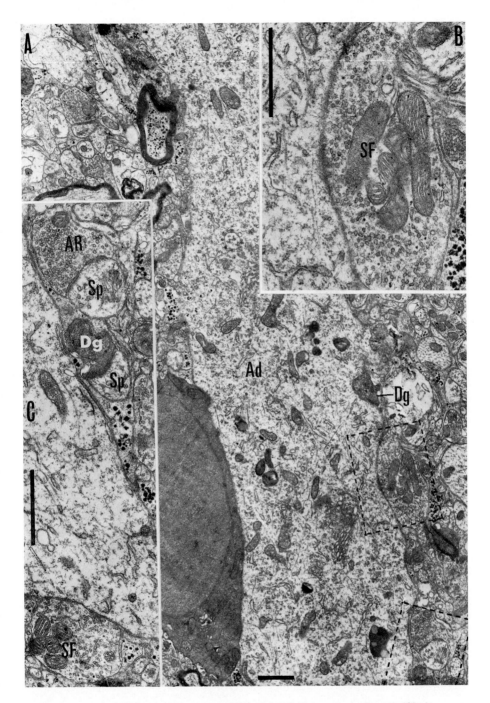

FIG. 5. Same material as in Fig. 4 (lamina III). Central electron micrograph **(A)** shows an apical dendrite **(Ad)** of pyramid cell. The two insets correspond to the upper **(B)** and to the lower **(C)** rectangular territory indicated in **A** (only part of the lower rectangular territory corresponding to **C** is indicated in micrograph **A**). Typical SF-type synapses persist along and in direct contact with the apical dendrite. From axon spine **(Sp)** some have degenerated **(Dg)**, while others intact **(AR)**, presynaptic contacts. Scale 1 μm.

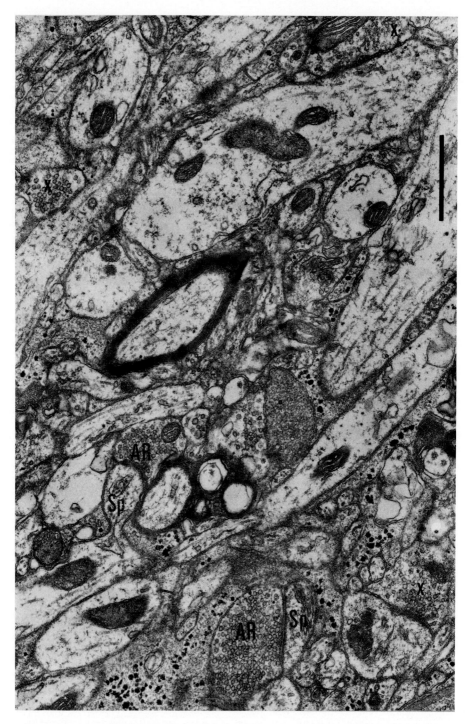

FIG. 6. Same material as in Figs. 4 and 5 (lamina I). The neuropil contains several typical AR-type axon–spine **(Sp)** synapses, but also some axodendritic synapses of various fine structure (indicated by **X**). The synaptic vesicles of the synapse **(X)** in the upper right corner have small pleomorphic vesicles; the others are roundish but not so densely arranged in the typical AR-type axon–spine synapses. Scale 1 μm.

cles becomes a much less reliable criterion, so that the identification of synapses has to be based mainly on characteristics of the postsynaptic membrane.

But even so a few facts were remarkable: (a) The typical "inhibitory" type of SF synapses have all but disappeared, a few persisting around cell bodies of lamina II, and upper lamina III pyramid cells may be the terminals of the small local basket cells of the second layer (28). From the characteristic double axon-spine synapses, from which one is an AR- and another an SF-type synapse, and from which the SF type was attributed (32) to the axonal tuft cells of Ramón y Cajal (18), some persisted. (b) The number of typical "AR" axon–spine synapses has radically decreased, apart from the most superficial layer of lamina I. This latter observation is in strong contradiction to our earlier impression (31) (gained from Golgi specimens of isolated fortical slabs) that pyramid-cell collaterals would practically not invade lamina I. It has to be checked also in view of the possibility that some very superficial tangential fibers escape destruction during the isolation.

A reason for the loss in typical axon–spine synapses may be a loss or shrinkage of the spines (Fig. 7), observed earlier in Golgi specimens (24) (see also Figs. 1 and 2), and also found in isolated cerebellar cortical slabs; so that earlier true axon–spine synapses might become simple axodendritic synapses. (c) What is most remarkable, however, is the large number of axodendritic synapses of various types that persist apparently unharmed in contact with both normal (or at least nondegenerating) and with degenerating dendrites (Fig. 8). On first sight, one might get the impression that these synapses were not present in the normal or even in the isolated total cortex slabs; however, on more careful comparison one finds that these synapses are present also in the normal material, but go unrecognized beside the more conspicuous axon–spine synapses of the usual AR and of the double synapses of the AR and SF types, as well as the axosomatic and axon–shaft dendrite SF-type synapses. The assumption that these inconspicuous axodendritic synapses would be the result of sprouting is hardly tenable, in view of the relatively short survival period; the lack of symptoms of sprouting was also apparent in earlier Golgi studies on isolated slabs with longer survival periods. Many of these (nonspine) axodendritic synapses, but certainly not all, might belong to pyramid cell collaterals. In spite of the distortion in this material of many terminals and especially of the synaptic vesicles, one gains the impression that the persisting synapses of such small isolated slabs belong to different types of local neurons. (d) A significant number, both in laminae I and II, of the double-spine synapses, having one AR and one SF contact (or sometimes two of either type), persists either completely or more often with a degenerated AR contact. This would be in agreement with earlier observations, and the conclusion that the SF-type contact has to originate from some local (probably inhibitory) interneurons, for which the axonal tuft cell of lamina II has been considered as the most

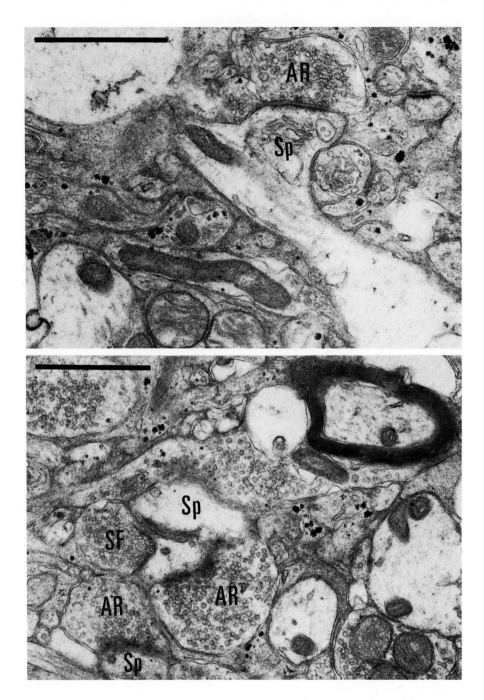

FIG. 7. Electron micrographs of neuropil details in small isolated cortical slabs (4 days after isolation; lamina I from visual cortex, adult cat). Shape and distribution of the synaptic vesicles are less well preserved than in isolated slabs of entire cortex. Upper electron micrograph shows persisting AR-type axon terminal in contact with short-necked spine **(Sp).** Lower micrograph shows one spine **(Sp, center)** possibly in early stages of degeneration with persisting double AR and SF presynaptic contacts. Another persisting AR spine **(Sp)** contact appears in lower left corner. Scales 1 μm.

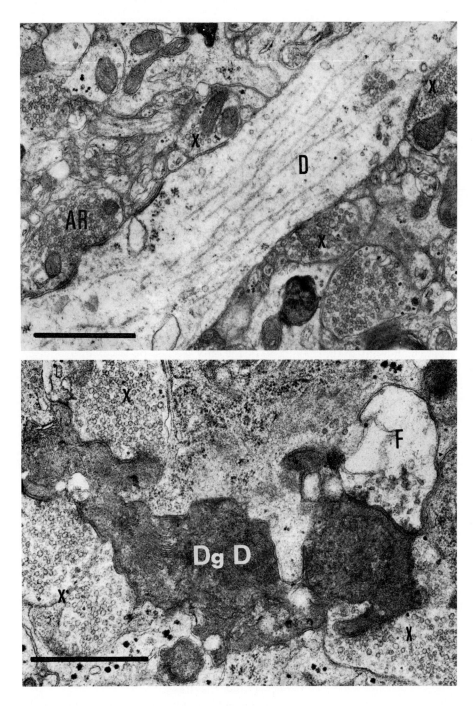

FIG. 8. Same material as in Fig. 7 (lamina II). Upper micrograph shows larger dendrite **(D)** with several persisting direct synaptic contacts, one of which appears to be a typical AR synapse (probably from pyramid axon collateral), the others **(X)** are of different fine structure. Lower micrograph shows degenerating dendrite **(DgD)** in contact with a F type probably also degenerating and several unidentified **(X)** axodendritic contacts. Scale 1 μm.

likely candidate (32). What is new is the persistence, in some cases, of the AR terminal (Fig. 7), which would indicate that not only distant afferents but also the pyramid axon collaterals might be involved in such contacts.

The main question that arises from these observations, particularly those listed under (c), is that of the origin of the persisting (nonspine) axodendritic synapses. Some of them might be pyramid axon collaterals contacting nonspiny interneurons. Some others might be earlier axon–spine synapses (also pyramid axons "translocated" in consequence of the atrophy of the spines). The first assumption would explain, if the nonspiny interneurons were inhibitory, the observation of inhibitory effects in the neighbourhood of active pyramid cells (2). But even if these assumptions were correct, we would have to account for a number of terminal axons that have round or pleomorphic vesicles but that do not fit into the picture — as concerns fine cytological details — of the pyramid axon collaterals. Indeed, there are in the upper cortical layers a considerable number of local Golgi type II cells, the terminals of which, so far, have not been even tentatively identified by electron microscopy. First, there are a considerable number of the general type of Golgi type II cells (according to the nomenclature proposed in ref. 31), which many authors think to be the only Golgi type II cell of the cortex. (One would wish that authors consult the classic description of the cerebral cortex by Ramón y Cajal (16,17) in which they would find almost all of the highly specific types of interneurons I have been trying to illustrate and to popularize over the last few years.) Although one occasionally finds the neurogliform cells of Ramón y Cajal also in the upper strata, they are probably much less frequent than in the deeper layers. There is, probably rarely, particularly one cell type that stains sufficiently in the Golgi material to be recognized. However, the large abundance of this type in some of our monkey material — mainly in parietal cortical regions — leads me to assume that it may be much more general than one might think from the lack of illustrations in the literature.

Some illustrations by Ramón y Cajal (16,18) show some resemblance to the cell shown in Fig. 9. This cell type has not been, so far, consciously observed (the same illustration and a brief description appears in ref. 33). It is a cell whose processes are usually arranged in a vertical columnar fashion, but what is remarkable is the strange honeycomb-like pattern caused by the side branches of the processes. It almost looks as though the "holes" of the honeycomb would accommodate cell bodies; on more close consideration, however, the "holes" are too small and much too densely arranged for such an assumption to be tenable. All the processes are apparently dendrites, but their arborizations show distinct axonal features.

In view of the rapidly increasing information in several regions of the central nervous system about amacrine-type anaxonal, or if not anaxonal, about cells having presynaptic dendrites (for information see ref. 15), we

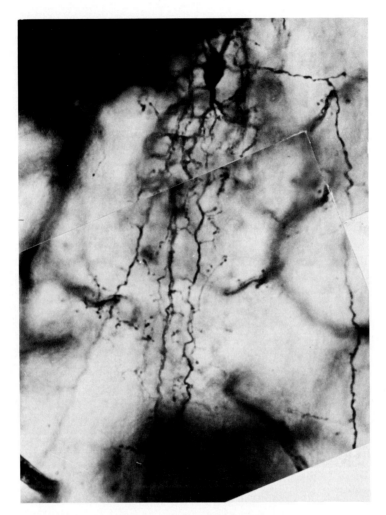

FIG. 9. Local interneuron with "axonal-like" arborization of the dendrites. Perfusion Golgi–Kopsch procedure, adult monkey parietal cortex, upper lamina III.

have to keep our minds open for the possibility that one or the other variety of these cells occurs also in the cerebral cortex. The apparent lack of the presynaptic dendrites in cortical structures, as compared with their abundance in thalamic and geniculate nuclei, and the scarcity of axoaxonal contacts does not rule out the possibility that other types of unconventional neurons do occur. The abundance of various unidentified types of synapses persisting in small isolated cortical slabs of the superficial layers (Figs. 7 and 8) would certainly point in this direction. In order to clarify this problem, one ought to have some direct electron microscopic observation on such cells (as shown in Fig. 9, for example, identified in Golgi-stained specimens) which might enable us to get some better information on their processes (i.e., whether they are presynaptic or postsynaptic).

The essential message that comes through from these observations and considerations is that there is a rather dense system of (autonomous) intrinsic connections in the upper $2\frac{1}{2}$ layers of the cerebral cortex (i.e., laminae I and II and the superficial part of lamina III) predominantly established over axodendritic (nonspine) synapses. A significant portion of these may be attributed to pyramid axon collaterals, but by no means all (probably even less than half). The relatively few persisting axon–spine synapses of the AR type with densely distributed relatively large, round synaptic vesicles can be identified on the basis of fine structural criteria, on analogy with the terminals of corticocortical, corticothalamic (geniculate), and corticosubcortical synapses with high confidence as being of pyramid axon collateral origin. By the same token, axodendritic synapses of similar structural features contacting dendrite surfaces proper are probably also of pyramid axon collateral origin. There is no reason whatsoever to assume that all of these dendrites are nonspiny parts of pyramid cell dendrites, although this has to be investigated by electron microscopic studies on Golgi-stained specimens of such isolated cortices.

But even if we would attribute half of the persisting synapses to pyramid cell axons, there would remain the other half of unidentified synaptic contacts. They have round or occasionally slightly pleomorphic vesicles, their membrane attachments are not clearly asymmetrical (A or I type of Gray), subsynaptic membrane thickenings or undercoatings are inconspicuous, the vesicles are of varying sizes in the several synapses, and much less densely distributed than in the terminals considered of pyramid cell origin. The scarcity of the typical SF-type synapses is apparent and suggests that only a few small basket cells of the upper layers and possibly some of the so-called "axonal tuft" cells of the second layer remain intact, which contribute the SF contacts of the persisting double axon–spine synapses.

The conclusion, therefore, is that a considerable number of local interneurons has to survive in the isolated upper layers of the cortex that have mainly axodendritic synapses lacking the usual criteria of the assumed conventional excitatory AS and putative inhibitory SF contacts.

We have seen in the preceding paragraph that there are several candidates for local (Golgi type II) cells that could be the sources of these contacts. It is worthwhile in this context to recall a recent imaginative approach to the general significance of so-called local circuit neurons in neural functions by Schmitt et al. (20), which gave much consideration to possible functional roles of such local neurons that would be radically beyond the functional roles hitherto attributed in the neural circuits to local neurons.

CONCLUSIONS

As discussed at some length in the first part of this paper, a very high degree of specific "wiring" prevails in most distant connexions of the cerebral cortex: both in corticocortical and subcorticocortical (and reverse) pathways. This specificity concerns both the types of neurons as well as of postsynaptic loci, and the relations between points that are connected. The "resolution" in topic connectivity is certainly within 300 μm (measured in tangential direction), but in reality probably much less (i.e., the resolution is much finer). An even more refined modus of connexion specificity is brought about in many types of local interneurons by a systematic spatial arrangement of axonal arborizations, termed the "modular" arrangement or construction principle of the cerebral cortex (32). Although there is nothing in cortical structure that might suggest any one-to-one (or true point-to-point) relation between two cortical neurons, the spatial resolution of this "modular system" may be as fine as 25 μm (in one dimension; in the other dimensions the modules are generally more extended).

But this is only one aspect of cortical connectivity. As seen in the example of the pyramid axon collaterals, there is also another system of connectivities that appears to be quasirandom within up to 3-mm-wide columns through the entire depth of the cortex. We cannot be sure at present whether there is any selectivity for types of neurons or for postsynaptic sites in the formation of contacts by the pyramid axon collaterals, but there seems to be no spatial selectivity for the location of synapses within the fairly rigidly determined arborization pattern of these collaterals. Even if one would find, with the aid of computer reconstruction of the true spatial arborization some anisotropy (i.e., some preferential direction in the horizontal plane—as shown, the general orientation in the vertical planes is determined by the sequence of origin—of the pyramid axon collateral arborizations, the spatial resolution in this type of connections is coarser by one order of magnitude at least, but possibly by two than that of the connexions mentioned in the preceding paragraph). Another possible source of randomness in spatial connectivity, probably on a finer scale, is introduced by some of the local interneurons: most probably by the so-called general type of Golgi type II cells, and possibly also by the hitherto little-considered type of cells illustrated in Fig. 9 which do not seem to have distinguishable axons, or, more correctly, whose dendritic arborizations bear many characteristics of axons. [Whether the so-called "neurogliform" cells of Ramón y Cajal (18) always have axons is not yet certain.] As judged from persisting synapses in isolated small cortical slabs, most of these interneurons establish axodendritic synapses with ill-defined fine structural characteristics, or at least with those that do not fit into the conventional picture of the assumed excitatory (AR-type) or putative inhibitory (SF-type) synapses.

Without wanting to enter into daring speculations about the possible significance of these two contrary aspects of cortical architecture, it appears intuitively acceptable that one would need something more in the cortex than an exactly predetermined blueprint of "wiring." In addition to such a predetermined specific connectivity, one would certainly want to have some "randomization" that would give room for the development of dynamic patterns, or some kind of cooperation in the neuronal network.

REFERENCES

1. Colonnier, M. (1968): Synaptic patterns of different cell types in the different laminae of the cat visual cortex. An electron microscope study. *Brain Res.*, 9:268–287.
2. Creutzfeldt, O. D., Garey, L. J., Kuroda, R., and Wolff, J. R. (1977): The distribution of degenerating axons after small lesions in the intact and isolated visual cortex of the cat. *Exp. Brain Res.*, 27:419–440.
3. Grant, G., Landgren, S., and Silfvenius, H. (1975): Columnar distribution of U-fibres from the postcruciate cerebral projection area of the cat's group I muscle afferents. *Exp. Brain Res.*, 24:57–74.
4. Hess, R., Negishi, K., and Creutzfeldt, O. (1975): The horizontal spread of intracortical inhibition in the visual cortex. *Exp. Brain Res.*, 22:415–419.
5. Jones, E. G. (1975): Varieties and distribution of non-pyramidal cells in the somatic sensory cortex of the squirrel monkey. *J. Comp. Neurol.*, 160:205–268.
6. LeVay, S., Hubel, D. H., and Wiesel, T. N. (1975): The pattern of ocular dominance columns in macaque visual cortex revealed by a reduced silver stain. *J. Comp. Neurol.*, 159:559–575.
7. Lund, J. S. (1973): Organization of neurons in the visual cortex area 17 of the monkey (*Macaca mulatta*). *J. Comp. Neurol.*, 147:455–496.
8. Lynch, G., Stanfield, B., and Cotman, C. W. (1973): Developmental differences in postlesion axonal growth in the hippocampus. *Brain Res.*, 59:155–168.
9. Lynch, G., Stanfield, B., Parks, T., and Cotman, C. W. (1974): Evidence for selective postlesion axonal growth in the dentate gyrus of the rat. *Brain Res.*, 69:1–11.
10. Marin-Padilla, M. (1970): Prenatal and early postnatal ontogenesis of the human motor cortex: A Golgi study. I. The sequential development of the cortical layers. *Brain Res.*, 23:167–184.
11. Oscarsson, O. (1973): Functional organization of spinocerebellar paths. In: *Handbook of Sensory Physiology, Vol. 2. Somatosensory System*, edited by A. Iggo, pp. 339–380. Springer Verlag, Berlin.
12. Palkovits, M., Magyar, P., and Szentágothai, J. (1971): Quantitative histological analysis of the cerebellar cortex in the cat. III. Structural organization of the molecular layer. *Brain Res.*, 34:1–18.
13. Peters, A., and Walsh, T. M. (1972): A study of the organization of apical dendrites in the somatic sensory cortex of the rat. *J. Comp. Neurol.*, 144:253–268.
14. Raisman, G. (1969): Neuronal plasticity in the septal nuclei of the adult rat. *Brain Res.*, 14:25–48.
15. Rakic, P. (1975): Local circuit neurons. *Neurosci. Res. Program Bull.*, 13:289–446.
16. Ramón y Cajal, S. (1899): Estudio sobrala cortezza cerebral humana. *Rev. Trim. Microscop.*, 4:1–63.
17. Ramón y Cajal, S. (1900): *Studien über die Hirnrinde des Menschen.* J. A. Barth, Leipzig.
18. Ramón y Cajal, S. (1911): *Histologie du Système Nerveux de l'Homme et des Vertébrés, Vol. 2.* Maloine, Paris.
19. Scheibel, M. A., and Scheibel, A. B. (1970): Elementary processes in selected thalamic and cortical subsystems—the structural substrates. In: *The Neurosciences Second Study Program*, Editor-in-Chief F. O. Schmitt, pp. 443–457. Rockefeller University Press, New York.
20. Schmitt, F. O., Dev, Parvati, and Smith, B. H. (1976): Electrotonic Processing of information by brain cells. *Science*, 193:114–120.

21. Schneider, G. E. (1970): Mechanisms of functional recovery following lesions of visual cortex or superior colliculus in neonate and adult hamsters. *Brain Behav. Evol.*, 3:295–323.
22. Schneider, G. E. (1972): Development of regeneration in the mammalian visual system. *Neurosci. Res. Program Bull.*, 10:287–290.
23. Schneider, G. E. (1973): Early lesions of superior colliculus: Factors affecting the formation of abnormal retinal projections. *Brain Behav. Evol.*, 8:73–109.
24. Szentágothai, J. (1965): The use of degeneration methods in the investigation of short neuronal connections. In: *Progress in Brain Research, Vol. 14. Degeneration Patterns in the Nervous System*, edited by M Singer and J. P. Schadé, pp. 1–32. Elsevier, Amsterdam.
25. Szentágothai, J. (1965): The synapse of short local neurons in the cerebral cortex. In: *Symposia Biologica Hungarica, Vol. 5. Modern Trends in Neuromorphology*, edited by J. Szentágothai, pp. 251–276. Akadémiai Kiadó, Budapest.
26. Szentágothai, J. (1967): The anatomy of complex integrative units in the nervous system. In: *Recent Development of Neurobiology in Hungary, Vol. 1. Results in Neuroanatomy, Neurochemistry, Neuropharmacology and Neurophysiology*, edited by K. Lissák, pp. 9–45. Akadémiai Kiadó, Budapest.
27. Szentágothai, J. (1968): Growth of the nervous system: An introductory survey. In: *Growth of the Nervous System*, edited by G. E. W. Wolstenholme and M. O'Connor, pp. 3–12. A Ciba Foundation Symposium. Churchill, London.
28. Szentágothai, J. (1969): Architecture of the cerebral cortex. In: *Basic Mechanisms of the Epilepsies*, edited by H. H. Jasper, A. A. Ward, and A. Pope, pp. 13–28. Little, Brown, Boston.
29. Szentágothai, J. (1970): Les circuits neuronaux de l'écorce cerébrale. *Bull. Acad. R. Med. Belg. 7 Sr.*, 10:475–492.
30. Szentágothai, J. (1972): The basic neuronal circuit of the neocortex. In: *Synchronization of EEG Activity in Epilepsies*, edited by H. Petsche and M. A. B. Brazier, pp. 7–24. Springer Verlag, Wien–New York.
31. Szentágothai, J. (1973): Synaptology of the visual cortex. In: *Handbook of Sensory Physiology, Vol. 7. Part 3B, Central Processing of Visual Information*, edited by R. Jung, pp. 269–324. Springer Verlag, Heidelberg.
32. Szentágothai, J. (1975): The "Module-Concept" in cerebral cortex architecture. *Brain Res.*, 95:475–496.
33. Szentágothai, J. (1976): Die Neuronenschaltungen in der Grosshirnrinde. *Verh. Anat. Ges.*, 70:S187–215.
34. Szentágothai, J., and Arbib, M. A. (1974): Conceptual models of neural organization. *Neurosci. Res. Program Bull.*, 12:307–510.
35. Szentágothai, J., and Rajkovits, K. (1955): Die Rückwirkung der spezifischen Funktion auf die Struktur der Nervenelemente. *Acta Morphol. Acad. Sci. Hung.*, 5:253–274.
36. Voogd, J. (1969): The importance of fiber connections in the comparative anatomy of the mammalian cerebellum. In: *Neurobiology of Cerebellar Evolution and Development*, edited by R. Llinás, pp. 493–514. American Medical Association, Chicago.
37. Woolsey, T. A., and Van der Loos, H. (1970): The structural organization of layer IV in the somatosensory region (S 1) of mouse cerebral cortex. The description of a cortical field composed of discrete cytoarchitectonic units. *Brain Res.*, 17:205–242.
38. Záborszky, L., Gallyas, F., and Wolff, J. R. (*in preparation*).

Architectonics of the Cerebral Cortex,
edited by M. A. B. Brazier and H. Petsche.
Raven Press, New York © 1978.

Cortical Architectonics: The Last 50 Years and Some Problems of Today*

Kurt Fleischhauer

Anatomical Institute, University of Bonn, Bonn, Federal Republic of Germany

As we learned from Brazier (*this volume*), correlation between certain architectonic subdivisions of the cerebral cortex—such as area giganto-pyramidalis—and functional centres—such as the precentral motor region—had been established during the 19th century. However, at the end of that century, as well as during the first half of this one, the power of resolution of morphological methods far exceeded that of the physiological techniques of the day. And since Nissl staining permitted better reproducibility and resolution than stainings for myelin or impregnations of neurofibrils, the Nissl technique became the method of choice and the main tool for architectonic studies of the cerebral cortex. Thus, cytoarchitectonics are predominant in the work of the Vogts as well as in that of von Economo and their respective co-workers and disciples (see refs. 16,17,56,69,71,72).

It should be emphasized, however, that both von Economo and the Vogts were aware of the fact that cyto- and myeloarchitectonic descriptions reveal only part of the picture. In programmatical form, particularly the Vogts (70) stressed the need for fibrillo-, glio-, angio-, and other forms of architectonic studies, and there were many early attempts to follow these suggestions. The investigations of Schröeder (60) into glioarchitectonics or of Pfeifer (49,50) into angioarchitectonics—to name but two of the more important authors—substantiated gross subdivisions arrived at with the cytoarchitectonic method but on the whole did not lead much further. And even researches carried out with more modern methods into chemoarchitectonics (20,22,35,58) and pigmentarchitectonics (5,6) have so far proved to be of limited value for a better functional understanding of cortical structure.

Apart from differences in interpretation and terminology, which were a permanent source of contention between von Economo and the Vogts, there were two major and, in my opinion, rather important differences between the methodological approaches of the two schools. The first concerns the plane of sectioning. Whereas von Economo strongly recommended the use of sections cut in a plane perpendicular to the long axis

---

* *Dedicated to Professor Gian Töndury, Zürich, on the occasion of his 70th birthday.*

of a gyrus, Oscar and Cecil Vogt based their cytoarchitectonic descriptions mainly on serial sections through an entire hemisphere usually cut in the frontal plane. After the untimely death of von Economo in 1931, the methods used by the Vogts prevailed, and almost all the cytoarchitectonic maps of the cerebral cortex that were prepared during the 1930s and in later decades are based on the study of frontal serial sections.

The other difference between the two schools relates to the fact that von Economo recognized the need for exact quantitative data to substantiate the quantitative descriptions. Although the measurements given in the book by von Economo and Koskinas (17) are based on too small a number of brains and must be criticized from a methodical point of view, the idea of von Economo to express the relation between neuropil and cell density in the form of the so-called "Grauzellkoeffizient" (15) proved to be an important new concept. Here, too, his untimely death curtailed a promising if cumbersome line of research. It was later taken up again with gradually improving methods by Shariff (61), Haug (24–26), Sholl (62,63), and others. However, today there is still a lack of sufficient quantitative data on the composition and variability of the neocortex, and much is expected to result from the increasing application of computer-aided methods.

The cytoarchitectonic investigations of both the Vogts and von Economo led to a subdivision of the cerebral cortex into many more fields than had originally been described by Brodmann (7). Whereas Brodmann's maps contain about 80 fields, in the work of von Economo and of the Vogts more than 200 different fields and subfields are discriminated, and this number was later even further increased by the work of Rose and others (see 56).

However, whereas gross cytoarchitectonic differences are obvious even to the uninitiated, the very numerous subdivisions proposed in the 1930s were based on minute morphological details, and the criteria used by the investigators lacked rigorous definition. No wonder, therefore, that these subdivisions were no longer accepted without opposition. This opposition was forcibly put forward in a paper by Lashley and Clark that appeared in 1946 and became widely known (36). In this paper the deficiencies of the definitions used in the field of cytoarchitectonics are clearly set out and attention is drawn to the fact that in many of the published studies and maps the extent of individual variations has not been sufficiently taken into account. The criticism raised in this well-argued paper is devastating; and in the discussion the first sentence under the heading "The problem of architectonics" runs as follows: "The charting of areas in terms of poorly defined and variable characters, in the hope that future physiologic studies may sometime reveal their significance, has contributed nothing to the knowledge of cerebral organization and gives no promise of better achievement in the future."

In the following years there appeared a series of atlases by Bailey, von

Bonin, and co-workers on the cortical architectonics of several primate brains, and in 1951 their monograph *The Isocortex of Man* was published (2). In these investigations many of the areas defined by previous workers were no longer accepted as being constant features of the cerebral cortex.

It is surprising that the architectonic studies of the German school as well as the criticism against it were based solely on the morphological findings obtained with the Nissl method and occasional myelin stainings. This is particularly astounding when one is reminded of the fact that between 1922 and 1938 Lorente de Nó (40–43) conducted important Golgi studies on the internal structure of the cerebral cortex and that at the same time our knowledge concerning the topographical relation between certain parts of the cerebral cortex and certain thalamic nuclei was greatly advanced, particularly by the degeneration studies of A. E. Walker whose book on the primate thalamus appeared in 1938 (73).

Yet it was not before 1948 that the question, "Does a cortical area which receives projection fibres from a specific thalamic element possess structural characteristics which permit its morphological delimitation?", was explicitly raised by Rose and Woolsey in a paper on the limbic cortex (53). Their careful experimental study suggests a high degree of correlation between the structure of a cortical region and the distribution of thalamic fibres. Thus, in the limbic region it was "possible to define three fields in structural terms and to show that they appear to be coextensive with the distribution fields of the anterior thalamic group." Such close correlation between cytoarchitectonic structure and the projection fields of individual thalamic nuclei was later also revealed in other regions of the cerebral cortex and has recently been visualized in a most elegant and strikingly convincing way by Jones and Burton (9,31) with the new method of autoradiographic tracing of cerebral connexions (see 12).

The morphological studies of Rose and Woolsey (53) clearly showed the criticism of Lashley and Clark (36) to be greatly exaggerated. They also indicated that by complementing cytoarchitectonic descriptions with experimental data on thalamocortical connexions, homologies between various cytoarchitectonic fields can be established with much greater certainty than by a purely morphological description of the cytoarchitectonic picture.

At about the same time, the electrophysiological method of recording evoked potentials had become a powerful tool for systematic studies of the topographic arrangement of afferent signals at high resolution. In conjunction with morphological investigations, this technique opened a new and important way for establishing correlations between functional representation and cytoarchitectonic structure (29,51,52,54,78, and others).

One of the most striking examples of such correlation is provided by the somatosensory region of the rodent brain, where each mystacial vibrissa of the contralateral snout is represented by a distinct cytoarchitectonic unit in layer IV, the so-called barrel. In the mouse, each barrel consists of a ring of cells, the side, which surrounds a less cellular central structure, the hollow (79). The total number of barrels in the posteromedial barrel subfield of each hemisphere equals the number of mystacial vibrissae on the contralateral side. It is of methodological interest to point out that by studying the conventional coronal sections, early authors had already noted certain cytoarchitectonic peculiarities of this region which was therefore duly singled out as T_1 by Rose in 1929 (55), but that they did not grasp the true form of the barrels or of the barrel field. This only became possible in 1970, when in an unconventional approach Woolsey and van der Loos (79) studied sections cut tangential to the surface of the brain. In such sections the pattern formed by the barrels is clearly revealed. It then also becomes obvious that due to an oblique arrangement of the rows of cells this pattern cannot properly be studied in the usual coronal or sagittal sections. However, once the true structure of the barrels had been revealed, the possible functional relation between the posteromedial barrel subfield and the mystacial vibrissae was obvious and could soon be confirmed by electrophysiological (74) and other experimental means. It was shown, for instance, that the barrels are formed during postnatal development and that a given barrel does not appear when its respective vibrissa is removed immediately after birth (68,75).

Although cortical representation of mystacial vibrissae in the form of clearly delineated cytoarchitectonic units is not seen in every species, its occurrence in a number of lissencephalic cortices (see 80) provided important new evidence for the heuristic value of cytoarchitectonic studies of the cerebral cortex.

However, cytoarchitectonic studies are no longer the predominant method of architectonic research. Electrophysiological findings obtained by recordings from single layers and single cells brought new aspects of cortical architectonics to the fore and gave rise to morphological problems which cannot be solved with the classic methods but require the combined application of light microscopy, electron microscopy, and quantitative methods as well as the study of sections cut in various unfamiliar planes.

When studying, in 1957, the properties of single neurones of the cat's somatic sensory cortex after mechanical deformation of some peripheral tissue, Mountcastle (45) made two important observations, namely (a) that a given neurone is responsive only to one of various forms of stimuli applied to a given site, or, in other words, that there is specificity with respect to stimulus modality subgroups, and (b) that on vertical penetration of the cortex, groups of neurones are found to be responsive to the same single submodality.

These observations led Mountcastle to the hypothesis that in the somatosensory cortex there is a mosaic-like organization made up of elementary units consisting of vertical groups or cylinders or columns of cells extending through all the cortical layers. As Mountcastle has stated, this hypothesis was not new, because a similar conclusion had been reached years ago by Lorente de Nó (41,43) as the result of his Golgi studies. But serious discussion of columnar organization of the cerebral cortex did not begin before the electrophysiological findings of Mountcastle and their confirmation by other authors and, in particular, by the studies of Hubel and Wiesel (27,28,30) on the visual system of the cat and of primates.

From a different angle, the importance of vertical structures was also evidenced by attempts to correlate normal and abnormal EEG phenomena with the electrical activity of single neurones. For instance, depth profiles of cortical potentials showed that at some point within the cortex there is a reversal of polarity. And since in the same region different types of cortical waves were found to have different depth profiles, many questions arose which are still difficult to solve (see 13,48). There is no doubt that one of the requirements for solution of these problems is a precise knowledge of the morphology of vertical structures in the cerebral cortex.

Thus, in recent years an increasing interest in vertical patterns of organization has superseded the earlier emphasis on cortical lamination and its regional variation. This interest in vertical structures has stimulated many physiological experiments, morphological investigations, and theoretical considerations concerning vertical columns or cylinders or modules in the cerebral cortex (1,4,10,66,67, and others). But despite all these efforts, many problems concerning the morphology and functional interpretation of vertical structures are far from being resolved. Therefore, in the second part of my paper, I should like to ask, "What is known anatomically?", and to explain why it is still difficult and dangerous to attempt generalizations.

In the first instance, a certain vertical organization of the entire cerebral cortex is brought about by the vertically polarized structure of pyramidal cells and by the distribution of their axon collaterals. As illustrated by the Scheibels (59, Fig. 6), Golgi impregnations show the pyramidal cells to be surrounded by a network of recurrent axon collaterals extending through all the layers. These collaterals form overlapping cylinders in which many thousand cells may be contacted. In contrast to the branches of the dendritic tree, which are distributed within a cylindrical space with a diameter of no more than 500 μm, the cylinder formed by the recurrent axon collaterals has a diameter of roughly 3 mm. Within it, many connexions both in the vertical and in the horizontal direction may be established by various types of interneurones or local circuit neurones. The characteristic connexion patterns formed by these neurones have recently been summarized by Szentágothai (66) and will not be considered here.

Another predominantly vertical structure, influencing many cells, is is formed by the terminal arborizations of the thalamocortical axons. Each axon ends in a vertical plexus with a diameter of about 500 μm, extending mainly through the middle layers of the cortex. The Scheibels (59) have assumed that all the cortical cells that are included in the field of arborization of a single thalamocortical fibre constitute a distinct module. This assumption would explain the observations of Mountcastle (45). It is in good agreement also with the finding of vertically discrete thalamic projections from the ventral posterior nucleus to the cortical barrels in the rat (34) and with the findings of Hubel and Wiesel (30) concerning the visual system of primates. By means of degeneration studies, these authors were able to show that in the monkey striate cortex the physiologically defined ocular dominance columns are generated by a spatial segregation of the afferents from the ipsilaterally and contralaterally innervated layers of the lateral geniculate nucleus. And in later studies the ocular dominance columns could actually be visualized in normal brains by transneuronal transport of radioactive molecules (76) and, very elegantly, by a simple method of silver impregnation (39). With the latter method it was shown that in tangential sections through layer IV the ocular dominance columns appear in the form of alternating bands of dense tangential fibres separated by narrow bands with slightly lower density of fibres. The dense bands have a width of about 300 μm which—if shrinkage is taken into account—corresponds well with a width of 0.5 to 1 mm arrived at in the electrophysiological studies.

In contrast to the comparatively small cylinders or narrow bands formed by the terminal arborizations of specific thalamocortical afferents, the terminal plexus of unspecific thalamocortical fibres are distributed over large and widely overlapping fields with diameters of between 1 and 3 mm (see 59).

Apart from vertical patterns generated by the radial orientation of pyramidal cells and their recurrent axon collaterals or by the terminal arborization of individual afferent thalamocortical axons, a different type of vertical pattern is caused by clustering or nonrandom arrangement of groups of cortical nerve cells or axons or dendrites. In this respect, three phenomena are to be considered.

(1) One of the main structures to be noted in a histological section stained for myelin are the so-called radial bundles of myelinated fibres extending from the white matter into the grey. These bundles, which may reach the third layer, have been known for over 100 years. Their appearance and regional differences were systematically studied and beautifully illustrated by Kaes as early as 1907 (33). But although the patterns formed by the radial bundles were of considerable interest for myeloarchitectonic studies, neither the exact origin nor the possible functional significance of the various fibres constituting such a bundle could be ascertained. With the increasing preponderance of cytoarchitectonic studies and emphasis on the layering of the cerebral cortex, the radial bundles received less and less attention from the morphologists, and up to now their composition has not been exactly analyzed.

(2) In addition to the radial bundles of myelinated fibres, a grouping of nerve cells in vertically oriented clusters or columns is also obvious in many sections and mentioned in early texts on the histology of the cerebral cortex. In the book of von Economo and Koskinas (17), for instance, we find a thorough discussion of this phenomenon under the heading "Radiäre Gliederung der Zellen und Rindenstreifung." In this discussion attention is drawn to the fact that the regionally varying, vertical arrangement of nerve cells cannot always be correlated with a corresponding arrangement of myelinated fibres. The authors explicitly state that there are regions in which the nerve cells are distinctly arranged in vertical columns so as to produce a striped appearance of the entire section, yet that in the same region a corresponding pattern of radial fibre bundles is absent. They therefore conclude that the vertical clusters of nerve cells and the radial bundles of axons need not be regarded as being two aspects of the same phenomenon. However, despite this observation of von Economo and Koskinas it seems likely that in many instances at least some relation exists between vertically arranged groups of nerve cells and radial bundles of nerve fibres. The most recent evidence which would support this assumption has been adduced by Jones et al. (32). With the method of anterograde transport of isotopically labelled proteins it was shown that commissural and, to a lesser extent, other corticocortical fibres arise from clusters of nerve cells, are arranged in bundles and terminate in discrete vertical groupings. Yet until today the relation between the clusters of cortical nerve cells and the radial bundles of fibres has not been analysed systematically and therefore remains a problem.

(3) A third vertical pattern is provided by the so-called vertical bundles of dendrites, i.e., by a nonrandom arrangement of apical dendrites of large layer V pyramids. The existence of bundles or clusters of dendrites in the cerebral cortex was discovered in 1972 independently and almost simultaneously by Peters and Walsh (47) in the rat and by Fleischhauer et al. (21) in rabbit and cat. There is little doubt that these bundles are of interest for the interpretation of a number of electrophysiological data (see 48 and *this volume*), and, since over the last few years the work of my own laboratory has been mainly concerned with the morphology and regional variations of vertical bundles of dendrites in the neocortex, I would like to discuss this pattern in some detail.

Figure 1A shows a horizontal section through layer IV of area parietalis of the rabbit. The cross-sectioned apical dendrites are seen to be distributed in distinct groups or clusters. Each cluster is the cross section of a vertical bundle comprising an average of six thick dendritic shafts originating from closely apposed large layer V pyramids (21,44). Above layer V, the bundles are joined by some smaller dendrites arising from cells of layer IV and by a number of very small dendrites and/or axons of unknown origin. The bundles traverse layer IV in a radial direction and break up in layer III/II where the larger dendrites bifurcate and assume an oblique course. Within

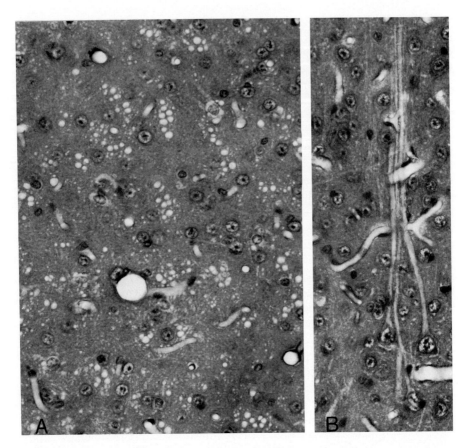

FIG. 1. A: Rabbit. Tangential section through layer IV of area parietalis to show cross sections of vertical bundles of dendrites. **B:** Cat. Section perpendicular to surface of visual cortex to show vertical bundle of dendrites. **A** and **B** are paraffin sections stained with Luxol fast blue followed by a periodic-acid-Schiff reaction and counterstaining with Ehrlich's hematoxylin. ×350.

layer IV, the individual dendrites of a bundle lie very close to each other, and frequently there are stretches of direct contact between the plasmalemmata of two or more adjacent dendrites.

A first quantitative analysis (37) of cross-sectioned bundles in layer IV of area parietalis of the rabbit has shown that out of a total of 819 dendrites no less than 308 dendrites, i.e., more than one in three, were in immediate contact with each other. The lengths of the contact stretches between the plasmalemmata of adjacent dendrites varied between 0.3 μm and more than 6 μm; and from a total of 167 contact stretches measured by Latz (37) an average length of 1.3 μm can be calculated. In the vertical direction, contact stretches could also be followed for a length of up to 5 μm but the number of measurements was not sufficiently large for calculating an average length.

The morphological details described here apply only to dendritic bundles in area parietalis of the rabbit. In other regions, for instance, the striate area, the average number of thick dendrites per bundle, the mean diameter of the thick dendrites and the relation between thick and thin cell processes are different. A clear picture of these variations can be obtained only by quantitative analysis. This is greatly facilitated if one uses automatic scanning devices and will be described in detail by Dr. Detzer (*this volume*).

In addition to variations in the numerical composition of the bundles there are other regional differences of a more fundamental nature (14,18,19). The gyrencephalic brain of the cat provides a particularly interesting instance.

In the visual cortex (area 17) of the cat, most vertical bundles consist of two and some of three or more thick apical dendrites of large layer V pyramids. As seen from Fig. 1B the cells which give rise to these dendrites are situated in close proximity to one another; and tangential sections reveal that the bundles are accompanied by numerous small cell processes (dendrites and/or axons) the origin of which is still unknown. Thus, the general pattern is similar to that described above for the parietal and striate region of the rabbit. But despite this similarity, which also applies to yet other regions and other species, it would be wrong to generalize and to assume that the formation of radial bundles of dendrites containing primary apical shafts arising from clusters of large layer V pyramids is a common feature of the entire neocortex. It would be wrong because in the agranular cortex of the motor region (areas 4 and 6) an entirely different pattern is found (18). In this region, most apical dendrites arising from large layer V pyramids bifurcate immediately above layer V and give rise to obliquely running secondary branches. These secondary branches cross one another and give off further small branches before turning upward and joining other dendrites to take part in the formation of vertical bundles. Figure 2 shows this pattern in a section cut perpendicularly to the surface of area 4 in the lower bank of the superior sigmoid gyrus of the cat. Recent and still unpublished observations indicate that the complicated geometry of the relations between the dendritic arborizations can only be understood if the tangential structure of the various layers in this area is also taken into account.

It is a truly surprising fact that for almost a century the structure and architecture of the cerebral cortex has been investigated almost exclusively in frontal or sagittal sections or, in the case of von Economo, in sections cut perpendicularly to the long axis of a gyrus, whereas sections cut in a tangential plane were apparently regarded as being of little interest. In the wake of the quantitative studies of Sholl (62,63), this deficiency in the customary approach of histological investigation was recognized by Colonnier

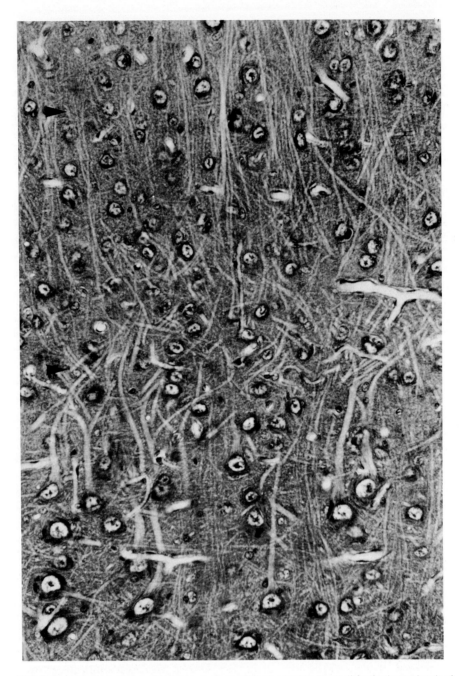

FIG. 2. Cat. Section perpendicular to surface of motor cortex (area 4) in the lower bank of the superior sigmoid gyrus. The figure is so arranged that the pial surface faces upward. Lower arrowhead indicates approximate position of tangential plane in which section Fig. 5A is cut; upper arrowhead indicates approximate plane of section Fig. 5B. For details see text. Staining as in Fig. 1. ×275.

in 1964 (11). In a careful study of the tangential organization of the visual cortex he found that "approximately twice as many nerve processes, axons and/or dendrites are oriented within a 30° angle bisected by the antero-posterior axis of the gyrus lateralis of the cat as in an 'average' oblique angle of the same size. In some layers a secondary increase in the number of fibres is found at right angles to the main anteroposterior direction." The paper of Colonnier (11) on the visual cortex was followed by studies of Mungai (46) on the somatic sensory and of Wong (77) on three auditory areas of the cat. But these investigations yielded less clear-cut results, and to my knowledge no further attempt has been made to find out more about preferential orientation in the tangential plane of the neocortex.

In my opinion, however, an exact knowledge of the structural organiza-tion in the tangential plane is almost as important for an understanding of the neocortex as of the cerebellar cortex. This will be evident from the last section of my communication.

If tangential sections through the superior sigmoid gyrus (area 4) facing the cruciate sulcus are investigated, a prominent preferential orientation of nerve cells as well as of axons and dendrites is revealed. In Fig. 3 the peri-karya of layer V pyramids have been outlined in a tangential section, i.e., in a section cut in a plane parallel to the cruciate sulcus. Most of the peri-karya are seen to be oval with their long axis preferentially oriented in one direction. In Bodian sections a similar preferential orientation of impreg-nated cell processes (axons and dendrites) is found. The direction of prefer-ential orientation is oblique with respect to the long axis of the superior sigmoid gyrus as it appears when seen from the outside of the brain. In Fig. 4 the direction of preferential orientation found in the lower bank of the superior sigmoid gyrus is indicated on the surface of the brain as seen from above, and found to be roughly parallel to the ansate sulcus. If in this plane sections are cut perpendicularly to the surface (Fig. 2), the complicated pattern formed by the apical dendrites arising from the layer-V pyramids is particularly well revealed. Investigation of tangential sections through the same region indicates that this is the consequence of a preferential orienta-tion of the bifurcations and decussations of apical dendrites. They are oriented in the same direction as the perikarya of the layer-V pyramids and the impregnated nerve fibres as indicated in Fig. 4.

The preferential orientation of the dendritic branchings and crossings is illustrated in Fig. 5A, which shows a tangential section through area 4 cut immediately above layer V in a plane indicated in Fig. 2 by the lower arrow-head. As seen from Fig. 2, immediately above layer V a distinct layer is formed by the decussations of obliquely running, mainly secondary or tertiary branches of apical dendrites of layer-V pyramids. In the tangential section through this layer (Fig. 5A), some apical dendrites are seen to be cross-sectioned, whereas many others are obliquely cut while crossing one another. Often several dendrites are seen to run close to each other while

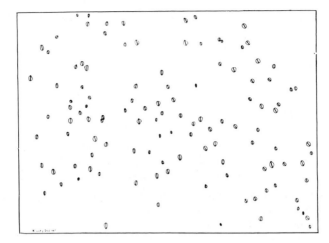

FIG. 3. Outline and long axis of perikarya of layer V pyramids in tangential section through area 4 of cat superior sigmoid gyrus. Tracing drawn from a photomontage at ×140 magnification to show preferential orientation of long axis of cell bodies.

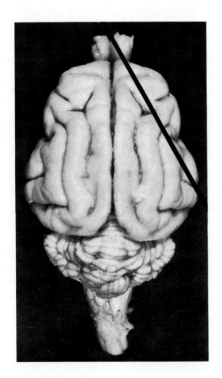

FIG. 4. Direction of preferential orientation of perikarya of layer-V pyramids and of cell processes in tangential plane of area 4 in the superior sigmoid gyrus, projected on the surface of the cat's brain. The perpendicular section Fig. 2 was cut in the oblique plane indicated by the dark line on the photograph. For details see text.

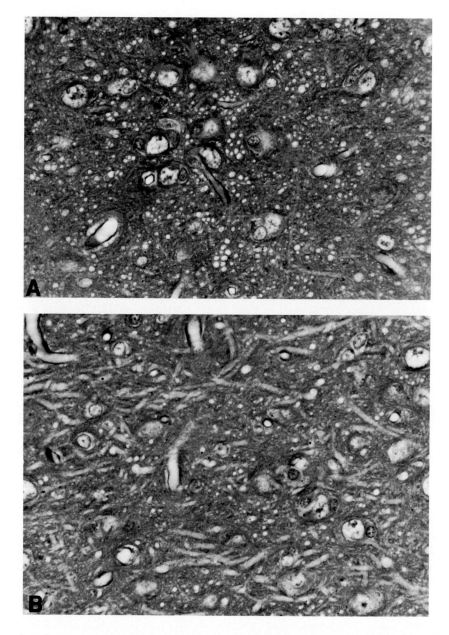

FIG. 5. Two tangential sections through area 4 in the lower bank of the superior sigmoid gyrus of the cat. **A:** The plane is in the layer of obliquely coursing and decussating dendrites, and is approximately indicated by the lower arrowhead in Fig. 2. **B:** Same region cut in a plane through the upper third of layer III, indicated by upper arrowhead in Fig. 2. For further details see text. Staining as in Fig. 1. ×560.

decussating and thus to form distinct clusters, which may also contain basal dendrites of layer-III pyramidal cells. In addition, the dendrites belonging to such a cluster are often preferentially oriented parallel to the lower margin of Fig. 5A. This direction is the same as that found for the preferential orientation of the perikarya and nerve cell processes and which in Fig. 4 is projected on the surface of the brain. Above the layer of crossings, the dendrites arrange themselves into more or less distinct vertical bundles. These are illustrated in Fig. 5B. The approximate plane in which this section was cut is indicated in the frontal section Fig. 2B by the upper arrowhead.

Unfortunately, I am not yet able to present electron microscopic pictures of the layer of dendritic crossings immediately above layer V. Close study of this region is likely to be of particular interest because in the monkey cortex Sloper (64) found that dendrodendritic synapses may be a particular feature of this layer.

According to the generally accepted nomenclature, which is based on the cyto- and myeloarchitectonic picture, both the layer of decussations (lower arrowhead in Fig. 2) and the layer of radial orientation and bundling of dendrites (upper arrowhead in Fig. 2) are part of layer III, because in the agranular motor cortex layer IV is thought to be lacking and layer III considered to begin immediately above layer V (23,57). This nomenclature has been attacked by von Bonin and Bucy (3,8) with the following words: "It is our belief that the usual omission of layer IV from the precentral agranular cortex is conducive to erroneous thinking. The importance on any structure resides in its function. The thalamocortical afferents terminate in the outer stripes of Baillarger. The region containing this stripe has been called layer IV in the postcentral but the lower part of layer III in the precentral cortex. It should, however, be referred to as layer IV in all areas of the neocortex, and we have done so in this chapter." Although this interpretation of von Bonin and Bucy has not been accepted in the more recent literature (see 23, 57, Fig. 3), it springs to mind when one sees the morphologically well-delineated layer in which the dendrites bifurcate, take a predominantly oblique course, and decussate. One might ask, therefore, whether there is reason to regard this conspicuous layer as an equivalent to layer IV in the sense of von Bonin and Bucy. In my opinion this is not so, and for the following reasons: (a) In all regions of the sensory cortex so far examined, the vertical bundles of dendrites in layer IV have been found to be formed mainly by primary apical dendrites of layer V pyramids and not by secondary or tertiary branches; and (b) because the investigations of Strick and Sterling (65) have shown that following lesions in the ventrolateral nucleus of the thalamus the great majority of degenerating synapses in the motor cortex are located in the upper two-thirds of layer III, whereas only extremely few degenerating synapses were found in the deep portion of layer III or in the upper part of layer V. Therefore, the assumption of von Bonin and Bucy that in the motor cortex the lower part of layer III corresponds to layer IV of the somatosensory cortex because the thalamocortical afferents terminate in this layer, does not apply to the morphologically conspicuous lower part of layer III in the cat. Thus, the finding, in area 4, of a well-delineated zone of branching and crossing dendrites does not necessitate any change in the accepted terminology.

The findings obtained in the cerebral cortex of the cat indicate that the relation between clusters of nerve cells and vertical bundles of dendrites is different in different regions, and that the relation is not always a simple one. This may have interesting functional implications. On the one hand, afferent fibres impinging on the dendrites of a bundle in the visual cortex presumably alter the excitatory state of nerve cells in a small and extremely well-localized spot. In the motor cortex, on the other hand, where bundles are composed of secondary branches of pyramidal cells belonging to several clusters, afferent impulses reaching the dendrites of a bundle would alter the excitatory state of nerve cells spread out over some distance in the horizontal plane. If a similar pattern exists in the monkey motor cortex, it would provide an explanation for the following puzzling electrophysiological findings. Whereas some experiments clearly indicate the existence of a columnar arrangement of efferent neurones with each column projecting to one or a few muscles, other experiments show that with respect to afferent input some cells in an efferent column may receive information from different peripheral zones. According to Lemon and Porter (38), this finding "suggests a variety of organizations which may be important in complex tasks where the activity or stability of a number of different joints is required." Perhaps the complex composition of the bundles in layer III of the motor cortex, i.e., in just that layer where the thalamocortical afferents impinge on the dendrites (65), represents the morphological basis for some of the variety of organizations deduced from the electrophysiological findings. However, anatomical investigation of the arrangement of the dendrites arising from large layer V pyramids in the monkey motor cortex and light and electron microscopical measurements are required to prove or disprove this assumption.

Space does not permit a discussion of other patterns of dendritic bundling. Nor is it possible to turn to embryology or to mention all the questions that remain open, such as, for instance: Are gap junctions to be found in vertical bundles of dendrites or in the layer of dendritic decussations in the motor cortex? Do dendrodendritic synapses exist between the dendrites forming a bundle? What are the relations between vertical bundles of dendrites and the radial bundles of myelinated fibres? What are the relations between bundles of dendrites and basal dendrites of layer III pyramids? However, I do hope to have given you at least an idea of the present state of affairs and of how during the last 50 years the gap between physiology and morphology has gradually become smaller and smaller and is now being bridged by much mutual stimulation and understanding and, fortunately, also by personal friendship.

ACKNOWLEDGMENT

This work was supported by the Deutsche Forschungsgemeinschaft and by a Twinning Grant of the European Training Programme in Brain and Behaviour Research.

REFERENCES

1. Asanuma, H. (1975): Recent developments in the study of the columnar arrangement of neurons within the motor cortex. *Physiol. Rev.*, 55:143–156.
2. Bailey, P., and Bonin, G. von (1951): *The Isocortex of Man.* University of Illinois Press, Urbana, Ill.
3. Bonin, G. von. (1949): Architecture of the precentral motor cortex and some adjacent areas. In: *The Precentral Motor Cortex,* edited by P. C. Bucy, Chap. 2, pp. 8–82. University of Illinois Press, Urbana, Ill.
4. Bonin, G. von, and Mehler, W. R. (1971): On columnar arrangement of nerve cells in cerebral cortex. *Brain Res.*, 27:1–9.
5. Braak, H. (1972): Zur Pigmentarchitektonik der Grosshirnrinde des Menschen. I. Regio entorhinalis. *Z. Zellforsch.*, 127:407–438.
6. Braak, H. (1976): On the striate area of the human isocortex. A Golgi and pigmentarchitectonic study. *J. Comp. Neurol.*, 166:341–364.
7. Brodmann, K. (1909): *Vergleichende Lokalisationslehre der Grosshirnrinde in ihren prinzipien Dargestellt auf Grund des Zellenbaues.* Barth, Leipzig.
8. Bucy, P. C. (Ed.) (1949): *The Precentral Motor Cortex.* University of Illinois Press, Urbana, Ill.
9. Burton, H., and Jones, E. G. (1976): The posterior thalamic region and its cortical projection in New World and Old World monkeys. *J. Comp. Neurol.*, 168:249–302.
10. Chow, K. L., and Leiman, A. L. (1970): The structural and functional organization of the neocortex. *Neurosci. Res. Program Bull.*, 8:153–220.
11. Colonnier, M. (1964): The tangential organization of the visual cortex. *J. Anat.*, 98:327–344.
12. Cowan, W. M., and Cuenod, M. (Eds.) (1975): *The Use of Axonal Transport for Studies of Neuronal Connectivity.* Elsevier, Amsterdam.
13. Creutzfeldt, O. (1974): The neuronal generation of the EEG. In: *Handbook of Electroencephalography and Clinical Neurophysiology, Vol. 2, Part C: The Neuronal Generation of the EEG,* edited by O. Creutzfeldt, pp. 2C-5–2C-55. Elsevier, Amsterdam.
14. Detzer, K. (1976): Course and distribution of apical dendrites of layer V pyramids in the barrel field and area parietalis of the mouse. *Anat. Embryol.*, 149:251–258.
15. Economo, C. von (1926): Ein Koeffizient für die Organisationshöhe der Grosshirnrinde. *Klin. Wochenschr.*, 5:593–595.
16. Economo, C. von (1927): *Zellaufbau der Grosshirnrinde des Menschen.* Springer, Berlin.
17. Economo, C. von, and Koskinas, G. N. (1925): *Die Cytoarchitektonik der Hirnrinde des erwachsenen Menschen (Textbuch und Atlas).* Springer, Berlin.
18. Fleischhauer, K. (1974): On different patterns of dendritic bundling in the cerebral cortex of the cat. *Z. Anat. Entwicklungsgesch.*, 143:115–126.
19. Fleischhauer, K., and Detzer, K. (1975): Dendritic bundling in the cerebral cortex. In: *Advances in Neurology, Vol. 12,* edited by G. W. Kreutzberg, pp. 71–78. Raven Press, New York.
20. Fleischhauer, K., and Horstmann, E. (1957): Intravitale Dithizonfärbung homologer Felder der Ammonsformation von Säugern. *Z. Zellforsch.*, 46:598–609.
21. Fleischhauer, K., Petsche, H., and Wittkowski, W. (1972): Vertical bundles of dendrites in the neocortex. *Z. Anat. Entwicklungsgesch.*, 136:213–223.

22. Friede, R. L. (1966): *Topographic Brain Chemistry*. Academic Press, New York.
23. Hassler, R., and Muhs-Clement, K. (1964): Architektonischer Aufbau des sensomotorischen und parietalen Cortex der Katze. *J. Hirnforsch.*, 6:377–420.
24. Haug, H. (1953): Der Grauzellkoeffizient des Stirnhirns der Mammalia in einer phylogenetischen Betrachtung. I. Theoretische, technische und mathematische Grundlage der Untersuchungen. *Acta Anat.*, 19:60–100.
25. Haug, H. (1956): Remarks on the determination and significance of the grey cell coefficient. *J. Comp. Neurol.*, 104:473–492.
26. Haug, H. (1958): *Quantitative Untersuchungen an der Hirnrinde*. Thieme, Stuttgart.
27. Hubel, D. H., and Wiesel, T. N. (1962): Receptive fields, binocular interaction and func tional architecture in the cat's visual cortex. *J. Physiol.*, 160:106–154.
28. Hubel, D. H., and Wiesel, T. N. (1963): Shape and arrangement of columns in cat's striate cortex. *J. Physiol.*, 165:559–568.
29. Hubel, D. H., and Wiesel, T. N. (1965): Receptive fields and functional architecture in two nonstriate visual areas (18 and 19) of the cat. *J. Neurophysiol.*, 28:229–289.
30. Hubel, D. H., and Wiesel, T. N. (1972): Laminar and columnar distribution of geniculocortical fibers in the macaque monkey. *J. Comp. Neurol.*, 146:421–450.
31. Jones, E. G., and Burton, H. (1976): Areal differences in the laminar distribution of thalamic afferents in cortical fields of the insular, parietal and temporal regions of primates. *J. Comp. Neurol.*, 168:197–248.
32. Jones, E. G., Burton, H., and Porter, R. (1975): Commissural and cortico-cortical "columns" in the somatic sensory cortex of primates. *Science*, 190:572–574.
33. Kaes, T. (1907): *Die Grosshirnrinde des Menschen in ihren Massen und ihrem Fasergehalt*. Fischer, Jena.
34. Killackey, H. P. (1973): Anatomical evidence for cortical subdivisions based on vertically discrete thalamic projections from the ventral nucleus to cortical barrels in the rat. *Brain Res.*, 51:326–331.
35. Krnjević, K., and Silver, A. (1965): A histochemical study of cholinergic fibres in the cerebral cortex. *J. Anat.*, 99:711–759.
36. Lashley, K. S., and Clark, G. (1946): The cytoarchitecture of the cerebral cortex of Ateles: A critical examination of architectonic studies. *J. Comp. Neurol.*, 85:223–305.
37. Latz, H. (1975): *Quantitative Messungen an Dendritenbündeln in der Hirnrinde des Kaninchens*. Inaugural Dissertation; Med. Fakultät; Bonn.
38. Lemon, R. N. and Porter, R. (1976): Are there restricted input-output columns in monkeymotor cortex? *J. Physiol.*, 258:109P–110P.
39. Le Vay, S., Hubel, D. H., and Wiesel, T. N. (1975): The pattern of ocular dominance columns in macaque visual cortex revealed by a reduced silver stain. *J. Comp. Neurol.*, 159:559–576.
40. Lorente de Nó, R. (1922): La corteza cerebral del ratón (primera contribución – la corteza acústica). *Trab. Inst. Cajal Invest. Biol.*, 20:41–78.
41. Lorente de Nó, R. (1933): Studies on the structure of the cerebral cortex. I. The area entorhinalis. *J. Psychol. Neurol.*, 45:382–438.
42. Lorente de Nó, R. (1934): Studies on the structure of the cerebral cortex. II. Continuation of the study of the ammonic system. *J. Psychol. Neurol.*, 46:113–177.
43. Lorente de Nó, R. (1938): Architectonics and structure of the cerebral cortex. In: *Physiology of the Nervous System*, 1st ed., edited by J. F. Fulton. Oxford University Press, Oxford.
44. Massing, W., and Fleischhauer, K. (1973): Further observations on vertical bundles of dendrites in the cerebral cortex of the rabbit. *Z. Anat. Entwicklungsgesch.*, 141:115–123.
45. Mountcastle, V. B. (1957): Modality and topographic properties of single neurons of cat's somatic sensory cortex. *J. Neurophysiol.*, 20:408–434.
46. Mungai, J. M. (1967): Dendritic patterns in the somatic sensory cortex of the cat. *J. Anat.*, 101:403–418.
47. Peters, A., and Walsh, T. M. (1972): A study of the organization of apical dendrites in the somatic sensory cortex of the rat. *J. Comp. Neurol.*, 144:253–268.
48. Petsche, H., Prohaska, O., Rappelsberger, P., and Vollmer, R. (1975): The possible role of dendrites in EEG synchronization. In: *Advances in Neurology, Vol. 12*, edited by G. W. Kreutzberg, pp. 53–70. Raven Press, New York.
49. Pfeifer, R. A. (1928): *Die Angioarchitektonik der Grosshirnrinde*. Springer, Berlin.

50. Pfeifer, R. A. (1940): *Die angioarchitektonische areale Gliederung der Grosshirnrinde.* Thieme, Leipzig.
51. Powell, T. P. S., and Mountcastle, V. B. (1959): The cytoarchitecture of the postcentral gyrus of the monkey *Macaca mulatta. Bull. Johns Hopkins Hosp.,* 105:108–131.
52. Powell, T. P. S., and Mountcastle, V. B. (1959): Some aspects of the functional organization of the cortex of the postcentral gyrus of the monkey: A correlation of findings obtained in a single unit analysis with cytoarchitecture. *Bull. Johns Hopkins Hosp.,* 105:133–162.
53. Rose, J. E., and Woolsey, C. N. (1948): Structure and relations of limbic cortex and anterior thalamic nuclei in rabbit and cat. *J. Comp. Neurol.,* 89:279–348.
54. Rose, J. E., and Woolsey, C. N. (1949): The relations of thalamic connections, cellular structure and evocable electrical activity in the auditory region of the cat. *J. Comp. Neurol.,* 91:441–466.
55. Rose, M. (1929): Cytoarchitektonischer Atlas der Grosshirnrinde der Maus. *J. Psychol. Neurol.,* 40:1–51.
56. Rose, M. (1935): Cytoarchitektonik and Myeloarchitektonik der Grosshirnrinde. In: *Handbuch der Neurologie,* Vol. I, pp. 589–778. Springer, Berlin.
57. Sanides, F. (1972): Representation in the cerebral cortex and its areal lamination patterns. In: *The Structure and Function of Nervous Tissue, Vol. V,* edited by G. H. Bourne, pp. 329–453. Academic Press, New York.
58. Scharrer, E., and Sinden, J. (1949): A contribution to the "chemoarchitectonics" of the optic tectum of the brain of the pigeon. *J. Comp. Neurol.,* 91:331–336.
59. Scheibel, M. E., and Scheibel, A. B. (1970): Elementary processes in selected thalamic and cortical subsystems—the structural substrates. In: *The Neurosciences,* Second Study Program, edited by F. O. Schmitt, pp. 443–457. The Rockefeller University Press, New York.
60. Schroeder, A. H. (1935): Gliaarchitektonik des Zentralnervensystems. In: *Handbuch der Neurologie,* Vol. I, pp. 791–810. Springer, Berlin.
61. Shariff, G. A. (1953): Cell counts in the primate cerebral cortex. *J. Comp. Neurol.,* 98:381–400.
62. Sholl, D. A. (1953): Dendritic organization in the neurons of the visual and motor cortices of the cat. *J. Anat.,* 87:387–406.
63. Sholl, D. A. (1956): *The Organization of the Cerebral Cortex.* Methuen, London.
64. Sloper, J. J. (1971): Dendro-dendritic synapses in the primate motor cortex. *Brain Res.,* 34:186–192.
65. Strick, P. L., and Sterling, P. (1974): Synaptic termination of afferents from the ventrolateral nucleus of the thalamus in the cat motor cortex. A light and electron microscope study. *J. Comp. Neurol.,* 153:77–106.
66. Szentágothai, J. (1975): The "module-concept" in cerebral cortex architecture. *Brain Res.,* 95:475–496.
67. Towe, A. L. (1975): Notes on the hypothesis of columnar organization in somatosensory cerebral cortex. *Brain Behav. Evol.,* 11:16–47.
68. van der Loos, H., and Woolsey, T. A. (1973): Somatosensory cortex: Structural alterations following early injury to sense organs. *Science,* 179:395–398.
69. Vogt, C., and Vogt, O. (1919): Allgemeine Ergebnisse unserer Hirnforschung. *J. Psychol. Neurol.,* 25:277–462.
70. Vogt, C. and Vogt, O. (1928): Die Grundlagen und die Teildisciplinen der mikroskopischen Anatomie des Zentralnervensystems. In: *Handbuch der Mikroskopischen Anatomie des Menschen, Vol. 4.* Springer, Berlin.
71. Vogt, O. (1903): Zur anatomischen Gliederung des Cortex cerebri. *J. Psychol. Neurol.,* 2:160–180.
72. Vogt, O. (1927): Architektonik der menschlichen Hirnrinde. *Z. Psychiatrie,* 86:247–266.
73. Walker, A. E. (1938): *The Primate Thalamus.* University of Chicago Press, Chicago.
74. Welker, C. (1971): Microelectrode delineation of fine grain somatotopic organization of SM I cerebral cortex in albino rat. *Brain Res.,* 26:259–275.
75. Weller, W. L., and Johnson, J. I. (1975): Barrels in cerebral cortex altered by receptor disruption in newborn, but not in five-day-old mice (Cricetidae and Muridae). *Brain Res.,* 83:504–508.
76. Wiesel, T. N., Hubel, D. H., and Lam, D. M. K. (1974): Autoradiographic demonstration

of ocular-dominance columns in the monkey striate cortex by means of transneuronal transport. *Brain Res., 79:273–279.*

77. Wong, W. C. (1967): The tangential organization of dendrites and axons in three auditory areas of the cat's cerebral cortex. *J. Anat.,* 101:419–433.

78. Woolsey, C. N. (1958): Organization of somatic sensory and motor areas of the cerebral cortex. In: *Biological and Biochemical Basis of Behavior,* edited by H. F. Harlow and C. N. Woolsey, pp. 63–81. University of Wisconsin Press, Madison.

79. Woolsey, T. A., and van der Loos, H. (1970): The structural organization of layer IV in the somatosensory region (SI) of mouse cerebral cortex. The description of a cortical field composed of discrete cytoarchitectonic units. *Brain Res.,* 17:205–242.

80. Woolsey, T. A., Welker, C., and Schwartz, R. H. (1975): Comparative anatomical studies of the Sm 1 face cortex with special reference to the occurrence of "barrels" in layer IV. *J. Comp. Neurol.,* 164:79–94.

Architectonics of the Cerebral Cortex,
edited by M. A. B. Brazier and H. Petsche.
Raven Press, New York © 1978.

Semi-Automatic Investigation of Composition and Structure of Vertical Bundles of Dendrites in Various Regions of Rabbit Neocortex

Klaus Detzer

Anatomical Institute, University of Bonn, Bonn, Federal Republic of Germany

In 1972 it was shown independently by Peters and Walsh in rat (6), by Fleischhauer et al. in rabbit and cat (3), and in 1975 by Detzer in mouse (2) that in layer IV the apical dendrites of large layer-V pyramids are not distributed at random. Instead, they form distinct bundles of dendrites that are orientated perpendicularly to the surface of the cerebral cortex. These bundles of dendrites may provide a morphological correlate of the vertically oriented, comparatively large generators postulated by Petsche et al. (7). The electrophysiological studies of these authors show distinct regional differences in the rabbit cerebral cortex. There are also marked regional variations in the structure of the dendritic bundles, as demonstrated in cat (4), rabbit (5), and mouse (2). Apart from regional variations, there are species-specific differences in the morphology of dendritic bundles. In contrast to the striking morphological differences between vertical bundles of dendrites in gyrus splenialis and in gyrus sigmoideus superior of the cat (4), less profound differences occur between parietal and striate cortex of the rabbit. Here the differences are related to the number of apical dendrites forming a bundle, the proportion of thicker to thinner fibres, and the variable propinquity of the dendrites within a bundle.

This chapter presents the method and the first results of a systematic quantitative investigation of dendritic bundles in the rabbit cerebral cortex.

The following preconditions are required for the use of automatic devices for quantitative examination of a number of different regions in the brain:

1. For comparison of several regions in one animal, as many tangentially cut sections as possible should be obtained.
2. It should be possible to identify exactly the original location of each sample.
3. It should be possible to compare the tangential sections with neighbouring sections cut frontally.
4. The majority of sections chosen for evaluation should be cut through one layer only.

5. Staining must be so that structures to be examined can be differentiated on the basis of varying grey values.

The following method goes most of the way to meeting these demands.

METHOD

Four-month-old male and female rabbits were subjected to thoracotomy under pentobarbitone sodium anesthesia and, after opening both jugular veins, were perfused via the left ventricle with a plasma expander followed by Bouin's solution. In order to prevent postmortem cellular damage (1), the brains were dissected out only after a lapse of 4 hr.

Figure 1A shows a trocar, as used by ophthalmic surgeons for removing corneal transplants. The knife has a diameter of 3 mm, which corresponds to a circular area of 7.069 mm². With such a knife, cylinders of cortical tissue exactly perpendicular to the pial surface are punched out at different regions. Before punching, the cortex needs to be undercut with a razor blade to avoid dislocation of the cylinder during removal of the trocar. The cylinders are washed free of the bore of the trocar using an injection syringe filled with Bouin's solution. The trocar is of a type long enough to penetrate all cortical layers from the pial surface to the white matter.

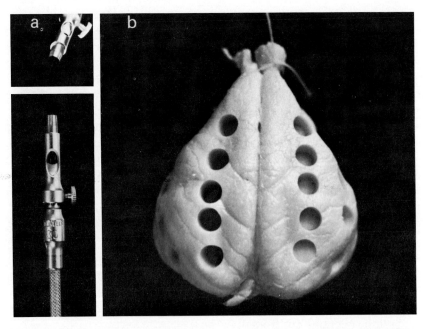

FIG. 1. a: Trocar as used to remove cylinders of cortical tissue. Diameter of the knife = 3 mm. **b:** Dorsal view of rabbit brain after removal of the tissue cylinders.

Sampling is performed symmetrically from the right and left hemispheres. For later topographical identification of the extracted tissue, the different sites of punching are noted on a diagram of the surface of the brain. After punching, the brain is photographed dorsally and from either side. Figure 1B shows such a brain. With some practice it is possible to punch out 30 cylinders from the rather flat regions of the rabbit cortex, i.e., from regions in the striate, parietal, and some temporal areas. Thus, 30 cylinders can be obtained from one brain, which, if favourably processed, can be cut exactly tangential to the pial surface. The photographs of the punched brains ensure an exact documentation of the sites of extraction. This facilitates a localisation and comparison with other brains or maps. The punched brain is embedded and cut frontally so that the tangential series can be compared with neighbouring frontal sections.

The punched-out cylinders are cut tangentially to the pial surface at a thickness of 8 μm and are brought onto microscopic slides, five sections per slide. The sections are deparaffinized and stained for 1.5 hr in Delafield's hematoxylin. The long staining period leads to overstaining of the sections. This is desirable because now the cross-sectioned cell processes stand out against the neuropil. Using suitable filters one obtains just the right contrast needed for evaluation. In addition, the staining method enables good reproducibility, which is essential in comparative studies.

The sections were evaluated with the apparatus for automatic picture analysis (Microvideomat). This apparatus permits programmed measurement and enumeration of structures that can be discriminated by their grey values. Figure 2A to D shows four photographs of the control monitor during the measuring procedure. Figure 2A shows the monitor screen before commencement. One can recognize cross sections of bundles of dendrites, cross-sectioned smaller cell processes running between the bundles, sectioned blood vessels on each side, and dark cell nuclei. The different degree of brightness between neuropil and cross-sectioned cell processes and blood vessels is made use of to select these structures preferentially. In the next step of the procedure, the bright areas are scanned and marked with tabs as shown in Fig. 2B. Now the individual structures can be automatically enumerated. To differentiate between bright structures of different diameters, an electronic shutter is superimposed. It moves in programmed, defined steps from left to right in the direction of the television lines. As soon as the superimposition by the shutter attains the diameter of a bright structure, this structure becomes eliminated. As seen in Fig. 2C, this is reflected on the monitor screen by a step-wise disappearance of the indicator tabs. In this particular case, those structures with a diameter of less than 3 μm have disappeared. With each step the remaining structures are automatically counted. In this way, the large blood vessels can be discriminated by their larger diameter, so that it is possible to enumerate only those cell processes with a diameter between, for instance, 1 and 10 μm. From

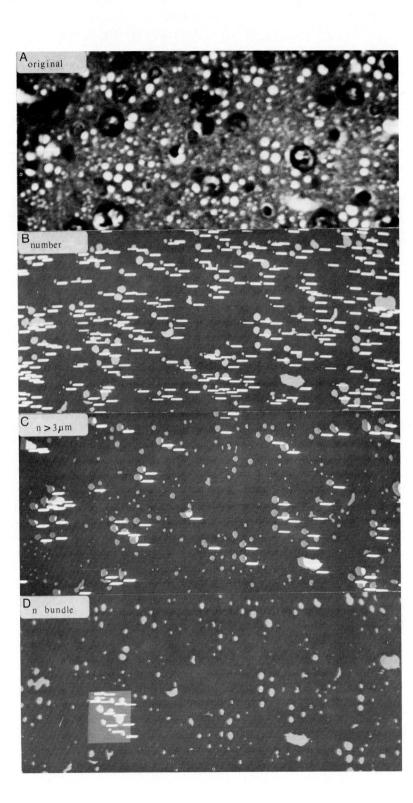

the summation obtained in this way, the computer calculates absolute frequencies for each type of structure, which can be expressed in the form of a histogram.

If the particulars of a specific bundle are to be measured (Fig. 2D), the histological section is scanned in meander fashion, and distinct bundles are circumscribed with an adjustable window. The evaluative process already described is now applied to the individual bundle as selected with the window. In addition, the area within the window is determined. In this process of measurement the decision as to which structures are to be classified as bundles rests on the subjective judgment of the investigator. This is a source of possible error which has to be tolerated until an objective criterion of what really constitutes a bundle has been worked out.

RESULTS

Before measurements of dendrites and dendritic bundles were made with this method, the same apparatus and a similar method were used to determine shrinkage of the tissue cylinder. It was found that, within a cylinder, the various cortical layers have different degrees of shrinkage. The results of measurement of 10 cylinders are documented in Fig. 3. Whereas the areas of sections close to the pial surface amount to 68% of the initial value, the area of a section from the fourth cortical layer is found to be 45% smaller than the original area. This difference in shrinkage of various layers must be taken into account when comparing results from different layers. Additional investigations are needed to find out whether such comparatively large differences in shrinkage are found only in the relatively small samples of tissue used in the present investigation or whether considerable layer-dependent differences in shrinkage have also to be taken into account when larger parts of the brain are processed in one tissue block. In addition, the length of the two axes at right angles of the tangential sections through the tissue cylinders were measured and interdivided. Cylinders in which the ratio thus obtained was not in the region of 1 were discarded, since they either had not been cut perpendicular to the long axis of the cylinder or had become crushed during cutting. With this method, optimal specimens were selected and in the next step bundles of dendrites of four selected regions were measured. In Fig. 4 the measurement of a single

---

FIG. 2. Control monitor of the picture analyser Microvideomat (Zeiss, Oberkochem, Fed. Rep. of Germany). **A:** Tangential section through area parietalis of rabbit cerebral cortex. Delafield's hematoxylin. ×500. **B:** Same section, bright structures of **A** marked with tabs for automatic enumeration. **C:** Same section, an electronic shutter is superimposed to differentiate between bright structures having different diameters. Only those structures with a diameter larger than 3 μm are marked with tabs and counted by the computer. **D:** Same section, a single bundle is selected by superimposition of a window the size of which can be altered. In this way measurement can be restricted to the components of a single bundle.

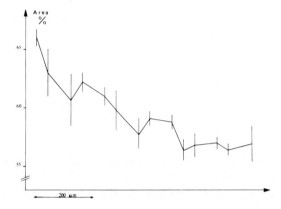

FIG. 3. The area of tangential sections through various cortical layers of 10 tissue cylinders after dehydration, embedded in paraffin and sectioned on a sliding microtome. Thickness, 8 μm. Mean area of the sections is expressed in percent of the size of the area before shrinkage as calculated from the diameter of the knife. Diameter, 3 mm = 7.069 mm^2 = 100%. **Abscissa:** Percentage of the sections measured. **Ordinate:** Depth below pial surface.

```
HISTOGRAM

RANGE:        .25    -      5.00  µm


nr        class         absolute          %
                        frequency


 1         5.00          .0             .00
 2         4.75          .0             .00
 3         4.50          .0             .00
 4         4.25          .0             .00
 5         4.00          .0             .00
 6         3.75          .0             .00
 7         3.50          .0             .00
 8         3.25          .5            4.82     XXXXX
 9         3.00         1.6           14.37     XXXXXXXXXXXXXX
10         2.75          .7            6.69     XXXXXX
11         2.50         1.2           11.33     XXXXXXXXXXX
12         2.25          .6            5.53     XXXXXX
13         2.00          .0             .00
14         1.75          .0             .08
15         1.50          .5            4.55     XXXXX
16         1.25          .9            8.21     XXXXXXXX
17         1.00          .6            5.98     XXXXXX
18         0.75         1.1            9.82     XXXXXXXXXX
19         0.50         1.8           16.07     XXXXXXXXXXXXXXXX
20         0.25         1.4           12.50     XXXXXXXXXXXXX

     n:    11.2      area:      422.92
```

FIG. 4. Protocol of measurement of a single bundle in area parietalis. Column 2 gives the upper limits of the diameter of the measured structures for each class in microns. Histogram columns on the right represent the percentage of measured structures in each class. *n* gives the absolute number of structures per bundle, area denotes the size of the window in square microns as shown in Fig. 2D. For details see text.

bundle of layer IV in area parietalis is shown as given by the computer. The first column gives the number of classes, each class indicating a step of 0.25 μm. The second column expresses the upper limits of each class as expressed in microns. The third column gives the absolute frequency of cross-sectioned cell processes in each class. In the fourth column these values are expressed as percentages of the total number of cell processes enumerated. These percentages are printed in the form of a histogram at the right-hand side of the figure. The last line of this figure gives the number of all cell processes participating in the evaluated bundle and the area of the measuring field in square microns, as delineated by the window. This area can be altered to accommodate the size of any given bundle. Figure 4 reveals that even in the lower part of layer IV the cell processes participating in a bundle have greatly differing diameters. Classes 8 to 12 are separated from the other classes by the free classes 13 and 14. These upper classes are likely to consist of apical dendrites from the large layer-V pyramids, which are known to take part in the formation of a bundle. Therefore, cell processes having a diameter larger than 2 μm and smaller than 5.5 μm were regarded as apical dendrites of large pyramidal cells of the fifth cortical layer. In classes 15 to 20 thin cell processes participating in a bundle are to be found. The applied method does not allow ascertainment of their nature and origin. These cell processes, therefore, may be axons and/or dendrites. In Fig. 5A to C the results of quantitative measurements in four different regions of the cortex can be compared. The histogram columns are marked with numbers corresponding to the numbers in the Fig. 5A denoting the sites of extraction. Figure 5B shows the results of investigation of single bundles. For each of the four areas the columns give the mean value for the number of all cell processes participating in a bundle. Large dots indicate the proportion of apical dendrites of layer-V pyramids, small dots that of thinner cell processes. The figure illustrates the striking differences between the numbers of dendrites per bundle in the four regions investigated. Attention is drawn to the finding that in two regions of the area striata, which according to Rose (8) is a cytoarchitectonically homogeneous field, the dendritic bundles differ with respect to their composition. Figure 5C gives the results if measurement is not restricted to single bundles but if, instead, all cross-sectioned cell processes in a larger field are measured so that the interspaces between the bundles are also taken into account. In this case, a higher proportion of vertically running thin cell processes is found. In three of the regions described in Fig. 5B, all vertically coursing structures in a field of 120,000 μm^2 were measured and are illustrated. The higher proportions of thinner cell processes in the fields indicate that considerable numbers of vertically running small cell processes course between the dendritic bundles.

The findings discussed in this communication are first results of attempts to quantify regional differences between bundles of dendrites. The measurements have been taken in samples of one brain only and must be enlarged to include individual variations in order to become significant. The main aim

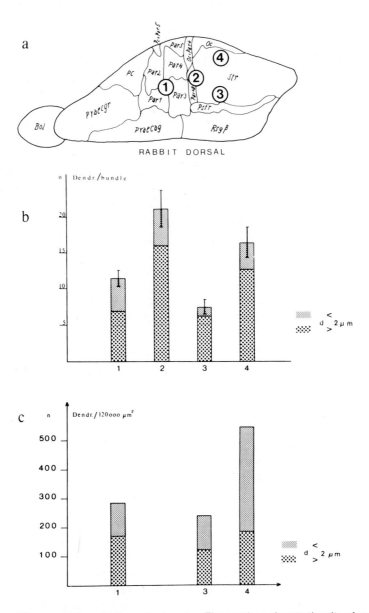

FIG. 5. a: Diagram of the rabbit cerebral cortex. The numbers denote the site of extraction of the tissue cylinders investigated. **b:** Composition of one bundle of apical dendrites (large dots) and thinner cell processes (small dots) in four different regions of cerebral cortex. $n = 40$. **c:** All vertically running cell processes within an area of 120,000 μm^2 are measured and classified. The higher proportion of thin cell processes indicates that a number of vertically running cell processes course between the bundles.

of this communication, however, is to present the newly developed method, because it is hoped that it facilitates exact comparisons between morphological and electrophysiological findings.

ACKNOWLEDGMENT

This work was supported by the Deutsche Forschungsgemeinschaft (F1 26/13) and by a Twinning Grant of the European Training Programme in Brain and Behavior Research.

REFERENCES

1. Cammermeyer, J. (1962): An evaluation of the significance of the "dark" neuron. *Ergeb. Anat. Entwicklungsgesch.*, 36:1–61.
2. Detzer, K. (1976): Course and distribution of apical dendrites of layer V pyramids in the barrel field and area parietalis of the mouse. *Anat. Embryol.*, 149:251–258.
3. Fleischhauer, K., Petsche, H., and Wittkowski, W. (1972): Vertical bundles of dendrites in the neocortex. *Z. Anat. Entwicklungsgesch.*, 136:213–223.
4. Fleischhauer, K. (1974): On different patterns of dendritic bundling in the cerebral cortex of the cat. *Z. Anat. Entwicklungsgesch.*, 143:115–126.
5. Fleischhauer, K., and Detzer, K. (1975): Dendritic bundling in the cerebral cortex. In: *Physiology and Pathology of Dendrites, Vol. 12*, edited by G. W. Kreutzberg, pp. 71–77. Raven Press, New York.
6. Peters, A., and Walsh, T. M. (1972): A study of the organisation of apical dendrites in the somatic sensory cortex of the rat. *J. Comp. Neurol.*, 144:253–268.
7. Petsche, H., Rappelsberger, P., and Frey, Z. (1971): Intracorticale Mechanismen bei der Entstehung der Penicillinspitzen. *EEG-EMG*, 2:176–180.
8. Rose, M. (1931): Cytoarchitektonischer Atlas der Großhirnrinde des Kaninchens. *J. Psychol. Neurol.*, 43:353–440.

Architectonics of the Cerebral Cortex,
edited by M. A. B. Brazier and H. Petsche.
Raven Press, New York © 1978.

Some Facts and Hypotheses Concerning Dendritic Spines and Learning

Almut Schüz

*Max Planck-Institut für biologische Kybernetik, 7400 Tübingen,
Federal Republic of Germany*

I want to begin with two statements:

1. I will limit myself to dendritic spines (10) in the cerebral cortex. Spines in different parts of the nervous system may have different functions.

2. By learning I mean the fixation of information from the environment in the fine structure of the brain. This, most likely, is achieved by a process which sets up or changes the connections between the nerve cells as a consequence of sensory stimulation.

In the course of the last 10 years several papers have appeared indicating that the growth of spines on pyramidal cells can be influenced by the environment. Surgical intervention (enucleation of one eye, severing the optic radiation, or section of the corpus callosum) in young animals resulted in a lower than normal number of spines on apical dendrites in the visual cortex (4,13). Even the simple procedure of rearing animals in the dark had an effect. The changes appeared in the number of spines (12), in the shape of the spines (5), or in the rate of the increase of the number of spines (14). "Enriched environments" gave results which went in the opposite direction to those of deprivation (3,8). The higher number of spines in the auditory cortex following visual or somatic deafferentiation (7) could perhaps be interpreted as a compensatory effect. These findings were especially interesting, since it had been shown (6) that spines are the sites of most synaptic connections on the dendritic tree of pyramidal cells. This led to the idea that spines could be the result of learning processes.

I shall first summarize a piece of work (11) that operated under this assumption and then reflect on some recent evidence in order to show that the idea of spines as memory traces is still very obscure.

VARIATIONS IN THE NUMBER OF SPINES ON PYRAMIDAL CELLS

In Golgi preparations of the mouse, pyramidal cells can occasionally be found with much fewer spines than their neighbours.

Various interpretations are possible:

1. The pyramidal cells, poor in spines, are not so healthy, perhaps atrophic or not well stained.

2. Under the assumption that spines are memory traces, perhaps some cells have learned more than others.

3. Possibly pyramidal cells do not mature synchronously, the cells with few spines perhaps being the immature ones.

There was no support of the first interpretation, that of pathology (11). In connection with a functional interpretation of the number of spines as a result of learning processes, it was interesting to establish that the spine density is a property of the entire neuron and not only of parts of it. The densities of spines on the apical and on the basal dendrites of the same neuron are correlated.

We may draw the conclusion that if spines are memory traces, the condition for the establishment of such an engram is not only a local condition but is also dictated by the entire neuron.

But are they really memory traces?

POSSIBLE ROLES OF SPINES IN LEARNING

Figure 1 shows some pyramidal cells of a newborn mouse. They have an apical dendrite but hardly any basal dendrites yet and practically no spines. The mouse at that time is quite helpless in its behaviour. So, the development of spines might coincide with the period of learning.

However, a look at the pyramidal cells of a newborn guinea pig (Fig. 2) casts some doubt on this. They have well-developed apical and basal dendrites, densely covered with spines, resembling the dendrites of a 13-day-old mouse. The behaviour of the newborn guinea pig is also more advanced than that of the newborn mouse. It can see, it walks around, and soon begins to eat solid food.

If we do not want to assume that guinea pigs do most of their learning in the womb, the presence of spines on their dendrites at birth suggests that spines are not the result of but the condition for learning. The 13-day-old mouse and the newborn guinea pig have in common that they are at an age when they begin to explore the environment. We may suppose that the appearance of spines inaugurates the critical period of learning. In fact, if we look at the mouse at the 13th day of life, when it just begins to open its eyes, we notice that it already has half of its spines in the visual cortex (14).

A spine, then, could represent, so to speak, the right to acquire a synapse, and only the decision as to which of the neighbouring axonal elements will become presynaptic to the spine could be made later on the basis of experience.

The following observation is compatible with this idea. Figure 3 shows two spines from the first layer of the mouse cortex. On serial sections we could convince ourselves that most of the spines (all the spines we analysed)

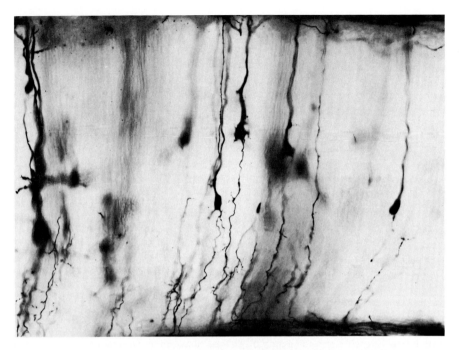

FIG. 1. Golgi-stained pyramidal cells of a 1-day-old mouse. ×164.

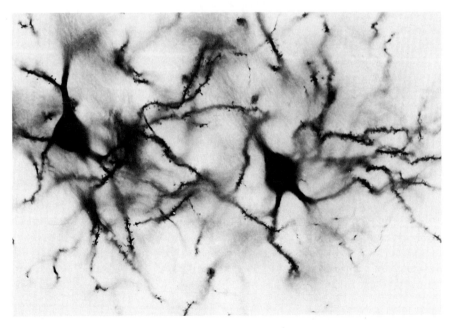

FIG. 2. Basal dendrites of Golgi-stained pyramidal cells of a newborn guinea pig. ×525.

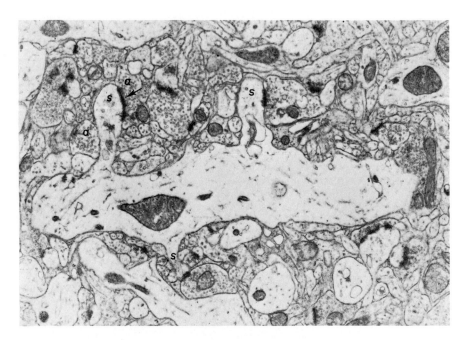

FIG. 3. Electron microscopic section of a series showing a piece of dendrite with three spines **(s)**. The spine to the left is touched by two axons **(a)** full of vesicles, but makes only one synapse **(arrow).** ×15,670.

have only one presynaptic terminal (see, however, ref. 2). It was also evident, however, that many if not all the spines are touched by more than one axon (e.g., the left spine in Fig. 3). Of the 10 spines which I followed on serial sections, six had their heads directly contiguous with one or two large axons full of vesicles with which they did not form synapses, besides the one which was presynaptic to them. In the other four cases, the additional neighbours were smaller segments of axons without vesicles or elements which could not be identified. This observation supports the assumption that the establishment of a synapse on a spine is a true choice of one out of several presynaptic candidates.

This idea leads to a new interpretation of the role of dendritic spines. The growth of spines provides a larger choice of presynaptic candidates available for the establishment of synapses. Actually, the number of axons touching a pyramidal cell may increase more than proportionally to the increase of the surface (which increases by about 70%[1]). Fibers that pass by the dendrite stay in contact with its surface for a longer stretch than they do on the spines, because of the stronger curvature of the spine head. This

---

[1] With 18 spines per 10 μm of dendritic length, a surface of 1.75 μm^2 on each spine and a dendritic diameter of 1.34 μm.

means that a given area on the surface of a spine can be touched by more elements than the same area on the surface of a dendrite. In the favorable case of a spine that can direct its tip toward a chosen axon, the number of reachable neighbours would be still higher than in the case of a rigid spine.

Nevertheless, we are not sure if the spines of the guinea pig at birth or those of the mouse at the beginning of its learning period are without synaptic contacts. In fact, the idea of the spine representing the right to acquire a synapse would imply that during the early learning period there should be many spines without synapses in the tissue. Nobody, to my knowledge, has given such a demonstration for the cortex. The increase in the number of synapses follows a curve which parallels that of the increase in the number of spines (Fig. 4). It is not possible yet to tell from the available data (1,9,14,15) whether or not the appearance of synapses lags behind that of spines.

In this connection I want to mention an interesting observation. In the rat, 10^9 synapses/mm^3 (1) or 6×10^{11} synapses in the whole cortex are established in 26 days. If the rat is awake half of the time, this means that 5×10^5 synapses must be established every second in the whole cortex. If the establishment of a synapse is a memory trace, it is difficult to imagine where this large amount of information comes from in the early days in the life of a rat.

DISCUSSION

If we consider the fact that spines can be influenced by the environment but that many of them appear before stimuli from the environment can have access to the brain, and if we do not want to assume that spines before birth are formed by a different mechanism than those after birth, there are two possibilities:

(1) Spines are formed at a certain time during the process of maturation. Synaptic contacts are made later as a result of sensory stimulation, or, if they are already present before, they might be provisional and wait for modification by neuronal activity. In any case, spines can be interpreted as the condition for learning. The results of deprivation experiments could be explained by supposing that spines with useless contacts disappear again, or that the further maturation of the cell and the increase in the number of spines is hindered or delayed by the deprivation (see also ref. 14).

(2) The formation of spines is not simply a consequence of the maturation of the cell but depends on neuronal activity. The formation of spines due to sensory stimulation—spines as memory traces—would be a special case, preceded by the formation of spines due to neuronal excitation induced by internal activity (the so-called spontaneous activity). For us it makes a great difference, because connections that can be influenced by the environment we call "learned," and connections that are established before stimuli from

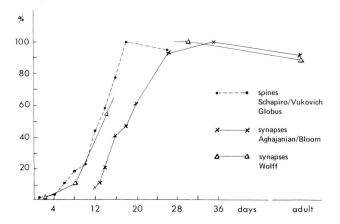

FIG. 4. Comparison between the increase with age in the number of spines and that of synapses in the cortex of the rat. The curve of spines **(broken lines)** shows the average number of spines on apical and basal dendrites in the visual cortex. The values of Wolff are taken from the uppermost tenth of the visual cortex, those of Aghajanian and Bloom from the first layer of the parietal cortex. The number of spines and synapses is expressed in percent of the maximal value.

outside can have access to the brain we call "inborn." It may be the same for the mechanism that makes spines and synapses.

We cannot yet decide between possibility (1) or (2).

ACKNOWLEDGMENT

I am very grateful to Prof. V. Braitenberg and to Dr. G. Palm for many discussions, to Mrs. D. Stoll and to Mr. H. Steffen for the Golgi preparations, to Mrs. K. Witte for the electron microscopical material, and to Miss G. Kurz for typing the manuscript.

REFERENCES

1. Aghajanian, G. K., and Bloom, F. E. (1967): The formation of synaptic junctions in developing rat brain: A quantitative electron microscopic study. *Brain Res.,* 6:716–727.
2. Colonnier, M. (1968): Synaptic patterns on different cell types in the different laminae of the cat visual cortex. An electron microscope study. *Brain Res.,* 9:268–287.
3. Globus, A., Rosenzweig, M. R., Bennett, E. L., and Diamond, M. C. (1973): Effects of differential experience on dendritic spine counts in rat cerebral cortex. *J. Comp. Physiol. Psychol.,* 82(2):175–181.
4. Globus, A., and Scheibel, A. B. (1966): Loss of dendrite spines as an index of pre-synaptic terminal patterns. *Nature,* 212:463–465.
5. Globus, A., and Scheibel, A. B. (1967): The effect of visual deprivation on cortical neurons: A Golgi study. *Exp. Neurol.,* 19:331–345.
6. Gray, E. G. (1959): Axo-somatic and axo-dendritic synapses of the cerebral cortex: An electron microscope study. *J. Anat.,* 93:420–433.
7. Ryugo, D. K., Ryugo, R., Globus, A., and Killackey, H. P. (1975): Increased spine density in auditory cortex following visual or somatic deafferentiation. *Brain Res.,* 90:143–146.

8. Schapiro, S., and Vukovich, K. (1970): Early experience effects upon cortical dendrites: A proposed model for development. *Science,* 167:292–294.
9. Schapiro, S., Vukovich, K., and Globus, A. (1973): Effects of neonatal thyroxine and hydrocortisone administration on the development of dendritic spines in the visual cortex of rats. *Exp. Neurol.,* 40:286–296.
10. Scheibel, M. E., and Scheibel, A. B. (1968): On the nature of dendritic spines—report of a workshop. *Commun. Behav. Biol., Part A,* 1:231–265 (*comprehensive discussion about dendritic spines*).
11. Schüz, A. (1976): Pyramidal cells with different densities of dendritic spines in the cortex of the mouse. *Z. Naturforsch.,* 31c:319–323.
12. Valverde, F. (1967): Apical dendritic spines of the visual cortex and light deprivation in the mouse. *Exp. Brain Res.,* 3:337–352.
13. Valverde, F. (1968): Structural changes in the area striata of the mouse after enucleation. *Exp. Brain Res.,* 5:274–292.
14. Valverde, F. (1971): Rate and extent of recovery from dark rearing in the visual cortex of the mouse. *Brain Res.,* 33:1–11.
15. Wolff, J. R. (1976): Quantitative analysis of topography and development of synapses in the visual cortex. In: *Proc. 7th Intern. Meeting of Neurobiology, Göttingen, Sept. 15–19, 1975. Exp. Brain Res.,* Suppl. 1.

Architectonics of the Cerebral Cortex,
edited by M. A. B. Brazier and H. Petsche.
Raven Press, New York © 1978.

On the Pigmentarchitectonics of the Human Telencephalic Cortex

H. Braak

Anatomisches Institut der Universitat Kiel, D-23 Kiel, Federal Republic of Germany

Most of the nerve cells of the human brain accumulate a great number of lipofuscin granules during their life span. The characteristics of the pigment within the various types of nerve cells vary considerably. Most of the lipofuscin granules in neurons are more or less intensely stained by the basic dye aldehydefuchsin, if—prior to staining—the pigment sulphur is transformed into strongly acidic SO_3H groups by means of a suitable oxidation, as for instance, an oxidation with performic acid. If the pH of the dye solution is low enough, the aldehydefuchsin stains neurolipofuscin granules selectively. Astonishingly enough, most of the pigment granules of the glial cells or the constituents of the blood vessels do not pick up any dye, or are only faintly tinged. Thus, the pigment staining with aldehydefuchsin marks nerve cell bodies very well and more or less selectively.

The appearance of pigment granules during ontogenesis varies considerably, if one compares different types of nerve cells. The neurons of the inferior olive, for example, accumulate masses of lipofuscin granules already during childhood, whereas those of the superior olive or the motor nuclei of the eye muscles remain more or less devoid of pigment inclusions, also in the brains of elderly people (4).

Besides these differences in the progress of pigmentation, there exist marked variations with respect to the amount of pigment accumulations. Some varieties of neurons are crammed with lipofuscin—such as for instance the basket cells of the Ammon's horn, whereas others store only a moderate amount of finely grained pigment, such as the majority of the pyramidal cells.

Hence, the characteristic pattern of pigmentation allows a clear determination of the various types of nerve cells. The differences in pigmentation are often more pronounced than those of the shape and size of the rough endoplasmic reticulum. Therefore, it is often easier to classify a nerve cell as belonging to a certain nucleus or a cortical layer with the aid of the pigment preparation than with that of the Nissl picture. As early as 1903, Obersteiner (25) drew attention to the fact that various types of nerve cells can frequently be better characterized by their distinguishing lipofuscin inclusions than by their appearance in the Nissl preparations (29).

Although lipofuscin accumulates in nerve cells to a certain degree with advancing age, this overall increase does not affect the marking pattern of pigmentation. Moreover, there are only little variations from individual to individual; thus, the pigmentation pattern may serve as an excellent criterion for the determination of nerve cells.

The fact that the staining is restricted to a single cytoplasmic component allows us to greatly enlarge the thickness of the sections, in contrast to the possibilities offered by the Nissl method. Depending on the dimensions and the possible irregularity of the structure to be investigated, we utilize frozen sections ranging from 500 to 1,000 μm. This is a considerable advantage in comparison with the classic Nissl preparations, which become increasingly indistinct with growing thickness, since innumerable nuclei of the glial and endothelial cells obscure the picture of the nerve cells.

The thick pigment preparations greatly facilitate the processing and examination of a great amount of material. Furthermore, the thick slices are especially adapted for low-power examination with the stereomicroscope — an indispensable instrument for architectonic studies, which mainly fill the gap between macroscopic and microscopic investigations. Moreover, the amplitude of accommodation of the eyes enables the student to pass the focus through the whole depth of the slice, getting in this way a direct impression of its three-dimensional structure. As a rule, the numberless superimposed dots, seen at a glance, allow one to determine with ease the limits of both the cellular layers and the cortical areas.

Figure 1 shows a low-power view of a coronal section through the temporal lobe in the latitude of the amygdala. The cortical band adjoining the amygdala belongs to the palaeopallium: to be more precise, to the entorhinal region (Brodmann's field 28) which is a particularly highly developed part of the palaeopallium. Thereafter follows a relatively primitively organized part of the temporal isocortex.

The transition zone between the palaeopallium on the one hand and the neopallium on the other is of particular interest. The outstanding feature is a strongly pigmented layer, which continues the palaeopallial layer alpha of the outer main stratum and runs obliquely through the outer isocortical laminae, leading to a mutual indentation of the allo- and isocortical layers (5). This peculiar construction of the transition zone has never been made out with the aid of the classic neuroanatomical methods, although the area is fairly large, extending several millimeters in breadth and centimeters in length. In pigment preparations it is already visible with the naked eye.

The new method does not only facilitate the outlining of nuclei and cortical layers but in addition allows us to analyse their composition. Cortical layers as well as most of the subcortical nuclei are composed of different varieties of nerve cells. Accordingly, they do not appear as homogeneously tinged areas, but display differently pigmented components. This can be most easily demonstrated by using the example of the Ammon's horn (Fig. 2).

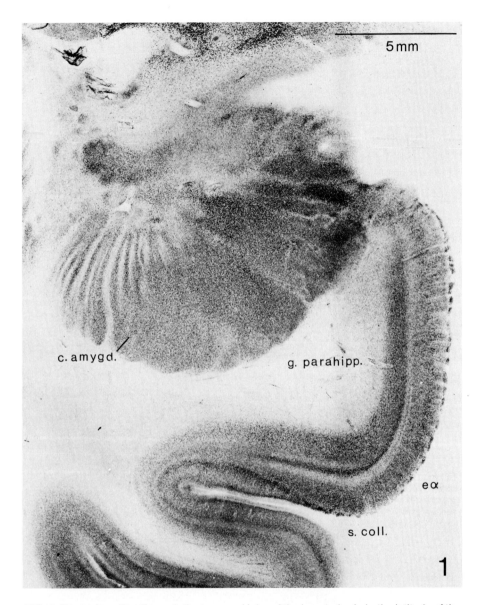

FIG. 1. Coronal section through the temporal lobe of the human brain in the latitude of the corpus amygdaloideum. The cortex covering the parahippocampal gyrus belongs to the entorhinal region. The intensely stained islands of its outermost cellular layer (lamina principalis externa alpha) coalesce in the vicinity of the collateral sulcus and run obliquely through the outer main stratum establishing an intimate indentation of the allocortical and isocortical layers. Pigment preparation: 1,000 μm, performic-acid aldehydefuchsin; **c. amygd.,** corpus amygdaloideum; **eα,** lamina principalis externa alpha; **g. parahipp.,** gyrus parahippocampalis; **s. coll.,** sulcus collateralis. (From ref. 11.)

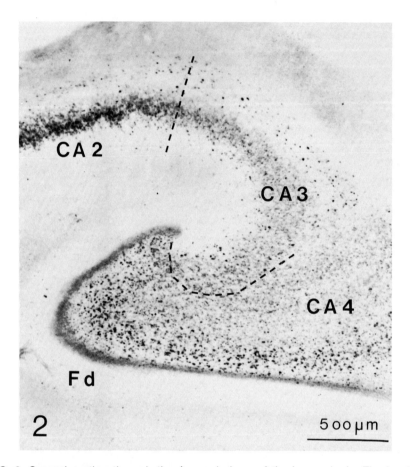

FIG. 2. Coronal section through the Ammon's horn of the human brain. The borders between the various sectors of the Ammon's horn are marked by dotted lines. Note the pigment-rich stellate cells within the stratum oriens of CA 2 and CA 3, and, in particular, the great number of these neurons in the immediate vicinity of the granular layer of the fascia dentata in CA 4. The pyramidal cells of CA 3 and the modified pyramids of CA 4 are only moderately pigmented. Pigment preparation: 500 μm, performic-acid aldehyde-fuchsin. **CA 2, CA 3, CA 4,** sectors of the Ammon's horn; **Fd,** fascia dentata. (From ref. 7.)

The subdivision of the Ammon's horn into four sectors, as proposed by Lorente de Nó (22), is confirmed by pigmentarchitectonics. The fourth sector of the Ammon's horn (CA 4) fills up the hilus of the oldest part of the archipallium, the fascia dentata (Fd). This survey already shows numerous dark spots which lie mainly in the vicinity of the granular layer of the dentate gyrus. They differ markedly from the only weakly tinged cells that build up the cortical band of sector 3 (CA 3) and the adjacent parts of the sector 4 (CA 4).

Figure 3 is a closer view of CA 4 in the vicinity of the fascia dentata.

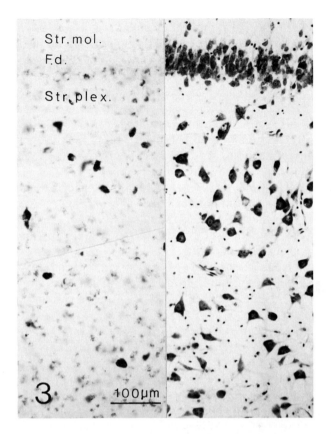

FIG. 3. Part of the sector CA 4 of the cornu ammonis of the human brain with adjacent portions ot the fascia dentata appearing along the upper margin. The left half shows a pigment preparation (400 µm, aldehydefuchsin). The large pigment-rich stellate cells are clearly distinguishable from the only faintly tinged modified pyramids of CA 4. The right half shows a similar area in the Nissl preparation (10 µm, cresyl violet). CA 4 is filled with multipolar nerve cells which form a seemingly homogeneous population. The differences between the modified pyramids and the stellate cells are not discernible. **F.d.,** stratum granulosum of the fascia dentata; **Str. mol.,** stratum moleculare of the fascia dentata; **Str. plex.,** Stratum plexiforme of the fascia dentata. (From ref. 7.)

The granular layer of the dentate gyrus is arranged along the upper margin. The right half shows a conventional Nissl staining opposed to a pigment preparation on the left. The Nissl staining shows only multipolar nerve cells of about the same size and shape which form a seemingly homogeneous population. The pigment preparation, on the contrary, shows gross differences. Besides a small population of nerve cells crammed with lipofuscin granules there exists evidently a majority of weakly tinged neurons.

In order to find other characteristics of the heavily and the faintly pigmented nerve cells—and to demonstrate that lipofuscin granules do not occur at random—we utilize another method which allows us to examine

successively both the Golgi and the pigment picture of individual neurons
(7). This method is explained in Fig. 4. The top picture on the left is a Golgi
picture of a large nerve cell, taken from the pyramidal layer of the Ammon's
horn (CA 1). The far-reaching slender and smoothly contoured dendrites
radiate in various directions. The axon ascends and splits up in the vicinity
of the parent soma. Hence, this cell belongs to the group of large stellate
cells. Cells of this sort which can be readily determined by their appearance
in the Golgi preparation are photographed a first time. Thereafter, the sections are firmly attached to specially prepared glass slides, counterstained
and photographed again (top right and bottom left). After notation of the
vernier, the preparations are bleached, oxidized, and restained with aldehydefuchsin and a weak nuclear stain. The approximate position of the cells
is determined with the aid of the vernier scale. Finally, the cells are reliably
identified by the characteristic pattern of the surrounding nuclei and then
photographed again (bottom right).

We have studied a great number of cortical neurons in this way. The most
important result of these examinations is that we can say with certainty that
there is a clear relation between the type of nerve cell and its pattern of
pigmentation.

The Golgi preparations of the fourth sector of the Ammon's horn, for
instance, show mainly large multipolar neurons that can be classified as
modified pyramids, because they have many traits in common with the
pyramidal cells of the third sector. The neurons are conspicuously marked
by extremely long-stalked appendages covering circumscribed areas of their
dendrites, establishing the contact zones with the mossy fibers. All of the
multipolar neurons of CA 4 having these long-stalked thorns come out to be
faintly tinged in pigment preparations. A few tiny lipofuscin granules are
more or less evenly distributed over large parts of the cytoplasm (Fig. 5,
upper third).

Now and then, multipolar nerve cells of similar size and shape appear
showing smoothly contoured dendrites without any thorns. As a rule, these
short-axoned stellate cells turn out to be strongly pigmented within the
archipallium. Their cell bodies are crowded with coarse and intensely
stained lipofuscin granules (Fig. 5, middle third).

Occasionally, some stellate cells occur and these are in contrast to the
pigment-laden variety almost devoid of lipofuscin granules (Fig. 5, lower
third). Structural details of the Golgi picture do not give any criteria for
distinguishing these two groups of stellate cells. The pigment-lacking type
is less frequently found within the archipallium than the pigment-rich
variety.

The question arises as to how to interpret these striking differences in
pigmentation. Can it be possible that neuropigments have something to do
with the transmitter substances of the neurons? If one looks at the neurons
containing neuromelanin such a relation has been established. The black

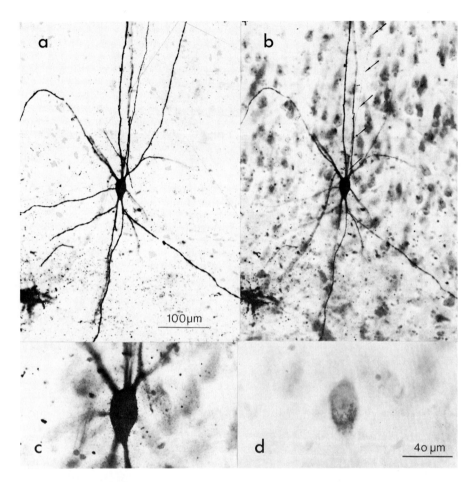

FIG. 4. Illustration of the methodical steps to establish a correlation between both the Golgi preparation and the pigment preparation by successive staining and examination of individual nerve cells. **a:** Neurons which can be readily determined in the Golgi preparation are photographed a first time. **b, c:** Thereafter, the sections are attached to glass slides, counterstained, and photographed again, their position being fixed by the vernier scale. **d:** Finally, the preparation is bleached, oxidized, and stained to bring out the pigment picture. The cell can be made out both with the aid of the vernier scale and the characteristic pattern of the surrounding nerve cell bodies and glial cell nuclei. (From ref. 7.)

cells of the human brain—for instance, those of the dorsal glossopharyngeus and vagus area, the locus coeruleus, the nucleus niger, the nucleus parabrachialis pigmentosus—produce catecholamines.

The nuclei of the raphe rhombencephali produce 5-hydroxytryptamin (15). In pigment preparations they are conspicuous by a vast and early accumulation of lipofuscin granules (3).

On the contrary, the Purkinje cells, the stellate, and the basket cells of

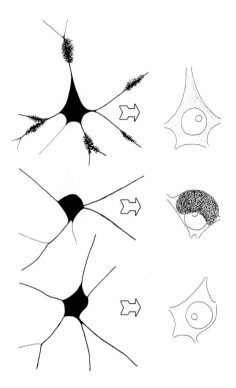

FIG. 5. Diagram of the three main cell types of CA 4. The modified pyramids **(upper third)** are conspicuously marked in Golgi preparations by a rich supply with long-stalked spines covering circumscribed areas of their dendrites. Cells with this characteristic are invariably only faintly tinged in pigment preparations, whereas the stellate cells with smooth dendrites are either richly endowed with lipofuscin granules **(middle third)** or almost devoid of pigment inclusions **(lower third).** The large pigment-rich stellate cells are more frequently found within the archipallium than the variety devoid of pigment.

the cerebellar cortex — known to produce γ-aminobutyric acid (18,27,28) — are almost devoid of lipofuscin inclusions which can be stained with aldehydefuchsin (6).

Hence, it would be tempting to suggest that the pigment-laden stellate cells of the Ammon's horn contain serotonin or serotonin-like substances, whereas those which are devoid of pigment granules utilize GABA or a related compound. From neurochemical investigations it is known that the Ammon's horn is particularly rich in both serotonin and GABA (1,14,17, 26). But, of course, this gives little support to this hypothesis. Obviously, it awaits confirmation by a topochemical demonstration of the respective transmitter substances within the cell bodies of the differently pigmented stellate cells.

Whatever may cause these different patterns of lipofuscin deposits, the pigment preparations enable us to classify the nerve cells of the cortex either with the various types of the pyramidal cells or with those of the stellate cells. What Fig. 6 shows is valid not only with respect to the various parts of the archipallium but also to those of the palaeopallium, the cortex derivatives claustrum and amygdala, and, above all, the entire neopallium.

Hence, the *qualitative* results of the precarious and capricious Golgi impregnations can be translated into the language of the pigment preparations, which give *quantitative* information about the distribution pattern and packing density of the pyramids and the different types of stellate cells.

A description of some details concerning the distribution of the pigment-rich stellate cells will serve as an illustration. The pigment-rich stellate cells can be subdivided into two classes: one of which is made up of the *small* or *minute* pigment-laden cells, and the other the *large* or *giant* ones.

The *large* pigment-rich stellate cell is a predominant constituent of the older parts of the telencephalon and is frequently found in the cortex derivatives, claustrum, and amygdala. Within the isocortex it is, in general, restricted to the inner main stratum and can be most frequently encountered within the lower reaches of the ganglionic layer and the adjacent parts of the multiform layer. In comparison with the archipallial and also the palaeopallial cortices, the large pigment-rich stellate cells are less densely arranged within the neopallium, and here again phylogenetically older parts are more richly endowed with these cells than younger ones.

To demonstrate this Fig. 7 shows two parts of the superior temporal gyrus, cut at the latitude of the anterior commissure. The one area, displaying a primitive cortex, lies in the vicinity of the insular circular sulcus; the other area lies not far from the lateral margin of the superior temporal plane and shows a highly differentiated isocortex (Fig. 7, inset). The primitively organized temporal cortex in the vicinity of the insula (Fig. 7, left half) displays numerous *large* and pigment-rich stellate cells scattered throughout the inner main stratum. They are loosely arranged with comparatively

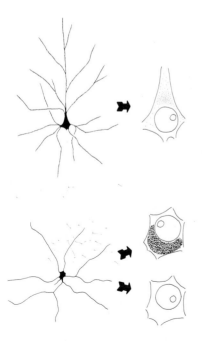

FIG. 6. Simplified diagram showing the characteristic pattern of pigmentation that can be found in the various types of allocortical and isocortical nerve cells. As a rule, the pyramidal cells contain finely grained, widely distributed and only weakly stained pigment, whereas the stellate cells are either crammed with coarse and intensely stained pigment granules or lack of pigmentation altogether.

large distances between the individual cells. Their number decreases gradually as one moves laterally from this area toward more refined isocortical fields. Such an area is shown in the right half of Fig. 7. The pigment-rich large stellate cells are hardly recognizable. Only a scarce number of dark spots are visible, mostly within the limits of layer Vb and the upper parts of layer VI. This is not merely a peculiarity of the temporal lobe, but can be shown in other parts of the telencephalic cortex as well. Again and again, one finds a greater number of large pigment-rich stellate cells in the older cortices and a lesser number in younger ones.

The other class of pigment-rich stellate cells, the *small* ones, show just the opposite. They are relatively infrequent in the older cortices and increase in number in accordance with the degree of development.

Two cortical areas, the one taken from the dorsal insular region the other from the lateral margin of the superior temporal plane (Fig. 8, inset) will illustrate this. In general, the *small* pigment-rich stellate cells populate the lower reaches of the corpuscular layer and the upper parts of the pyramidal layer. The insular field (Fig. 8, left side) displays a particularly broad pyramidal layer and above it a small corpuscular layer consisting almost totally of minute pyramidal cells. In general, the small and slender pyramids

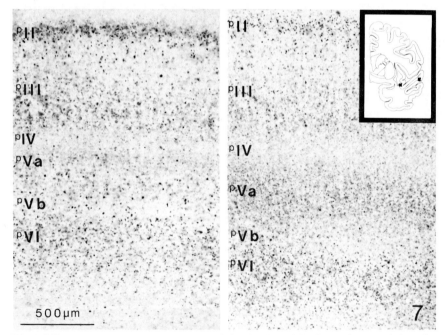

FIG. 7. Differences in number and pattern of distribution of the *large* pigment-rich stellate cells. The figure shows two parts of the superior temporal gyrus, cut at the latitude of the anterior commissure. The inset shows the location of the two cortical areas. The primitively organized field in the vicinity of the insula, shown on the left, displays a great number of large pigment-rich stellate cells distributed over the whole of the inner main stratum (PVa to PVI). By comparison, large and intensely stained cells are rarely encountered within the more refined temporal area, shown on the right.

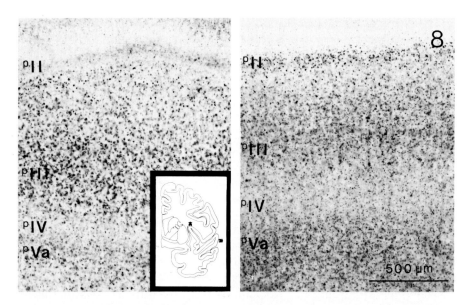

FIG. 8. Differences in number and pattern of distribution of the *small* pigment-rich stellate cells. The inset shows the location of the two cortical areas given in this picture. The primitively organized field from the dorsal insular region, shown on the left, displays a second layer composed of extremely sparsely pigmented tiny pyramidal cells. The layer is almost devoid of small pigment-rich stellate cells. Only the upper parts of the pyramidal layer are populated by moderately large pigment-rich stellate cells. The highly developed isocortex from the facies superolateralis of the superior temporal gyrus, shown on the right, displays by contrast a second layer which is particularly rich in the minute heavily pigmented stellate cell variety. A dense concentration of these cells giving the second layer a band-like appearance is a distinguishing mark of highly differentiated isocortical fields, as for instance the postcentral and temporal association areas. Pigment preparation: 800 μm, performic-acid aldehydefuchsin.

of the second layer are extremely sparsely pigmented and therefore hardly discernible. The dark spots of the larger pigment-rich stellate cells which occur in the upper reaches of the pyramidal layer are still recognizable, but the corpuscular layer is almost devoid of the tiny pigment-rich stellate cells which may also vanish completely. This is, of course, an extreme variation of the corpuscular layer, but it can be found, although less pronounced, also in other primitively organized cortical fields as well. The right half of Fig. 8 shows a refined isocortex. Apart from a moderate number of larger pigment-rich stellate cells in the upper reaches of the pyramidal layer, there exists a wealth of small stellate cells that are particularly densely packed along the lower limit of the corpuscular layer. The second layer may appear in pigment preparations as a dark band owing to the existence of innumerable superimposed pigment-rich stellate cells. This band-like appearance of the second layer is a distinguishing mark of the postcentral and temporal association areas. It disappears more and more as the field moves from the highly differentiated isocortical fields toward more primitively organized ones. These marked variations in distribution may give rise to the assumption that the small pigment-rich stellate cells are of a particular significance for the higher functions of the brain.

Figure 9 shows the main differences in the pattern of distribution of the pigment-rich stellate cells in the phylogenetically older and younger cortical areas. The left half shows a primitively organized field with numerous large stellate cells in the inner main stratum and only a few small ones in the corpuscular layer, whereas the right half displays a highly developed field with only a scarce number of large stellate cells and the characteristic band-like appearance of the second layer.

The small pigment-rich stellate cells have spindle-shaped or polygonal cell bodies from which a few slender and smoothly contoured dendrites originate. The dendrites are bush-like and for the most part oriented toward the cortical surface. The axon splits up in the vicinity of the parent soma (8). The cell body is filled with coarse lipofuscin granules that can serve as an excellent internal marker to identify these stellate cells in material prepared for electron microscopical investigations (2). In contrast to the grid-like arrangement of the pyramidal cells (20), the small pigment-rich stellate cells are arranged at random, as is revealed in sections that have been cut tangentially to the cortical surface (8).

The variations in the distribution pattern of the large and the small pigment-rich stellate cells alone open up a new field in architectonics. But there are still more structural details revealed in pigment preparations. The method shows, for instance, cortical layers that cannot be made out reliably with the aid of the classic neurohistological methods.

To exemplify this, one can cast a short glance at the striate area (Fig. 10). In this context a detailed description of its various layers can be omitted, because most of them resemble more or less the corresponding layers of other isocortical fields. I would therefore like to focus attention on the broad stripe which is conventionally termed the "internal granular layer" of the striate area, although in reality it is to a large extent not comparable with the fourth layer of other isocortical fields. The zone appears in pigment preparations as composed of a broad pale stripe which is followed by a narrow and sharply outlined dark one, and, again, a narrow pale band and another dark one. In pigment preparations the most striking component of the striate area is an intensely stained narrow band in the lower reaches of the fourth layer ($IVc\beta$, Fig. 10). This does not occur in other isocortical areas and turns out to be only a part of the small-celled layer IVc of the Nissl preparation (9).

The right half of Fig. 11 shows a pigment preparation with a thickness of about 800 μm. This was photographed and then embedded in epoxy resin. From this block, sections stained with methylene blue to get a Nissl preparation were cut at 7 μm; this can be seen on the left. In this way a comparison of the pigment picture and the Nissl picture of the same area is possible. One half of this combination is reproduced as the mirror image of the other;

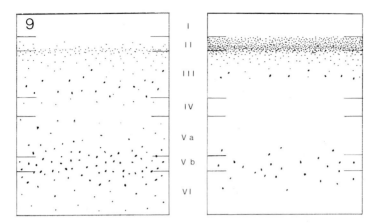

FIG. 9. Diagram of the main differences which can be found in the distribution of the large and the small pigment-rich stellate cells in phylogenetically older and younger cortical fields. The primitively organized field **(left)** shows numerous large and only a few small pigment-rich stellate cells, whereas the highly developed field **(right)** displays only a scarce number of large and a wealth of small pigment-rich stellate cells.

thus, the left-hand margin of the pigment picture corresponds exactly with the right-hand margin of the Nissl picture. If one compares the pigment and the Nissl picture, it becomes apparent that the cell-rich lower reaches of the "internal granular layer," which in the Nissl preparation are termed "IVc" (13), are at least divisable into four subunits (the pale IVcα, the sharply outlined IVcβ, the pale IVd, and the moderately pigmented Va) in the pigment preparation. This ties in with the results of the examinations of Golgi preparations which show different varieties of small nerve cells, as for instance tiny pyramids and minute stellate cells which are not arranged at random but form definite sublayers within the cell-rich lower third of the internal granular layer (23,24). Hence, the cellular components of this cell-rich stripe have only one trait in common, that is their small size. It is one of the pitfalls of the Nissl preparation that heterogeneously composed accumulations of small cells appear to be a uniform layer.

Golgi impregnations reveal that the striking IVcβ, for instance, is composed of a wealth of small stellate cells with slender and relatively short dendrites endowed with a moderate number of thorns (Fig. 12). The perikarya of this variety of stellate cells contain a few coarse agglomerations of lipofuscin granules with light vacuoles (9). Neurophysiological investigations have shown that these cells receive the bulk of projection fibers originating from the small-celled layers of the lateral geniculate body (19). The clear advantage of the pigment preparation is that it distinctly displays this main entrance of the visual radiation into the cortex.

Finally, a rough survey of the appearance of the different varieties of pyramidal cells in the pigment preparation can be given. Figure 13 shows

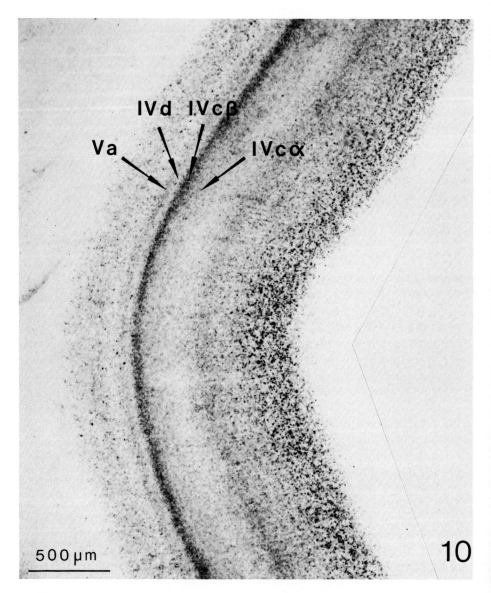

FIG. 10. The striate area of the human brain, cut perpendicular to the cortical surface. Note the four narrow differently pigmented layers, indicated by the arrows **(IVcα, IVcβ, IVd, Va)**. These layers form a cell-rich stripe which is in Nissl preparations termed "IVc." Pigment preparation: 800 μm, performic-acid aldehydefuchsin.

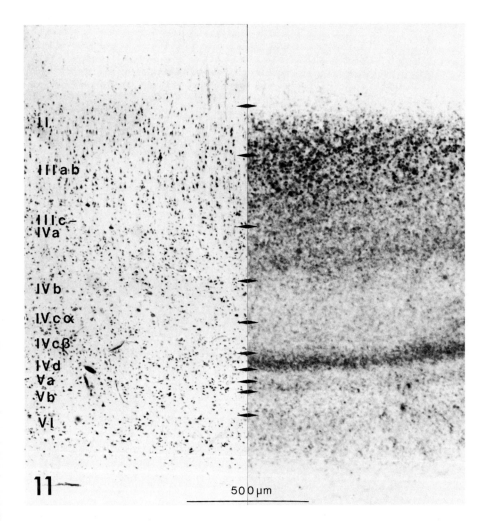

FIG. 11. Area striata of the human brain. The right half of the picture shows a pigment preparation (800 μm). In order to get the micrograph, shown on the left, the pigment preparation was embedded in epoxy resin. Sections (7 μm) were cut from this block and stained with methylene blue. To facilitate the comparison between the pigment and the Nissl preparation, one half is reproduced as the mirror image of the other. The left-hand margin of the pigment picture corresponds exactly with the right-hand margin of the Nissl picture. The picture demonstrates that it is almost impossible to subdivide the cell-rich lower reaches of the internal granular layer in the Nissl preparation. The heterogeneously composed accumulation of small cells **(IVcα to Va)** appears to be a uniform layer in the Nissl preparation.

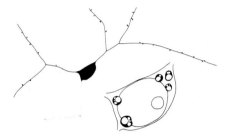

FIG. 12. Diagram of the typical small stellate cell variety of layer IVcβ. The cell body generates a few slender dendrites which are covered with a moderate number of thorns. The cell body contains coarse agglomerations of lipofuscin granules with light vacuoles.

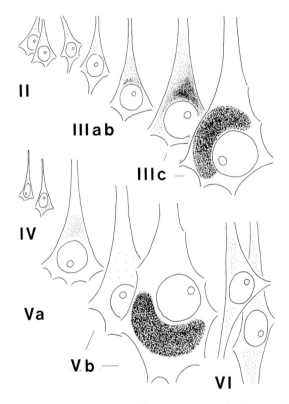

II

III a b

III c —

IV

Va

V b —

VI

FIG. 13. Simplified diagram showing the different patterns of pigmentation which can be found in the various types of pyramidal cells. Second-layer pyramids are sparsely pigmented. The third-layer pyramids show an increase in pigmentation from top to bottom. Within a restricted number of association areas unusually large pyramids occur in the lower reaches of the third layer which contain large and compact masses of pigment granules in circumscribed portions of their cell body. The small pyramids of the granular layer are sparsely pigmented. The ganglionic layer pyramids have finely grained pigment which can be only weakly stained. A restricted number of cortical areas show giant pyramids of Betz in layer Vb. They are marked by compact and rounded masses of lipofuscin granules. The pyramidal and triangular cells of the sixth layer contain only a scarce number of pigment granules.

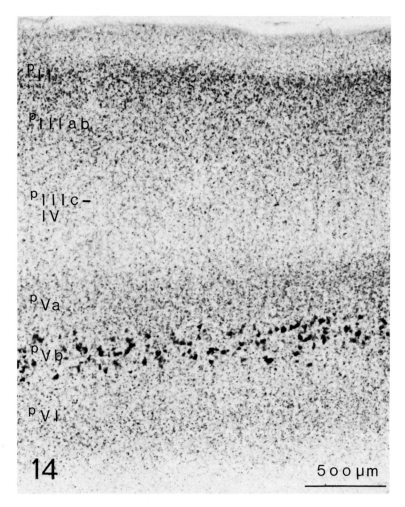

FIG. 14. The precentral gigantopyramidal area of the human brain. The pigment preparation shows a clear lamination also in this highly modified motor cortex. The giant Betz pyramids stand out by their compact pigment accumulations. The layers are indicated along the left-hand margin. Pigment preparation: 800 μm, performic-acid aldehyde-fuchsin.

the typical pigmentation which is in general achieved from the pyramidal cells of the various cortical layers. As a rule, the pigment in pyramidal cells is finely grained and less intensely stained by aldehydefuchsin than that of the pigment-rich stellate cells. The small pyramids of the second layer, as well as those of layers IIIa, IV, and Vb, are scarcely pigmented. A moderate amount of pigment is encountered within the pyramids of layers IIIb and Va. The large pyramids of layer IIIc are generally richly endowed with lipofuscin granules. Two varieties of pyramidal cells show extremely large

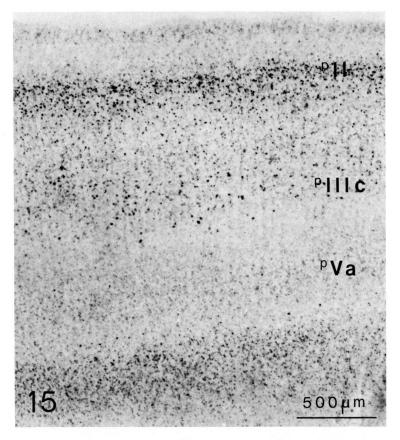

FIG. 15. The sensory speech area (Wernicke center) of the human brain. The pigment preparation shows unusually large pyramids in the lower reaches of the third layer which contain compact and rounded masses of lipofuscin granules. The layers are indicated along the right-hand margin. Pigment preparation: 800 μm, performic-acid aldehyde-fuchsin.

pigment accumulations, but these cell types exist only in a restricted number of isocortical areas.

The strongly pigmented pyramids belong either to the giant pyramidal cells of Betz, which can be found in the lower half of the ganglionic layer in various isocortical fields, or to the large pyramids scattered throughout the lower reaches of the pyramidal layer in certain association areas. In contrast to the scattered distribution of the pigment in pyramids found elsewhere, the lipofuscin granules in these two types form compact and rounded masses which are concentrated in one part of the cell body. Hence, this characteristic pattern allows us to distinguish these cells from others.

Figure 14 shows a pigment preparation of the gigantopyramidal area (Brodmann's field 4). Its dominating constituents are the giant pyramids of

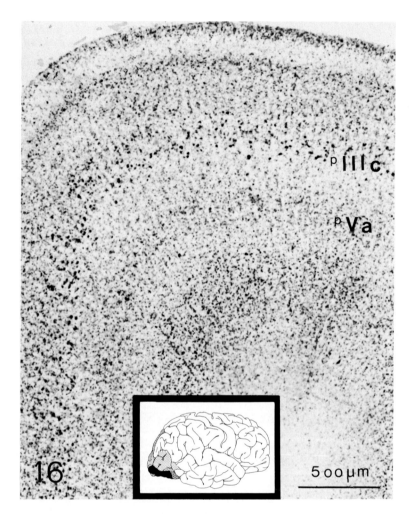

FIG. 16. The magnopyramidal field of the peristriate region of the human brain. The inset shows the location of the area in black. Numerous large and pigment-rich pyramids are distributed over the lower reaches of the third layer. The layers are indicated along the right-hand margin. Pigment preparation: 800 μm, performic-acid aldehydefuchsin.

Betz that are scattered throughout the lower half of the ganglionic layer. The Betz cells stand out because of their large pigment accumulations and contrast greatly with the other constituents of layer Vb which are particularly scarcely pigmented. Thus, they can be easily determined and so it is also possible to identify small or only moderately large Betz cells which can be found – apart from in the gigantopyramidal area – also in other isocortical fields (10,16).

The unusually large pyramids populating the lower reaches of the pyramidal layer and subjacent parts of the granular layer as well show a similar pattern of pigmentation (12). These large pyramids can be found only in a limited number of highly developed association areas, such as the sensory temporal speech area (Wernicke center) which is shown in Fig. 15. Moreover, the sudden appearance of the strange pigment-rich pyramidal cells in the lower reaches of the third layer allows one to delineate reliably the speech area from the surrounding fields covering other parts of the superior temporal gyrus.

Besides the sensory speech area, a few other association areas are also richly endowed with large IIIc pyramids of the pigment-laden variety. Some of these association areas have, to date, not been described, for instance a small field in the peristriate region (Brodmann's field 19). The magnopyramidal field within this region occupies the edge between the facies inferior and the superolateral facies of the occipital lobe, shown in the inset of Fig. 16. The sharply outlined field differs from the surrounding peristriate areas in that the layer IIIc is crowded with unusually large and pigment-rich pyramidal cells (12). This particular feature gives the field a close resemblance to the sensory speech area—and for this reason it would be tempting to suggest that the possible functional significance of this occipital area might be that of a special visual association area. In any case, this magnopyramidal field represents, from a morphological point of view, the most highly differentiated isocortex of the peristriate region and may well be of particular importance for the more advanced processing of visual impressions.

ACKNOWLEDGMENT

The author wishes to thank Sybille Piontek for her excellent technical assistance. He would also like to express his sincere appreciation to Prof. Wanke (Pathol. Inst., Rendsburg) for kindly providing him with autopsy material. This work was sponsored by the Deutsche Forschungsgemeinschaft.

REFERENCES

1. Bogdanski, D. F., Weissbach, H., and Udenfried, S. (1957): The distribution of serotonin, 5-hydroxytryptophan decarboxylase, and monoamine oxidase in brain. *J. Neurochem.*, 1:272–278.
2. Braak, E. (1976): On the fine structure of the small, heavily pigmented non-pyramidal cells in lamina II and upper lamina III of the human isocortex. *Cell Tissue Res.*, 169:233–245.
3. Braak, H. (1970): Über die Kerngebiete des menschlichen Hirnstammes. II: Die Raphekerne. *Z. Zellforsch.*, 107:123–141.
4. Braak, H. (1971): Über das Neurolipofuscin in der unteren Olive und dem Nucleus dentatus cerebelli im Gehirn des Menschen. *Z. Zellforsch.*, 121:573–592.
5. Braak, H. (1972): Zur Pigmentarchitektonik der Großhirnrinde des Menschen. I. Regio entorhinalis. *Z. Zellforsch.*, 127:407–438.
6. Braak, H. (1974): On the intermediate cells of Lugaro within the cerebellar cortex of man. A pigmentarchitectonic study. *Cell Tissue Res.*, 149:399–411.

7. Braak, H. (1974): On the structure of the human archicortex. I. The cornu ammonis. A Golgi and pigmentarchitectonic study. *Cell Tissue Res.*, 152:349–383.
8. Braak, H. (1974): On pigment-loaded stellate cells within the layer II and III of the human isocortex. A Golgi and pigmentarchitectonic study. *Cell Tissue Res.*, 155:91–104.
9. Braak, H. (1976): On the striate area of the human isocortex. A Golgi and pigmentarchitectonic study. *J. Comp. Neurol.*, 166:341–364.
10. Braak, H. (1976): A primitive gigantopyramidal field buried in the depth of the cingulate sulcus of the human brain. *Brain Res.*, 109:219–233.
11. Braak, H. (1976): Zur Pigmentarchitektonik der Endhirnrinde des Menschen. *Verh. Anat. Ges.*, 70:1003–1006.
12. Braak, H. (1977): The pigment architecture of the human occipital lobe. *Anat. Embryol.*, 150:229–250.
13. Brodmann, K. (1903): Beiträge zur histologischen Lokalisation der Großhirnrinde. Der Calcarinatypus. *J. Psychol. Neurol.*, 2:133–159.
14. Curtis, D. R., Felix, D., and McLennan, H. (1970): GABA and hippocampal inhibition. *Br. J. Pharmacol.*, 40:881–883.
15. Dahlström, A., and Fuxe, K. (1964): Evidence for the existence of monoamine containing neurons in the central nervous system. I. Demonstration of monoamines in the cell bodies of brain stem neurons. *Acta Physiol. Scand.*, 62, Suppl. 232:1–55.
16. Economo, C. von, and Koskinas, G. N. (1925): *Die Cytoarchitektonik der Hirnrinde des erwachsenen Menschen.* Springer, Berlin.
17. Fonnum, J., and Storm-Mathisen, J. (1969): GABA synthesis in rat hippocampus correlated to the distribution on inhibitory neurons. *Acta Physiol. Scand.*, 76:35A–37A.
18. Hökfelt, T., and Ljungdahl, Å. (1970): Cellular localization of labeled gamma-aminobutyric acid (^{3}H-GABA) in rat cerebellar cortex: an autoradiographic study. *Brain Res.*, 22:391–396.
19. Hubel, D. H., and Wiesel, T. N. (1972): Laminar and columnar distribution of geniculocortical fibers in the macaque monkey. *J. Comp. Neurol.*, 146:421–450.
20. Koelliker, A. (1896): *Handbuch der Gewebelehre des Menschen. Bd. II Nervensystem des Menschen und der Thiere.* 6. Aufl. Engelmann, Leipzig.
21. Lasher, R. S. (1974): The uptake of (^{3}H)GABA and differentiation of stellate neurons in cultures of dissociated postnatal rat cerebellum. *Brain Res.*, 69:235–254.
22. Lorente de Nó, R. (1934): Studies on the structure of the cerebral cortex. II. Continuation of the study of the ammonic system. *J. Psychol. Neurol.*, 46:113–177.
23. Lund, J. S. (1969): Non pyramidal cells of layers I-IV of the monkey striate cortex. *Anat. Rec.*, 166:339 (*abstract*).
24. Lund, J. S. (1973): Organization of neurons in the visual cortex, area 17, of the monkey (*Macaca mulatta*). *J. Comp. Neurol.*, 147:455–496.
25. Obersteiner, H. (1903): Über das hellgelbe Pigment in den Nervenzellen und das Vorkommen weiterer fettähnlicher Körper im Centralnervensystem. *Arb. Neurol. Inst. Wien,* 10:245–274.
26. Paasonen, M. K., McLean, P. D., and Giarman, N. J. (1957): 5-hydroxytryptamine (serotonin, enteramin) content of structures of the limbic system. *J. Neurochem.*, 1:326–333.
27. Schon, F., and Iversen, L. L. (1972): Selective accumulation of (^{3}H)GABA by stellate cells in rat cerebellar cortex *in vivo. Brain Res.*, 42:503–507.
28. Sotelo, C., Privat, A., and Drian, M. J. (1972): Localization of (^{3}H)GABA in tissue culture of rat cerebellum using electron microscope radioautography. *Brain Res.*, 45:302–308.
29. Vogt, C., and Vogt, O. (1942): Morphologische Gestaltungen unter normalen und pathogenen Bedingungen. *J. Psychol. Neurol.*, 50:1–524.

Architectonics of the Cerebral Cortex,
edited by M. A. B. Brazier and H. Petsche.
Raven Press, New York © 1978.

Ontogenetic Aspects of Cortical Architecture: Lamination

J. R. Wolff

*Department of Neurobiology, Neuroanatomy, Max Planck-Institute for Biophysical
Chemistry, 3400 Göttingen, Federal Republic of Germany*

The internal architecture of the adult neocortex is characterized by variations of the packing density and orientation of its neuronal components, mainly in two directions, vertical and horizontal, respectively. The vertical arrangement has gained considerable attention, since so-called functional "columns" were described (8,21) and since the mode of cell migration into the cortical plate was suggested to produce the columnar arrangement of neurons (25,30).

On the other hand, there is little information about the development of the horizontally oriented laminae. The laminar structure develops gradually over a long period of time. It begins with the appearance of the marginal zone during early stages of the cortical development and is said to end with a late, postnatal differentiation of neurons in lamina II (see ref. 23). Consequently, the laminar differentiation could be induced and influenced by many of the processes participating in the development of the cortex, such as proliferative activity of the underlying ventricular zone, migration of neurons to their final position within the cortical plate, sprouting, growth, and arborization of dendrites and axons, as well as the formation of synapses by axons of intra- or extracortical origin.

In Reeler mice, it has been shown that the date of birth of cortical neurons corresponds to that of normal animals, although no orderly lamination is formed (7). Also, the presence of a lateromedial and a caudorostral time gradient of cell origin (23) and a scatter of the inside-out layering (5) suggest that the date of birth and probably also the time of migration of neurons do not have a crucial influence on the development of laminae. On the other hand, Lund and co-workers (18) have pointed out that the specific afferent fibers reach the visual cortex only after the neurons of lamina IV have been formed and do not enter the cortex before the middle layers have started differentiation. Finally, although afferent axons are destroyed, in explants of newborn cerebral cortex a lamination is formed *in vitro,* which resembles that of intact neocortex (27).

Thus, there is little evidence in favour of a hypothesis that axons of subcortical origin cause directly the formation of the neocortical lamination.

Only axons originating within the cortex might be involved in the development of four layers corresponding to laminae I, II–III, IV–V, and VI (27). The time and site of origin of such axons have yet to be detected. It is also unknown whether the development of cortical laminae corresponds to initial variations of synaptogenesis, and if so, which postsynaptic sites are responsible for such variations.

This chapter will concentrate on:

1. A special group of horizontal neurons, which according to the time of appearance, to their shape, orientation, and laminar position seem to be intimately linked to the beginning of the laminar development.

2. The structure and distribution of synapses forming in the occipital cortex of the rat.

3. Some angioarchitectonic characteristics of the neocortex, which suggest that the initial development of the cortical laminae seems to be accompanied by a horizontal metabolic compartimentation.

MATERIAL

The brains of albino rats (age: between 11 days postconception, "p.c.," and 30 days after birth, "p.n.," as well as adults) were either prepared according to chloralhydrate-Golgi-impregnation methods (70-μm-thick sections) or fixed by a mixture of aldehydes, osmicated and embedded in Epon (thin sections for electron microscopy, semithin sections in coronal and tangential series for light microscopy). In a postnatal series of anesthesized animals the vascular system was infused with an ink-gelatine mixture (see refs. 4,35). Our observations on the synaptogenesis were confined to the visual cortex and to its presumptive precursor field in the embryonic brain, while angioarchitecture and Golgi preparations were evaluated in larger parts of the occipital cortex. The date of birth of neurons was determined in a series of autoradiograms, which were prepared from adults after ^{3}H-thymidine injections 11 to 21 days p.c.

The quantitative analysis of the synaptogenesis included 3 (six hemispheres) to 15 animals per stage, from which 15 to 30 tissue blocks containing prospective or identified visual cortex were selected. In each block, three to six electron micrographs were taken randomly within each of 10 equidistant bands which added up to the total cortex. Synapses were counted on pictures (final magnification: 24,500:1), which represented an area of 177 μm^2.

EARLY DIFFERENTIATING HORIZONTAL NEURONS

In the neocortex, the so-called Cajal-Retzius cells in lamina I seem to be the first neurons to undergo their last mitosis and start differentiation (23,24). Our autoradiographic studies confirm that the first neurons of the rat's occipital cortex can be labeled by ^{3}H-thymidine during day 13 p.c. They migrate to the marginal surface and only 1 day later one to several processes can be impregnated, which are mainly orientated in parallel to the marginal surface. For simplicity, this orientation is called "horizontal." Already on day 16 p.c., processes of Cajal-Retzius cells may reach a length of about 100 μm. In coronal sections most of the horizontal neurons appear bipolar. However, from tangential sections one observes these cells sending dendrites in various directions within the horizontal plane, suggesting that many are multipolar neurons.

On day 15 p.c., the first neurons form a row below the marginal zone, i.e., the cortical plate begins to develop. Below these plate neurons dispersed cells are present with nuclei that resemble those of Cajal-Retzius cells. They have a more differentiated appearance than the plate neurons and the longer axis of their nuclei is oriented horizontally. Such horizontal cells could be impregnated at the lower border of the cortical plate and even within the intermediate zone, from day 16 p.c. onward. These horizontal neurons closely resemble the horizontal cells in the intermediate zone of the scheme drawn by Rakic (36).

On day 17 p.c. another set of horizontal neurons appears somewhat within the cortical plate. These are situated at the lower margin or within the middle zone of the prospective lamina VI, i.e., at the lower border of the bipolar part of the cortical plate (Fig. 1A). In the multipolar part of the cortical plate, horizontal neurons show one to five processes, most of them being much longer than the primitive precursors of the basal dendrites of neighbouring pyramidal neurons. These processes emerge primarily from two poles of the perikaryon, the result being essentially a bipolar cell.

Between days 18 and 20 p.c., horizontal neurons occur in several cortical levels corresponding to lamina I, lamina II-III (near the upper surface of and within the bipolar cortical plate, Fig. 1B and C), lamina IV-V (near the lower surface of the bipolar cortical plate), and at least at two different levels in lamina VI (Fig. 1D).

After day 20 p.c., no further levels are created by horizontal neurons. Postnatally, a proliferation of new dendrites and dendritic branches transforms many of the horizontal into stellate neurons (Fig. 2). This transformation coincides with the thickening of the respective laminae. Other cells retain their fusiform shape in regions where the tangential growth exceeds that of the depth, e.g., lamina VI. Postnatally, the tangential growth of the cortex increasing the surface area by an approximate factor of four results in a strong dilution of prenatally formed horizontal neurons. We therefore have to expect that many nonpyramidal neurons, but in particular the small stellate cells, must begin their differentiation postnatally.

It is widely accepted that in most areas of the brain the principal neurons which project from that area develop earlier than the local circuit neurons, "which are usually the last neurons to appear and differentiate" (see Jacob-

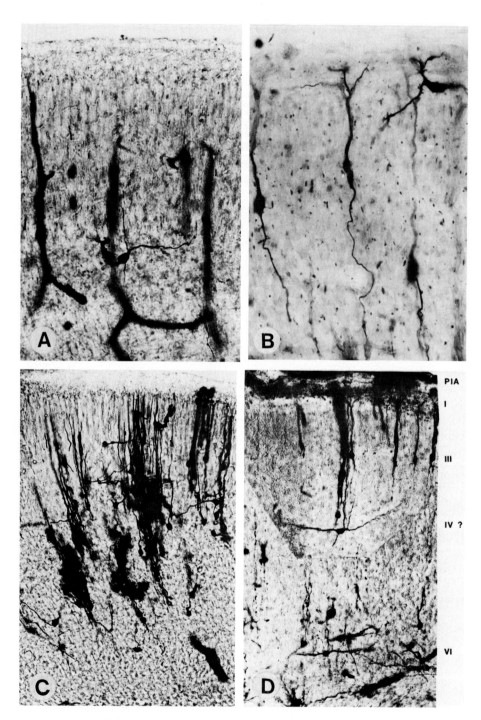

FIG. 1. Neurons with more or less horizontally oriented dendrites occur in several levels of the cortical plate. **A:** Lamina VI, 17 days p.c., **B:** Lamina II, 20 days p.c., **C:** The uppermost neuron is situated in the bipolar part of the cortical plate, e.g., in the prospective lamina III. **D:** Twenty days p.c.

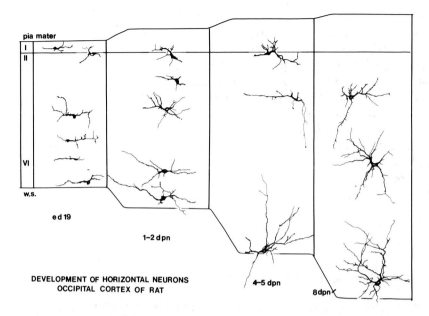

pia mater

I
II

VI

w.s.

ed 19

1–2 dpn

DEVELOPMENT OF HORIZONTAL NEURONS
OCCIPITAL CORTEX OF RAT

4–5 dpn

8dpn

FIG. 2. Summary of observations in Golgi impregnations. Prior to birth, horizontal neurons exist in at least six levels. Lamina II seems to be the last layer in which horizontal neurons arise. Postnatally, these cells seem to be transformed predominantly into stellate neurons, but also into fusiform neurons (not shown).

son in ref. 26). If this statement is valid with regard to the neocortex, then the described horizontal neurons can be assumed to be projection neurons. It is known, for instance, that Cajal-Retzius cells project very long axons to neighbouring cortical areas, even though these fibres remain in lamina I (6). Improperly oriented pyramidal neurons may show corticofugal axons (29). In addition, it has been shown that some nonpyramidal neurons can be labeled with horseradish peroxidase from subcortical regions and ipsi- or contralateral cortical areas (14,17,18). Further studies are necessary to determine whether labeled nonpyramidal projection neurons correspond to the old horizontal neurons, for if they do not, we may then presume an early differentiation of some local circuit neurons within the neocortex. More information about the final structure and fate of early differentiating horizontal neurons is needed, before they can be discussed in terms of cell types in adult cortex. However, from the present results it is clear that prenatally not all neurons possess vertical processes, as stated earlier (20,22).

A surprising observation was that horizontal neurons may develop their processes in the compact bipolar part of the cortical plate. Semithin sections (1 μm) through the bipolar plate reveal small lightly stained, loosely packed avascular zones. In horizontal sections, these zones appear as elongated channels free of vessels and cell nuclei, which may be interconnected to form two-dimensional networks. In more advanced parts of the cortex, these isolated horizontal channels fuse and form layers containing large amounts of neuropil. Thus, the dendrites of horizontal neurons seem to represent a very early differentiation product, which precedes the differentiation of the cortical plate and the separation of laminae.

Throughout all developmental stages the dendrites of horizontal neurons were longer and more elaborated than corresponding basal dendrites of pyramidal cells. If the development of horizontal dendrites is accompanied by the formation of postsynaptic sites, then the dendrites of horizontal cells might be superior competitors for synapses with ingrowing axons throughout their respective levels of the cortical plate. On the other hand, in the intervening layers that lack horizontal neurons, the probability to form synapses would be smaller. This would lead to a hypothesis that synaptogenesis in the cerebral cortex does not follow a continuous gradient from deeper and superficial layers, but shows periodical variations.

EARLY STAGES OF SYNAPTOGENESIS

To test this hypothesis, we investigated the *distribution* of synapses during pre- and postnatal synaptogenesis in coronal and tangential sections of the visual cortex by electron microscopy. The first isolated synapses have been observed on day 16 p.c. in the marginal zone and near the border zone between cortical plate and intermediate zone (see also ref. 15). The early synapses are connected to relatively large and horizontally oriented dendrites. On days 17 to 20 p.c. the density of synapses increases slowly above and below the bipolar cortical plate, i.e., in laminae I and VI. Their intralaminar distribution is characterized by clusters of several synapses separated by regions containing no or very few isolated synapses. Toward the end of the gestation period, single synapses can also be found on horizontal and vertical dendrites within the bipolar part of the cortical plate.

On day 2 p.n., the number of synapses has increased significantly enough to allow for a quantitative evaluation in a topographical manner. In lamina I most of the synapses now are restricted to the superficial half of the layer. They are situated not only on large horizontal, but also on smaller obliquely ascending dendrites. The latter probably represent peripheral branches of apical dendrites of pyramids, which develop axoshaft synapses before spines are formed during the following days (1). In coronal sections of the multipolar plate, synapses appear concentrated in small clusters, in larger zones of irregular shape, and in horizontal and vertically oriented bands, while in the surrounding regions only occasional synapses can be found (Fig. 3). Somata and vertical (apical?) and horizontal dendrites serve equally as postsynaptic sites.

The packing density of synapses has been determined in random samples, which were collected from horizontal bands each representing one-tenth of

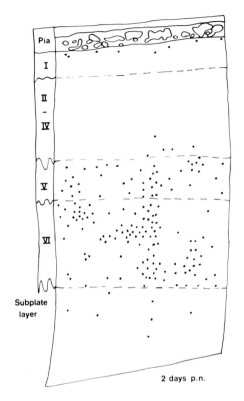

FIG. 3. Dots mark the position of synapses in a coronal section of the occipital cortex of rat. Note the varying density in deeper layers of the cortical plate in contrast to the rather uniform distribution in the superficial level of lamina I, and a few synapses in subcortical levels.

the cortical thickness. A separate analysis of these sets of samples revealed that the average density of synapses is not equal in all levels of the multipolar cortical plate. There is a larger number of synapses in 5/10 and around 8/10 than in the neighbouring levels (Fig. 4). At this time, the multipolar part of the cortical plate corresponds mainly to lamina VI, only the most superficial zone seems to develop into lamina V. Synapses, therefore, seem to accumulate in the middle of laminae VI and V, while their density decreases toward the intermediate zone, between laminae VI and V and in the bipolar part of the cortical plate. On day 8 p.n., a fourth maximum arises in the deep part of lamina I and in lamina II, which is again separated from the neighbouring maximum by a zone of lower density (Fig. 4).

On day 14 p.n., further synaptogenesis has compensated most of the laminar differences except for a gradient rising toward the cortical surface. The most rapid formation of synapses takes place in 1/10, i.e., the upper half of lamina I. It starts during the second postnatal week, continues at least for the third week and produces an overshoot of the density of synapses at about 1 month after birth (Fig. 4, top; ref. 2). It is notable that this overshoot is confined to the first tenth and does not include the rest of lamina I, which in later developmental stages and in adults includes a major part of the

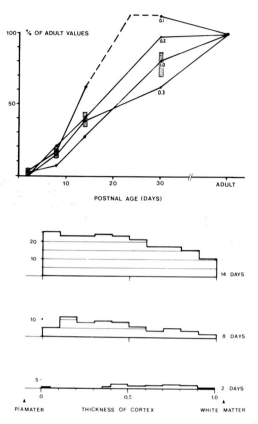

FIG. 4. The relative number of synapses has been determined in horizontal bands (= one-tenth of the total cortical thickness). **Top:** The vertical bars include the values of 0.4 to 0.9. Note the laminar heterochronicity of postnatal synaptogenesis. **Bottom:** The periodical variations of the number of synapses per 177 μm² (abscissa) vanish after 8 days p.n.

second tenth. Thus, not only various laminae show a different time course of synaptogenesis, but also different levels of the same lamina (sublaminae) may show a heterochroneous development (Fig. 4; refs. 3, 32, 34).

Two structurally different types of synapses (symmetrical and asymmetrical) can be recognized from almost the onset of synaptogenesis. Therefore, the *morphogenesis* of synapses has been studied with special attention to possible laminar differences. As early as day 17 p.c., in the shaft of some dendrites dense zones have been observed along the plasma membrane, although no axon or presynaptic element was attached to this site. More often intermediate stages between free postsynaptic elements and complete attachment were found. In these type-I synapses (10), presynaptic dense projections and vesicle aggregates become visible only after the attachment between the pre- and postsynaptic element is completed. Hence, the formation of asymmetric or type-I synapses can start with a free postsynaptic element, which is in agreement with the findings of several authors for various parts of the CNS (see ref. 12). Their relatively small number within the visual cortex of rats suggests that free postsynaptic elements may either become attached to presynaptic elements soon after formation or degraded. After birth, free postsynaptic elements are very seldom seen. In other synapses, presynaptic vesicles are aggregated along ill defined postsynaptic densities. This type of symmetrical synapses probably represents immature type-I synapses (11,12). It is seldom found during the prenatal period, but becomes rather numerous during the first and second postnatal weeks. Prenatally, Gray's type-II synapses (10) can be followed back to symmetrical densities without any vesicles being attached to either side. It seems, therefore, that structures comparable to free postsynaptic elements do not exist or cannot be detected during the formation of type-II synapses.

Finally, we studied *the distribution of the two types of synapses* during cortical development. The first synapses appearing on day 16 p.c. in the marginal zone and near the lower border between the cortical plate show the characteristic postsynaptic density of asymmetrical or type-I synapses of Gray, but contain a relatively small number of dispersed and aggregated presynaptic vesicles and ill-defined presynaptic dense projections. Such immature synapses have been found in all stages of development and in all layers. According to their relative frequency, it seems, however, that in later stages maturation proceeds more rapidly, particularly after the first postnatal week.

As early as day 17 p.c., some symmetrical synapses appear in lamina I. In lamina VI they appear 1 or 2 days later. Two days after birth, 23% of the synapses in lamina I and 20% in lamina VI are symmetrical synapses. Toward the upper part of the multipolar plate, which probably develops into lamina V, the fraction of symmetrical synapses amounts to less than 10%, but increases during the following days. About 4 days p.n., symmetrical synapses are present in all layers of the occipital cortex. Between birth and day 14 their percentage increases to values greater than in adults. This overshoot coincides exactly with the rapid multiplication of type-I synapses and is probably due to the temporary dominance of their immature precursors. In the adult cortex, there are only insignificant variations of the packing density of type-II synapses; however, their percentage increases gradually from 17% in lamina I to 28% in lamina VI.

The present observations on early stages of synaptogenesis in the visual cortex of rat may be *concluded* as follows:

(1) Synapses appear initially on dendrites, which probably belong to horizontal neurons. The first synapses of the various laminae arise in a similar temporospatial sequence as horizontal neurons: first in lamina I, immediately followed by lamina VI, then in lamina V, and progressively to lamina II. Synapses were observed 1 to 3 days after dendrites of horizontal neurons could be impregnated for the first time. In agreement with the dis-

tribution of horizontal neurons during early developmental stages, layers containing many synapses alternate with layers in which the synaptic activity is low. The intervals between the stages in which synapses were counted are too large to decide whether the maxima represent snapshots of a moving wave or mark levels of initially high synaptogenic activity. However, the coincidence between levels of high synaptic density and levels that contain horizontal neurons and the fact that the first synapses occur mainly on horizontal dendrites seem to support the latter possibility.

After the first postnatal week, the differences in synaptic density vanish due to the rapid formation of axospine synapses, most of which seem to be formed by axons of intracortical origin (9,28). Later stages of synaptogenesis do not show a laminar character, but are dominated by a high synaptogenic activity in the superficial half of the cortex, which results in a gradient of roughly decreasing synapse density from the cortical surface to deeper layers (32,34). Synaptogenesis proceeds heterochroneously not only in different laminae, but also in different levels of the same lamina.

(2) The first type-I synapses in the occipital cortex seem to develop from free postsynaptic densities on dendritic shafts of horizontal neurons. Type-II synapses appear very soon (several hours to 1 day) after type-I synapses on the same postsynaptic neurons. The spatial sequence is equal for both synaptic types: laminae I, VI, V to II. By 4 days p.n., significant numbers of type-II synapses are present in all layers of the cortex. When synaptogenesis is strongly accelerated during the early postnatal period, immature type-I synapses form a major fraction of the symmetrical synapses. However, prenatally symmetrical synapses mainly represent type-II synapses. No laminar differences have been found with respect to morphogenesis or quantitative relation of the two types of synapses during development. Type-II synapses seem to appear much earlier during the laminar development than would be expected from the literature on the development of interneurons (13). If the structural discrimination of type-I and II synapses is equivalent to functional and biochemical differences of the corresponding axons, then we have to look not only for the origin of one type of axon, but of two, which are involved in the early events of laminar differentiation.

DEVELOPMENT OF CORTICAL ANGIOARCHITECTURE

Before the cortical plate is formed, vascular sprouts enter the pallium from the meningeal plexus between days 11 and 13 p.c. The cortical plate initially lacking capillaries, therefore, is penetrated by vertically oriented vascular trunks, which elongate as the cortical plate thickens. In the adult cortex these old vessels give rise to only a few, short branches on their way through all layers.

There is a general tendency of the neuroblasts of deeper layers to be formed earlier than those of superficial layers ("inside-out layering," ref. 5).

The differentiation of neuroblasts follows a similar, although not steady, gradient (19). Consequently, all vascular sprouts arising from meningeal vessels have to penetrate an undifferentiated part of the cortical plate, before they form terminal branches in deeper levels. The thickness of this undifferentiated stratum is gradually reduced as development proceeds.

Tangential growth causes additional vascular sprouts to enter the newly formed cortical surface. Dependent on the time of formation, these sprouts terminate in different levels of the cortex (old = deep; young = superficial). At the same time, the terminal branches of older vessels multiply and expand their terminal territory in all deeper levels. This dual effect of tangential growth has the result that, in the adult cortex, the earliest vessels not only possess longer trunks, but also a wider terminal territory than lately formed vessels (Fig. 5).

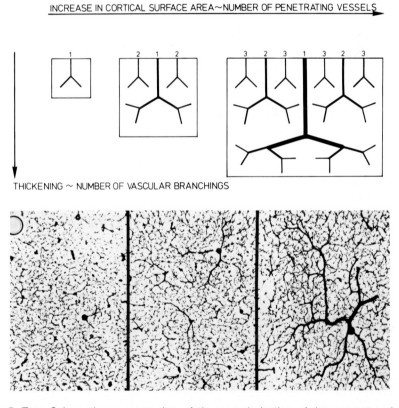

FIG. 5. Top: Schematic representation of the vascularization of the neocortex. **1:** the oldest preterminal vessels supply deep layers and extensive territories, while the youngest vessels **(3)** branch in the most superficial level and form only small terminal territories. **Bottom:** Tangential sections through superficial **(left)**, middle, and deep **(right)** layers of the adult occipital cortex of a rat after ink-gelatin injection. Note the increasing diameter of preterminal branchings.

Thickening of the cortex also has a differential effect on the arrangement of intracortical microvessels according to the type of growth. If new layers are added, the trunks of preexisting vessels are elongated. If, however, existing layers merely increase their thickness, then the vertical extension of the terminal branching territory of the corresponding vessels increases also. These different effects can be observed during early developmental stages, when the preterminal branches are formed. Subsequent development of capillaries is governed by metabolic and spatial factors, but not by laminar boundaries (4,33,35).

The adult cortical angioarchitecture consists of (a) a continuous three-dimensional network of capillaries and (b) at least three sets of vascular modules feeding and draining the capillary system (see ref. 16). Being the largest, the oldest modules supply mainly to lamina VI and connect to the meningeal surface by long trunks. These are superimposed by concentrically arranged, smaller modules supplying the middle cortical layers. A third set of even smaller vessels is connected to the capillaries of laminae I to III (31). These sets of vascular modules can only remain separated, if there is some limiting mechanism preventing sprouting from deeper vessels into more superficial layers during early developmental stages. It is tempting to speculate that this phenomenon might be related to the existence of levels without horizontal neurons and with a low density of synapses during pre-natal and early postnatal periods. Similar laminar variations can be shown by histochemical techniques that demonstrate the enzymatic activity of the energy metabolism (see Chap. 12). Such speculation would be encouraged by the fact that the laminar differences of the synaptic density are compensated after the first postnatal week, i.e., before most intracortical capillaries develop (32).

SUMMARY

Golgi studies in the occipital cortex of rats have demonstrated that horizontal neurons are the first to form horizontal dendrites of considerable length. These neurons do not only occur in lamina I as so-called Cajal-Retzius cells, but appear sequentially in several other distinct levels between laminae VI and II before birth.

An electron microscopical analysis has revealed a similar temporospatial sequence for the development of synapses in the visual cortex. One to three days after following the first demonstration of horizontal dendrites the first synapses were seen. During early developmental stages, layers with high and low densities of synapses alternate within the cortex. These laminar differences vanish during the rapid development of axospine synapses. Type-I synapses may develop from preexisting free postsynaptic elements or via a "symmetrical" transitional stage. These two modes do not show laminar differences, but differ in frequency during pre- and postnatal periods.

Type-II synapses develop rather early and are present in all layers by day 4 p.n. Type-I and II synapses are differently distributed in the cortex.

Cortical pre- and postcapillary microvessels show a modular arrangement. Older vessels supply a deeper and more extensive territory than the younger vessels. Two other sets of vascular modules exist in the rat's cortex, one supplying the middle layers and another laminae I to III. Each set is separate, being interconnected only by capillaries.

It is concluded that the induction and development of neocortical laminae is not a uniform process. At least two phases can be distinguished. The first and earliest is the differentiation of horizontal neurons, dendrites, and synapses resulting in a preliminary laminar pattern. This "original" lamination is subsequently lost during a postnatal developmental stage, characterized by (a) further growth, which substantially reduces the packing density of early horizontal neurons, and (b) rapid synaptogenesis, which compared to prenatal stages changes its structural, spatial, and dynamic properties. This is the time when more and more cortical neurons differentiate and the characteristic cytoarchitectonic features of the adult cortex are produced. In contrast, the early transitory lamination does not show any lamina-typic differences, but seems to mark out the later position of laminae and a few sublaminae within the neocortex.

ACKNOWLEDGMENT

I should like to thank my co-workers for providing some of the material: B. Chronwall (neuronal differentiation), M. Rickmann (neurogenesis), Dr. Th. Bär (synaptogenesis and vascularization), and Dr. S. Eins (stereology). The skillful technical assistance of E. Nicksch and B. Brandt and the preparation of the manuscript by G. Kotte are gratefully acknowledged. Special thanks are devoted to my wife who conducted a large part of the quantitative evaluation concerned with the synaptogenesis. This study was supported by Deutsche Forschungsgemeinschaft, SFB 33, Proj. E 3.

REFERENCES

1. Adinolfi, A. M. (1971): The postnatal development of synaptic contacts in the cerebral cortex. In: *Brain Development and Behavior,* edited by M. B. Sterman, D. J. McGinty, and A. M. Adinolfi, pp. 71–88. Academic Press, New York.
2. Aghajanian, G. K., and Bloom, F. E. (1967): The formation of synaptic junctions in developing rat brain—a quantitative electron microscopic study. *Brain Res.,* 6:716–727.
3. Bär, T.: Wirkung chronischer Hypoxie auf die postnatale Synaptogenese im Occipitalcortex der Ratte. *Anat. Anz., (in press).*
4. Bär, T., and Wolff, J. R. (1973): Quantitative Beziehungen zwischen der Verzweigungsdichte von Kapillaren im Neocortex der Ratte während der postnatalen Entwicklung *Z. Anat. Entwicklungsgesch.,* 141:207–221.
5. Berry, M., and Rogers, A. W. (1965): The migration of neuroblasts in the developing cerebral cortex. *J. Anat.,* 99:691–709.
6. Cajal, Ramón y, S. (1891): Sur la structure de l'écorce cérébrale de quelques mammifères. *La Cellule,* 7:125–176.

7. Caviness, V. S., and Sidman, R. L. (1973): Time of origin of corresponding cell classes in the cerebral cortex of normal and Reeler mutant mice: An autoradiographic analysis. *J. Comp. Neurol.*, 148:141–151.

8. Chow, K. L., and Leiman, A. L. (eds.) (1970): The structural and functional organization of the neocortex. *Neurosci. Res. Program Bull.*, 8:153–220.

9. Creutzfeldt, O. D., Garey, L. J., Kuroda, R., and Wolff, J. R. (1977): The distribution of degenerating axons after small lesions in the intact and isolated visual cortex of the cat. *Exp. Brain Res.*, 27:419–440.

10. Gray, E. G. (1959): Axo-somatic and axo-dendritic synapses of the cerebral cortex. An electron microscope study. *J. Anat.*, 93:420–433.

11. Hinds, J. W., and Hinds, P. L. (1976): Synapse formation in the mouse olfactory bulb. I. Quantitative studies. *J. Comp. Neurol.*, 169:15–40.

12. Hinds, J. W., and Hinds, P. L. (1976): Synapse formation in the mouse olfactory bulb. II. Morphogenesis. *J. Comp. Neurol.*, 169:41–62.

13. Jacobson, M. (1975): Development and evolution of type II neurons: Conjectures a century after Golgi. In: *Golgi Centennial Symposium: Perspectives in Neurobiology*, edited by M. Santini, pp. 147–151. Raven Press, New York.

14. Jacobson, S., and Trojanowski, J. (1974): The cells of origin of the corpus callosum in rat, cat and rhesus monkey. *Brain Res.*, 74:149–155.

15. Kostovic, I., and Molliver, M. E. (1974): A new interpretation of the laminar development of cerebral cortex: synaptogenesis in different layers of neopallium in the human fetus. *Anat. Rec.*, 178:395 (*abstract*).

16. Lazorthes, G., Espano, J., Lazorthes, Y., and Zadeh, J. O. (1968): The vascular architecture of the cortex and the cortical blood flow. *Prog. Brain Res.*, 30:27–32.

17. Lund, R. D.: The development of laminar connections in the mammalian visual cortex. *Exp. Brain Res.*, (*in press*).

18. Lund, J. S., Lund, R. D., Hendrickson, A. E., Blunt, A. H., and Fuchs, A. F. (1975): The origin of efferent pathways from the primary visual cortex, area 17, of the macaque monkey, as shown by retrograde transport of horseradish peroxidase. *J. Comp. Neurol.*, 164:287–304.

19. Marin-Padilla, M. (1970): Prenatal and early postnatal ontogenesis of the human motor cortex: A Golgi Study. I. The sequential development of the cortical layers. *Brain Res.*, 23:167–183.

20. Marin-Padilla, M. (1971): Early prenatal ontogenesis of the cerebral cortex (neocortex) of the cat (Felis domestica): A Golgi Study. *Z. Anat. Entwicklungsgesch.*, 134:117–145.

21. Mountcastle, V. B. (1957): Modality and topographic properties of single neurons of cat's somatic sensory cortex. *J. Neurophysiol.*, 20:408–434.

22. Peters, A., and Feldman, M. (1973): The cortical plate and molecular layer of the late rat fetus. *Z. Anat. Entwicklungsgesch.*, 141:3–37.

23. Raedler, A., and Sievers, J. (1975): The development of the visual system of the albino rat. *Adv. Anat. Embryol. Cell Biol.*, 50:3–88.

24. Raedler, A., and Sievers, J. (1976): Light and electron microscopical studies on specific cells of the marginal zone in the developing rat cerebral cortex. *Anat. Embryol.*, 149:173–181.

25. Rakic, P. (1974): Mode of cell migration to the superficial layers of fetal monkey neocortex. *J. Comp. Neurol.*, 145:61–84.

26. Rakic, P. (ed.) (1975): Local circuit neurons. *Neurosci. Res. Program Bull.*, 13:393–415.

27. Seil, F. J., Kelly, J. M., and Leiman, A. L. (1974): Anatomical organization of cerebral neocortex in tissue culture. *Exp. Neurol.*, 45:435–450.

28. Szentágothai, J. (1973): Synaptology of the visual cortex. In: *Handbook of Sensory Physiology, Vol. III/3B*, edited by R. Jung, pp. 267–324. Springer, Berlin.

29. van der Loos, H. (1965): The "improperly" oriented pyramidal cell in the cerebral cortex and its possible bearing on problems of neuronal growth and cell orientation. *Bull. Johns Hopkins Hosp.*, 117:228–250.

30. von Bonin, G., and Mehler, W. R. (1971): On columnar arrangement of nerve cells in cerebral cortex. *Brain Res.*, 27:1–10.

31. Wolff, J. R. (1976): An ontogenetically defined angio-architecture of the neocortex. *Drug Res.*, 26:1246 (*abstract*).

32. Wolff, J. R. (1976): Quantitative analysis of topography and development of synapses in the visual cortex. *Exp. Brain Res., Suppl.* 1:259–263.
33. Wolff, J. R., and Bär, T. (1974): Ontogenesis of the terminal vascular bed in CNS. In: *Pathology of Cerebral Microcirculation,* edited by J. Cervós-Navarro, pp. 15–19. De Gruyter, Berlin-New York.
34. Wolff, J. R., and Bär, T.: Die Morphometrie der postnatalen Synaptogenese im Occipital-cortex der Ratte. *Anat. Anz., (in press).*
35. Wolff, J. R., Goerz, C., Bär, T., and Güldner, F. H. (1975): Common morphogenetic aspects of various organotypic microvascular patterns. *Microvasc. Res.,* 10:373–395.
36. The Boulder Committee (1970): Embryonic vertebrate central nervous system: Revised terminology. *Anat. Rec.,* 166:257–261.

Architectonics of the Cerebral Cortex,
edited by M. A. B. Brazier and H. Petsche.
Raven Press, New York © 1978.

A Topographical Study of Enzyme Maturation in Human Cerebral Neocortex: A Histochemical and Biochemical Study

* E. Farkas-Bargeton and ** M. F. Diebler

*Laboratoire de Neuropathologie, Hôpital St. Vincent de Paul,
75674 Paris Cedex 14, France*

Until the present time, only conventional histological methodology has been utilized for the study of the morphological maturation of the neocortex of the child. The data obtained indicate that the migration of the majority of neurons toward the cortical plate is almost terminated by the fifth foetal month (37) and from this age onward the cortex, in terms of actual formation, is unchanged.

Studies of later periods have been concerned essentially with the growth in size of neurons, the differentiation of their perikaryon, the growth of dendrites and of axons as well as the formation of dendritic spines. Neuropil development, the myelinization and growth of the overall thickness of the cortex as well as of its different layers have also been studied (9,22–25,31–34,50). The results obtained indicate that cortical maturation in the child, already largely initiated during the second half of foetal life, continues during several years following birth.

In spite of this considerable amount of morphological data which has been accumulated concerning the different stages of the maturation of the child's neocortex, it remains nevertheless difficult to specify the age at which a given cortical region or layer reaches maturity. The only valid criterion for the evaluation of this maturity would be the existence of mature-type synaptic junctions in a quantity and distribution comparable to the adult. This evaluation requires an ultrastructural investigation which is impossible with autopsy material because of swelling and rapid bursting of structures following death. It was thus performed only on young foetuses on whom removal of cortical samples could be done immediately following abortion (16,26).

Since the activities of certain enzymes remain stable for several hours following death, while intermediary metabolites in general are rapidly degraded, we thought that a histochemical study of regional enzymatic maturation of the child's cerebral cortex, complemented by quantitative biochemical

* *Directeur de Recherche à l'INSERM.*
** Attaché de Recherche à l'INSERM.

studies, would enable us to evaluate the activities of certain metabolic cycles at this level during development.

Adult-type functioning of the nervous system has high energy requirements. Since, in the normal adult this energy is provided exclusively by the utilization of glucose, especially by aerobic glycolysis, we undertook a study of the evolution of the activities of several enzymes (12,13) which intervene in energy metabolism. We hoped by this approach to determine with better precision the ages at which the different cortical regions and layers reach their maturity.

For enzymes having a purely mitochondrial localization and not diffusing into the incubation medium, the investigation was both histochemical and biochemical. For partially or completely soluble enzymes, only biochemical methodology was utilized.

The material employed in these studies came from abortions or from early autopsies (samples taken 5 to 6 hr after death) of children who died from nonneurological illnesses and who experienced neither severe anoxia nor ischemia. The cortical areas studied were chosen according to the neocortical regions defined by von Economo (11):

1. The motor cortex of gyrus centralis anterior – area FA – which is an agranular heterotypic isocortex, taken in the region of the hand.
2. The visual cortex – area OC – and the somatosensory cortex of gyrus centralis posterior in area PB, each of which is a granular heterotypic isocortex.
3. A purely associative region, the gyrus supramarginalis – area PF – which is a parietal homotypic isocortex in which the large neurons of the third layer are as large or larger than those in the fifth layer.

Five different enzymes were studied: two Kreb's cycle enzymes, succinate dehydrogenase (SDH) and malate dehydrogenase (MDH); two enzymes of anaerobic glycolysis, pyruvate kinase (PK) and lactate dehydrogenase (LDH); and one enzyme participating in the NAD/NADH cycle and in lipid metabolism, mitochondrial α glycerophosphate dehydrogenase (α-GPDH).

POSTMORTEM STABILITY OF THE ENZYMATIC ACTIVITIES STUDIED

Since our work mostly involved material sampled at early autopsies, and since only the relatively great stability of SDH has been reported in the literature (41), we undertook a systematic study of the postmortem stability of all the other enzymatic activities studied in the present work. The test system chosen was the rat brain. Animals were decapitated and assays were performed on each of the enzymes in the crude brain homogenate, either immediately after death or after having left the heads intact at ambient temperature for 3 hr, followed by an additional 3, 4, 5, and 13 hr at 4°C. This modality was chosen to mimic actual conditions, where cadavers are usually refrigerated only 2 to 3 hr after death and remain at 4°C until autopsy. No noticeable differences in activities were observed, even after 16 hr postmortem; the only exception was MDH activity, which decreased progressively and regularly, losing 10% of its activity after 6 hr and 25% of its activity after 16 hr following death.

HISTOCHEMICAL STUDIES OF REGIONAL ENZYMATIC MATURATION OF THE CEREBRAL NEOCORTEX

For the enzyme histochemical study the cortical areas chosen were quickly removed and frozen. Cryostat sections were then prepared at −10°. The activity of two bound mitochondrial enzymes, whose activities could be well localized, SDH and menadione-dependent α-GPDH (6) were demonstrated. The identification of cortical layers in histoenzymological preparations was done by staining serial sections with cresyl violet and then ascribing the respective depths of the layers in relation to the surface with an ocular micrometer.

Motor Cortex of Gyrus Centralis Anterior (Area FA)

In a 27-week-old fetus, there is only a very weak SDH activity in the perikarya of the immature cortical neurons, and some activity can be detected in the more mature neurons in the fifth layer (Fig. 1a).

In the premature baby of 36 to 38 weeks and the newborn, in whose cortex the subdivision into six layers is clearly recognizable (22), there is high SDH activity only in the neuronal bodies and the neuropil of the fifth layer, where the neurons are more advanced in their maturation (23,31,33), and a somewhat lower activity in the deeper portion of the third layer. There is practically no activity in the other layers.

Between 1.5 and 3 postnatal months, SDH activity becomes more marked in the third and fifth layers (Fig. 2b), especially in the perikarya, which become clearly distinct from the neuropil; the superficial and fourth layers still remain only slightly active. At about 4.5 months, detectable activity appears in the two superficial layers, with an intensity which decreases toward the surface and in the fourth and the sixth layers.

The SDH enzyme architectony is qualitatively the same at about 7 and 9 months as it is at 4.5 months but quantitatively more intense.

Between 1.5 and 2.5 years, SDH enzymoarchitectony is the same with a comparable activity in all the layers with the exception of a higher activity in the third layer (Fig. 1c). Adult-type enzymoarchitectony is not reached even at the age of 11 years; at this time, the most intense activity encompasses the superficial portion of the third and the second layers, whereas

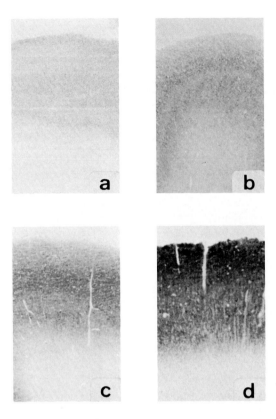

FIG. 1. Maturation of succinate dehydrogenase in the motor cortex of gyrus centralis anterior (Area FA). **a:** Twenty-seven-week-old foetus; very weak activity at the borderline between the molecular and the second layer where the immature neurons are densely packed and in the more mature neurons of the fifth layer. **b:** Two and a half-month-old baby; activity is prominent in the fifth and the third layers. **c:** One and a half-year-old child; activity is mostly the same in all the layers with the exception of the third layer where it is slightly more intense. **d:** Adult; very intense activity in the three superficial layers and in the large pyramidal cells of the fifth layer.

in the adult this very intense activity involves the three superficial layers (Fig. 1d). In the mature subjects, the activity in these layers is the same in the neuropil and in the neuronal perikarya. In the deeper layers most of the neurons have a higher activity than that of the neuropil and can thus be clearly distinguished. α-GPDH activity evolves quite differently from that of SDH. Fetal neuroblasts exhibit a highly intense activity and, at about term, activity is localized in the neuropil as well as in neuronal perikarya of all the layers. From 1 month onward the sixth layer becomes more active, while the activity in the other layers sharply decreases. In the grown child and in the adult, a notable activity in neuronal perikarya and the neuropil persists only at the level of the sixth layer, the neuronal perikarya at the other layers being completely devoid of activity.

Visual Cortex (Area Striata OC)[1]

SDH activity in a 27-week-old foetus is barely detectable at this level, as in area FA at the same age (Fig. 2a).

---

[1] Nomenclature for delimitation of layers is after Spatz et al. (39).

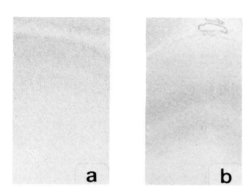
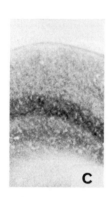
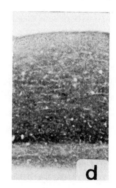
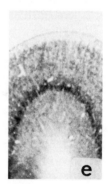

FIG. 2. Maturation of succinate dehydrogenase in the visual cortex (area striata OC). **a:** Twenty-two-week-old foetus; very weak activity in the borderline between the molecular and the second layer where the immature neurons are densely packed. **b:** Newborn; activity is prominent in the fourth and the sixth layers. **c:** One and a half-month-old baby; intense activity in the fourth layer and to a lesser degree in the sixth layer. Activity in the fifth layer is weaker than that of fourth and sixth layers. The molecular layer is almost inactive. **d:** Nine-month-old baby; enzyme architectony as previously but activity increased in all the layers. **e:** Adult; activity of the fifth layer is similar to that of the sixth layer. The molecular layer has the lowest activity.

Up to 36 weeks and in the newborn, the difference in relation to the FA becomes obvious, with activity appearing in the fourth layer and to a lesser degree in the sixth layer (Fig. 2b) and not in the fifth and third layers as in the motor cortex. The fourth layer will retain an activity greater than that of all the other layers during the whole duration of maturation and also in the adult. From 1.5 months onward, the activity progressively increases in the third, second, and first layers, reaching the pial surface at about 4.5 months, but the activity of the molecular layer will always remain less than in the underlying layers (Fig. 2c, d, and e). The fifth layer remains distinctly less active than the fourth and sixth layers (Fig. 2c and d) until the age of 3 years. Nevertheless, adult-type enzymoarchitectony is reached neither at this age nor at 5 years of age, since the SDH staining intensity of the two

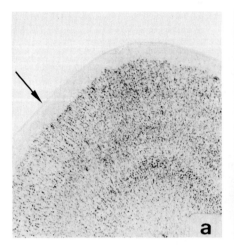 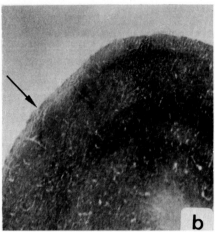

FIG. 3. Serial sections of the visual cortex areas OC and OB of a 9-month-old baby. **a:** Nissl staining. Cytoarchitectony changes abruptly between areas OC and OB (arrow). **b:** SDH activity. Enzyme architectony of area OC differs from that of area OB (arrow at the boundary zone between the two areas).

supragranular layers (third and second) is more intense than that of the two deep layers (fifth and sixth). On the contrary in an 11-year-old child and in the adult these latter layers have the same activity as the supragranular layers (Fig. 2e). It should be noted that the enzymoarchitectony, as the cytoarchitectony, of the visual cortex (area OC) becomes abruptly modified at the level of passage toward the area OB (Fig. 3).

The activity of α-GPDH evolves as at the FA level: contrary to that of SDH, it is very intense in the foetus and the newborn until the age of 1 month (Fig. 4a and b1); the activity subsequently decreases but remains higher in the two deep layers having weak SDH activity than in the superficial layers until the age of 5 years (Fig. 4a2 and d2). In the child of 11 years and in the adult, the activity of the deep layers is less than that observed in young children and almost equal to the activity of the superficial layers.

Gyrus Centralis Posterior (Area PB)

SDH maturation at this level begins as it does in the visual cortex in the fourth and, to a lesser extent, in the sixth layers, and then evolves in the same fashion. At 2.5 years of age, the third and second layers do not have activities equal to that of the fourth layer, as in the 11-year-old child and in the adult. In these latter, the band of high activity is not confined to the fourth layer, as in the visual cortex, but encompasses the third and second layers as well (Fig. 5a). Contrary to the visual cortex, the fifth layer remains slightly less active than the sixth in the mature subject.

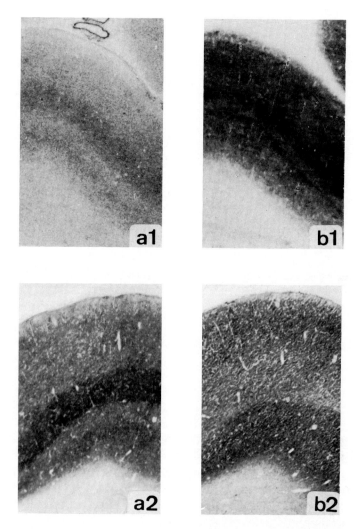

FIG. 4. Visual cortex area OC. **a:** Succinate dehydrogenase. **b:** Mitochondrial α-GPDH. **a1:** Thirty-six-week-old foetus. Very weak SDH activity except in layers IV and VI. **b1:** Thirty-six-week-old foetus. α-GPDH activity is more intense. Band of lower activity in the deep part of the fourth layer and the molecular layer. **a2:** Nine-month-old child. Band of high SDH activity in the fourth layer. The fifth layer is less active than the sixth layer. **b2:** Nine-month-old child. α-GPDH is less active in the fourth and the molecular layers and this activity is very high in the two deep layers.

The evolution of α-GPDH is comparable to that observed in the visual area, but the band of high activity is only localized in the sixth layer after the first year; prior to this time, it also encompassed the fifth layer, in which only rare active neuronal perikarya are noticed.

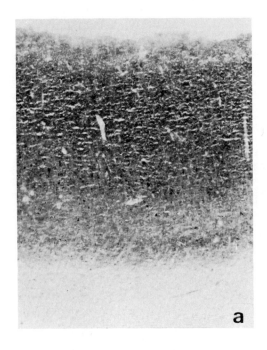

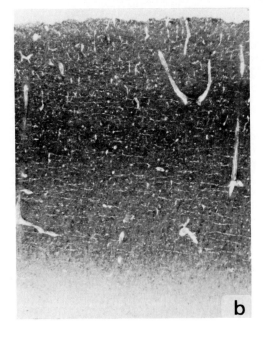

FIG. 5. Succinate dehydrogenase. **a:** Adult; somatosensory cortex. Gyrus centralis posterior area PB. Band of high activity in layers II, III, and IV. **b:** Adult gyrus supramarginalis area PF. The deep part of the third layer is more active than the other layers.

Gyrus Supramarginalis (Area PF)

During the precocious maturation of SDH in this cortical region, no layer is more active than another. Only at the age of 7 months can a slightly greater activity be detected in the deep part of the third layer in relation to the rest of the cortex. This enzymoarchitectony, although quantitatively increasing in all the layers, subsequently remains unchanged during maturation and can be found in the adult (Fig. 5b).

The intensity of α-GPDH activity will diminish during maturation, but later than in the other areas studied. Although the activity is identical in all the layers in the newborn, from 7 months onward, and at the adult stage activity is predominant at the level of the sixth layer as well as in the FA and PB fields.

BIOCHEMICAL STUDIES

Immediately after sampling of the cortical areas studied, the cortex was separated from white matter by dissection at 4°C and frozen in liquid nitrogen. Before enzyme assays were performed, the samples were weighed and homogenized in the cold at high speed in 0.25 M sucrose. SDH and mitochondrial α-GPDH were assayed as described by Arrigoni and Singer (4), PK was assayed by the technique of Beisenherz (7) as modified by Wiesmann et al. (46), LDH was assayed by the method of Wroblewski et al. (49), and mitochondrial MDH by the method of Thorne (43). The results obtained are expressed on wet weight and tissue DNA bases.

RESULTS

From foetal life (18 weeks) to the adult stage, SDH activity increases 12 to 25 times on a fresh weight basis, depending on the cortical area studied. Adult values seem to be reached at 11 years with the exception of the motor cortex (FA) and perhaps also the gyrus supramarginalis (PF) (Table 1). It should be noted that adult values are obtained in the visual cortex at the end of the first year, and that the activity at 11 years is greater than that of mature adults, which we studied (Table 1). The other Kreb's cycle enzyme examined, MDH, also undergoes an increase in activity during maturation, of the order of three to six times between birth and adult age. The results obtained are variable, however, and this can perhaps be explained by the lower stability of this enzyme after death.

The activity of PK increases five to sevenfold between the 18-week-old foetus and the 11-year-old or the adult (Table 2). LDH evolution is comparable to that of PK with nevertheless the particularity of being higher in the cortex of a foetus of 18 weeks than in one of 27 weeks (Table 2). The highest values of PK and LDH at 11 years are found in the two primary sensory receptive areas, the visual and somatosensory cortex.

TABLE 1. *Activity of succinate dehydrogenase in different areas of the neocortex in the child*

	FA	PA	GSM	OC
△OD/g wet weight/min				
Foetus 18 weeks	2.0	2.0	2.3	4.4
Foetus 27 weeks	4.1	3.7	3.4	3.9
Newborn 1	12.2	6.2	9.6	2.9
Newborn 2	10.8	11.5	5.7	6.7
10 days	9.1	15.0	5.7	3.7
1 month	15.1	12.2	7.6	8.6
7 months	22.8	19.9	15.4	30.0
9 months	23.6	19.6	16.7	36.0
11 years	36.0	37.4	28.6	55.7
Adult 1	53.0	44.2	30.7	34.6
Adult 2	44.5	31.6	65.2	36.4
△OD/mg DNA/min				
Foetus 18 weeks	1.55	1.55	1.83	3.50
Foetus 27 weeks	3.36	2.72	2.25	1.95
Newborn	19.8	19.9	9.8	9.8
10 days	16.8	38.4	13.2	8.5
1 month	41.6	23.1	25.2	24.0
7 months	51.3	95.7	73.8	51.0
9 months	60.7	54.4	64.7	100.0
Adult 1	104.7	116.2	58.5	60.1
Adult 2	91.0	71.8	183.1	87.7

Each value is the mean of three measures.
FA: Gyrus centralis anterior in the region of the hand.
PA: Gyrus centralis posterior in the region of the hand.
GSM: Gyrus supramarginalis of lobus parietalis.
OC: Area striata of lobus occipitalis.

The evolution of mitochondrial α-GPDH activity is different from the preceding. This activity is rather high in the foetus, increases until the age of 1 month and subsequently declines at the end of maturation to reach values close to those found in the 27-week-old foetus (Table 3). The evolution is different in the associative cortex, maximum values seeming to be reached only around 9 months, and probably even later, as indicated by our histochemical preparations.

When expressed on a DNA basis, our results show a much greater increase in enzymatic activities than when expressed on a wet-weight basis (Table 1).

DISCUSSION

Our regional histochemical study indicates that each of the cortical regions studied has an enzymoarchitectony particular to it. These enzymoarchitectonic regions correspond exactly to the cytoarchitectonic areas as they were described by Constantin von Economo (11).

TABLE 2. *Activity of lactic dehydrogenase and pyruvate-kinase in different areas of the neocortex in the child*

	FA	PA	GSM	OC
LDH				
$\triangle$OD/g wet weight/min				
Foetus 18 weeks	111.8	111.8	86.6	116.5
Foetus 27 weeks	60.5	37.2	57.3	60.5
Newborn	141.7	—	108.0	94.5
10 days	187.1	133.2	192.8	223.3
7 months	223.6	236.2	245.7	223.6
11 years	283.0	554.0	313.0	428.0
Adult	630.0	531.7	—	—
P.K.				
$\triangle$ OD/g wet weight/min				
Foetus 18 weeks	43.8	43.8	39.0	51.0
Foetus 27 weeks	61.1	50.0	49.1	63.4
Newborn	53.6	48.7	39.3	40.6
10 days	157.9	74.1	102.4	74.9
7 months	160.3	149.5	118.5	188.2
11 years	156.0	301.0	203.0	348.0
Adult	329.0	254.8	139.1	212.5

Each value is the mean of three measures.
FA: Gyrus centralis anterior in the region of the hand.
PA: Gyrus centralis posterior in the region of the hand.
GSM: Gyrus supramarginalis of lobus parietalis.
OC: Area striata of lobus occipitalis.

TABLE 3. *Activity of α-glycerophosphate dehydrogenase in different areas of the neocortex in the child ($\triangle$OD/g wet weight/min)*

	FA	PA	GSM	OC
Foetus 18 weeks	14.4	14.4	9.3	12.4
Foetus 27 weeks	19.2	17.4	15.6	15.3
Newborn 1	26.4	21.6	18	21.6
Newborn 2	28.0	32.4	24.5	26.0
10 days	28.5	28.1	27.0	32.2
1 month	56.0	34.5	31.8	37.8
7 months	31.8	21.8	32.1	24.6
9 months	32.2	29.2	44.7	32.2
11 years	21.6	21.8	19.0	30.1
Adult 1	24.9	24.9	42.0	16.2
Adult 2	21.6	20.1	41.6	22.3

Each value is the mean of three measures.
FA: Gyrus centralis anterior in the region of the hand.
PA: Gyrus centralis posterior in the region of the hand.
GSM: Gyrus supramarginalis of lobus parietalis.
OC: Area striata of lobus occipitalis.

Thus, SDH activity in the adult subject is the highest in the first three layers of the motor cortex, but is highest in the fourth layer of the visual cortex, is predominant at the level of the second, third, and fourth layers in the somatosensory cortex and is highest in the third layer in the associative cortex.

Considerable modifications occur during development in the relative intensities of the activities studied histochemically in the different cortical layers. Thus, SDH activity initially appears in the fifth and third layers in the motor cortex, whereas the maturation begins in the fourth and sixth layers in the two primary sensory receptive areas. Maturation begins in a diffuse fashion in the associative cortex studied, but there as everywhere else SDH activity develops later in the superficial layers (IIIb, IIIa, II, and I), progressing from deeper layers toward the surface. This retarded enzymatic maturation of the superficial layers depends upon the retarded cytological development of these layers (9,24,31), where neurons migrate later toward the cortical plate (3).[2]

Consistent with cytological data (9,24,25,31,33) the layers which mature first are those that receive specific sensory thalamocortical radiations such as the fourth layer of the visual cortex and of the somatosensory cortex, or those that emit projections for subcortical centers, as the fifth layer of FA. On the contrary, the layers which emit or receive corticocortical associative fibers, such as layers I, II, III, and V of the visual cortex (39) and layers I, II, and III of the frontal cortex (31,42) mature more belatedly.

The distribution and the evolution of α-GPDH activity in the different layers is often the opposite of that of SDH. This activity is localized equally well in the neuronal perikarya as in the neuropil in the foetus and the newborn. It disappears afterward progressively from the neuronal bodies during evolution except at the level of the sixth and, in some places, the fifth layer.

The overall increase of SDH activity, a marker of oxidative activity during development, which was observed in our histochemical preparations, was confirmed by biochemical assays. The increase in this activity, already considerable when expressed on a wet-weight basis (Table 1), is even more marked when expressed on a DNA basis (Table 1), due to the massive decrease in cellular density during maturation. However, if the values obtained do not show overlapping for the different age ranges during the first year of life, in the three subjects beyond this age important individual variations seem to occur. These data for the grown child and the adult are only preliminary and have to be confirmed by the study of many more cases.

Our results on the increase of SDH during maturation agree with the data obtained in various mammals (18,36) and also with the postnatal increase in oxygen consumption of the cortex in different species (8,44). Until the present time, the development of oxygen consumption in the infant has

---

[2] Bisconte, J. L. (1973): Histogenèse du Systeme Nerveux Central Chez le Rat. Thèsis, Paris.

only been studied in the fetus (17) and has already exhibited an increase before term.

The augmentation in MDH activity in the cortex of our subjects is less than that of SDH and on the order of that found in the rat (21).

The increase in activity of anaerobic glycolysis enzymes (PK and LDH) shown in the present work is comparable to results obtained in the rat (47) and is indicative of the postnatal evolution of the rate of glycolysis in the cortex. In spite of its growth in absolute value, its relative importance in energy production decreases during maturation (40). The high value of LDH activity found in the youngest foetus examined is similar to that found during the proliferation phase of neuroblasts in tissue cultures.[3]

The inverse evolution of α-GPDH activity in relation to the other enzymes studied in the present work shows that the immature cortex of the infant has a metabolic activity different from that of the adult: it has in fact already been demonstrated that the immature brain utilizes substrates other than glucose, acetoacetate, and 3-hydroxybutyrate (27,30). The inverse evolution of the two mitochondrial enzymes studied, SDH and α-GPDH, also suggests a mitochondrial heterogeneity, as indicated by the ultrastructural cytochemical studies of Kerpel-Fronius et. al. (19), or a modification of their enzymatic content during development.

Our histochemical and biochemical data show that the enzymatic maturation of the cortex of the child continues with certainty for quite a few years after birth: certain cortical areas, such as FA, seem not to have reached maturity, even at 11 years. Thus, certain regions seem to undergo maturation for a very long time (FA) and others, as the associative cortex (GSM), start developing later, as shown by the delay in SDH increase and the advanced age at which α-GPDH activity begins to decline in this area. This temporal disparity of the maturation of various cortical regions during the postnatal period is dependent on the disparity of their histological development (9,14,22,31,33,34,50).

The long-lasting enzymatic maturation of the neocortex of the child is consistent with the observations of Conel (9), who noticed morphological modifications of certain cortical regions, even after 6 years. Research on the increase in overall thickness of the cortex also indicates that this process continues beyond the 8th year in the motor cortex and in a prefrontal associative cortex (34), although this growth is arrested toward the end of the first year in the visual cortex (34). Other observations which showed that area 45, which is involved in the organization of speech, reached its maximum surface dimensions only toward the age of 12 years (20) are in good agreement with our data.

The completion of maturation in a given cortical layer is characterized essentially by an increase in SDH activity in the neuropil, as indicated by

[3] Ciesielsky-Treska, J. (1976): Recherches sur la Régulation de la Différenciation des Cellules du Neuroblastome en Culture. Thèsis, Strasbourg.

our histochemical preparations. This increase, which is in relation to either a larger number of mitochondria or their higher enzyme titer, indicates a high functional level of the energy-yielding Kreb's cycle. Some arguments permit the belief that this modification is essentially associated with the existence of a large number of functional synapses. Thus, the zones which are rich in synaptic junctions, such as the glomerules of the internal granular layer of the cerebellum (29) or the barrels of the sensorimotor cortex of the mouse (45,48), have elevated SDH activity (2,15).[4] In addition, adult-type synapses are particularly rich in mitochondria (28), and it is mitochondria isolated from the synaptosomal fraction that have the highest SDH activity (5,35). It has also been shown that nerve terminals have a higher-affinity glucose transport system than brain slices, to support a higher rate of energy production (10).

Altman (1) demonstrated that synaptogenesis in the molecular layer of the cerebellar cortex develops from deeper portions toward the surface in parallel to the development of SDH activity at this level. A comparison done in our laboratory, between the development of dendritic branching of Purkinje cells and their spines and the development of SDH in the molecular layer of the cerebellum in the child and in the rat, indicates that the formation of dendrites and their spines distinctly precedes the appearance of SDH activity in the neuropil. Thus, the formation of dendritic spines cannot, in fact, be considered as the terminal step in maturation, since spines can appear in a given zone before or without the formation of synaptic junctions (1,38), and especially before the development of oxidative metabolism necessary for adult-type functioning.

The long postnatal cortical maturation in the child permits one to believe that there is a long period of plasticity during which environmental stimuli could be especially important for the child's development.

ACKNOWLEDGMENT

This work was supported by the National Institute for Health and Medical Research (INSERM) and DGRST Paris, France.

REFERENCES

1. Altman, J. (1972): Postnatal development of the cerebellar cortex in the rat. II. Phases in the maturation of Purkinje cells and of the molecular layer. *J. Comp. Neurol.*, 145:399–464.
2. Altman, J. (1972): Postnatal development of the cerebellar cortex in the rat. III. Maturation of the components of the granular layer. *J. Comp. Neurol.*, 145:465–514.
3. Angevine, J. B., and Sidman, R. L. (1961): Autoradiographic study of cell migration during histogenesis of cerebral cortex in the mouse. *Nature,* 192:766–768.
4. Arrigoni, O., and Singer, T. P. (1962): Limitations of the phenazine methosulfate assay for succinic and related dehydrogenases. *Nature,* 193:1256–1258.

[4] Farkas-Bargeton, E.: *Unpublished data.*

5. Balazs, R., Dahl, D., and Harwood, J. R. (1966): Subcellular distribution of enzymes of glutamate metabolism in rat brain. *J. Neurochem.*, 13:897–907.
6. Barka, T., and Anderson, P. J. (1963): Histochemistry. Oxidative enzymes. Harper & Row, New York.
7. Beisenherz, G., Boltze, H. J., Bucher, T., Czok, R., and Garbade, K. H. (1953): Diphosphofructose-Aldolase, Phosphoglyceraldehyd-dehydrogenase, Milchsäure-dehydrogenase, Glycerophosphat dehydrogenase und Pyruvat-Kinase aus Kaninchenmuskulatur in einem Arbeitsgang. *Z. Naturforschg.*, 8:555–577.
8. Chesler, A., and Himwich, H. E. (1944): Comparative studies of the rates of oxidation and glycolysis in the cerebral cortex and brain stem of the rat. *Am. J. Physiol.*, 141:513–517.
9. Conel, J. (ed.) (1939–1967): The Postnatal Development of the Human Cerebral Cortex. Harvard University Press, Cambridge, Mass.
10. Diamond, I., and Fishman, R. A. (1973): High affinity transport of 2-deoxyglucose in isolated synaptic nerve endings. *Nature*, 242:122–123.
11. Economo, C. von, and Koskinas, G. N. (eds.) (1925): *Die Cytoarchitektonik der Hirnrinde des erwachsenen Menschen.* Springer, Wien.
12. Farkas-Bargeton, E. (1974): Histochemical study of the developing neo-cortex in children. In: *Ontogenesis of the Brain, Vol. 2,* edited by L. Jilek and S. Trojan, pp. 423–429. Universitas Carolina, Prague.
13. Farkas-Bargeton, E. (1974): Etude histo-enzymologique de la maturation du métabolisme énergétique dans le néo-cortex de l'enfant. In: *Pre- and Postnatal Development of the Human Brain, Vol. 13,* edited by S. R. Berenberg, M. Caniaris, and N. P. Masse, pp. 91–103. Karger, Basel.
14. Flechsig, P. (1920): Anatomie des menschlichen Gehirns und Rückenmarks auf myelogenetischer Grundlage. G. Thieme, Leipzig.
15. Friede, R. L. (ed) (1966): *Topographic Brain Chemistry.* Academic Press, New York.
16. Gruner, J. E. (1974): Sur la synaptogenèse vue en microscopie électronique. In: *Pre- and Postnatal Development of the Human Brain, Vol. 13,* edited by S. R. Berenberg, M. Caniaris, and N. P. Masse, pp. 57–67. Karger, Basel.
17. Himwich, W. A., Benaron, H. B. W., Tucker, B. E., Babuna, C., and Stripe, M. (1959): Metabolic studies on perinatal human brain. *J. Appl. Physiol.*, 14:873–877.
18. Himwich, W. A., Pennelle, D. K., and Tucker, B. E. (1963): Comparative biochemical development of fetal human, dog, and rabbit brain. In: *Recent Advances in Biological Psychiatry, Vol. 5,* edited by J. Wortis, pp. 263–278. Plenum Press, New York.
19. Kerpel-Fronius, S., and Hajos, F. (1971): Attempt at structural identification of metabolic compartmentation of neural tissue based on electron histochemically demonstrable differences of mitochondria. *Neurobiology*, 1:17–26.
20. Kononova, E. P., cited by S. Sarkisov (1964): The evolutionary aspect of the integrative function of the cortex and subcortex of the brain. In: *Growth and Maturation of the Brain, Vol. 4,* edited by D. P. Purpura and J. P. Schadé. pp. 30–38. *Progress in Brain Research,* Elsevier, Amsterdam.
21. Kuhlmann, R. E., and Lowry, O. H. (1956): Quantitative histochemical changes during the development of the rat cerebral cortex. *J. Neurochem.*, 1:173–180.
22. Larroche, J.-C. (1966): The development of the central nervous system during intrauterine life. In: *Human Development,* edited by F. Falkner, pp. 251–276. Saunders, Philadelphia.
23. Marin-Padilla, M. (1970): Prenatal and early postnatal ontogenesis of the human motor cortex: A Golgi study. I. The sequential development of the cortical layers. *Brain Res.*, 23:167–183.
24. Marin-Padilla, M. (1970): Prenatal and early postnatal ontogenesis of the human motor cortex: A Golgi study. II. The basket pyramidal system. *Brain Res.,* 23:185–191.
25. Marin-Padilla, M. (1974): Three dimensional reconstruction of the pericellular nests (baskets) of the motor (area 4) and visual (area 17) areas of the human cerebral cortex. A Golgi study. *Z. Anat. Entwicklungsgesch.*, 144:123–135.
26. Molliver, M. E., Kostovic, I., and van der Loos, H. (1973): The development of synapses in cerebral cortex of the human fetus. *Brain Res.*, 50:403–407.
27. Mourek, J. (1970): Oxidative metabolism of nervous tissue during ontogeny in rat. In: *Developmental Neurobiology,* edited by W. A. Himwich, pp. 370–390. Thomas, Springfield, Ill.

28. Palay, S. L. (1958): The morphology of synapses in the central nervous system. *Exp. Cell. Res.*, 5:275–293 (suppl.).
29. Palay, S. L., and Chan-Palay, V. (1974): *Cerebellar Cortex.* Springer, New York.
30. Patel, M. S., Johnson, C. A., Rajan, R., and Owen, O. E. (1975): The metabolism of ketone bodies in developing human brain. *J. Neurochem.*, 25:905–908.
31. Poliakov, G. I. (1961): Some results of research into the development of the neuronal structure of the cortical ends of the analysers in man. *J. Comp. Neurol.*, 117:197–212.
32. Purpura, D. P. (1975): Morphogenesis of visual cortex in the preterm infant. In: *Growth and Development of the Brain: Nutritional, Genetic, and Environmental Factors,* edited by M. A. B. Brazier, pp. 33–49. Raven Press, New York.
33. Rabinowicz, T. (1964): The cerebral cortex of the premature infant of the 8th month. *Prog. Brain Res.*, 4:39–92.
34. Rabinowicz, T. (1974): Some aspects of the maturation of the human cerebral cortex. In: *Pre- and Postnatal Development of the Human Brain,Vol. 13,* edited by S. R. Berenberg, M. Caniaris, and N. P. Masse, pp. 44–56. Karger, Basel.
35. Salganicoff, L., and de Robertis, E. (1965): Subcellular distribution of the enzymes of the glutamic acid, glutamine and y-aminobutyric acid cycles in rat brain. *J. Neurochem.*, 12:287–311.
36. Seiler, N. (1969): Enzymes. In: *Handbook of Neurochemistry, Vol 1,* edited by A. Lajtha, pp. 325–468. Plenum Press, New York.
37. Sidman, R. L., and Rakic, P. (1973): Neuronal migration with special reference to developing human brain: A review. *Brain Res.*, 62:1–35.
38. Sotelo, C. (1973): Permanence and fate of paramembranous synaptic specialisations in mutants and experimental animals. *Brain Res.*, 62:345–351.
39. Spatz, W. B., Tigges, J., and Tigges, M. (1972): Subcortical projections, cortical associations and some intrinsic interlaminar connections of the striate cortex in the squirrel monkey. *J. Comp. Neurol.*, 140:155–173.
40. Swaiman, K. F. (1970): Energy and electrolyte changes during maturation. In: *Developmental Neurobiology,* edited by W. A. Himwich, pp. 311–330. Thomas, Springfield, Ill.
41. Swanson, P. D., Harvey, F. H., and Stahl, W. L. (1973): Subcellular fractionation of post mortem brain. *J. Neurochem.*, 20:465–476.
42. Szentagothai, J. (1969): Architecture of the cerebral cortex. In: *Basic Mechanisms of the Epilepsies,* edited by H. H. Jasper, A. A. Ward, and A. Pope, pp. 13–28. Little, Brown, Boston.
43. Thorne, C. J. R. (1961): Properties of mitochondrial malate dehydrogenases. *Biochim. Biophys. Acta.*, 59:624–633.
44. Tyler, D. B., and Harreveld, A. van (1942): The respiration of the developing brain. *Am. J. Physiol.*, 136:600–603.
45. White, E. L. (1976): Ultrastructures and synaptic contacts in barrels of mouse SI cortex. *Brain Res.,* 105:229–251.
46. Wiesmann, U., Tonz, O., Richterich, R., and Verger, P. (1965): Die erythrocyten Pyruvat-Kinase bei gesunden und bei nichtsphärocytärer, hämolytischer Pyruvat-Kinase-Mangel-Anämie. *Klin. Wochenschr.*, 43:1311–1318.
47. Wilson, J. E. (1972): The relationship between glycolytic and mitochondrial enzymes in the developing rat brain. *J. Neurochem.*, 19:223–227.
48. Woolsey, T. A., and van der Loos, H. (1970): The structural organization of layer IV in the somatosensory region (SI) of mouse cerebral cortex. *Brain Res.*, 17:205–242.
49. Wroblewski, F., and Ladue, J. S. (1955): Lactic dehydrogenase activity in blood. *Proc. Soc. Exp. Biol. Med.*, 90:210–213.
50. Yakovlev, P., and Lecours, R. (1964): Myelination as a macroparameter of maturation. In: *Regional Maturation of the Nervous System in the Foetus and the Newborn,* edited by A. Minkowski. UNESCO, Paris.

Architectonics of the Cerebral Cortex,
edited by M. A. B. Brazier and H. Petsche.
Raven Press, New York © 1978.

Laminar Distribution of Cortical Field Potentials in Relation to Neuronal Activities During Seizure Discharges

E.-J. Speckmann, H. Caspers, and R. W. C. Janzen

Physiologisches Institut der Universität,
4400 Münster, Federal Republic of Germany

The relation of cortical field potentials and bioelectric activities of single cortical neurons has been studied extensively (4–6). Most of these investigations were performed to elucidate the mechanisms responsible for the generation of slow potential fluctuations, such as EEG waves and DC shifts in neuronal networks. In general, the results revealed some fundamental similarities between changes of field potentials and of neuronal membrane potentials (MP) in a variety of experimental conditions. These observations led to the conclusion that the slow bioelectric phenomena may originate, in principle, from a summation of neuronal MP fluctuations evoked, for instance, as EPSP or IPSP in synaptic regions. In many recordings, however, essential dissimilarities between variations of field potentials and neuronal events can also be found (19). They do not necessarily disprove the conclusion mentioned above, for such differences may have several other explanations.

One important reason seems to be that the response of the single element, from which the comparative intracellular recording is taken, may not be representative for the average activity changes of the neuronal population by which the field potential in question is built up. This difficulty may be partly overcome by forcing the greatest possible number of neurons involved in producing a slow wave into synchronized action. In this sense seizure activity can be regarded as a favourable experimental model. A further point, however, is that field potentials and unit activities are frequently recorded from different regions or structures. Thus, in studies on the cerebral cortex MP changes of pyramidal tract (PT) cells are often related to slow potential fluctuations led from the cortical surface. In the latter case the epicortical field potentials may well originate from generator structures other than the PT cell bodies in a deeper layer (19). The aim of the present investigations was to study this problem in more detail. To this purpose the MP changes of PT cells were compared with field potentials recorded from the surface and from various depths of the cortex. Both the AC waves of the conventional EEG and the DC component of the bioelectric activity served as indicators. For the reason mentioned above, seizure activity was chosen as an experimental model.

METHODS

The experiments were carried out on cats weighing 2 to 4 kg. The animals were anaesthetized initially either by 15 to 20 mg/kg pentobarbital i.p. after 5 to 10 mg diazepam had been administered 12 hr before or by 20 to 35 mg/kg pentobarbital i.p. alone. In both cases additional doses of 10 mg pentobarbital i.v. were applied during the experiments if necessary. The animals were paralyzed by gallamine and ventilated artificially with the body temperature kept constant at 37°C. Seizure activity was elicited by repeated i.v. applications of pentylenetetrazol (PTZ).

Electrophysiological recordings were taken from the gyrus sigmoideus anterior and posterior. After trepanation of the skull, the cortex was exposed and covered with paraffin oil. Pulsations of the cortex were minimized by aid of a pressure foot and by opening the cisterna cerebellomedullaris. Local Po_2 measured by platinum microelectrodes was found to remain unchanged after the pressure foot had touched the cortical surface. DC potentials with the EEG waves superimposed were led from the cortical surface by AgAgCl electrodes located in the pressure foot against a reference point in the nasal bone. Laminar DC recordings were performed by semimicroelectrodes filled with Ringer–Agar. The position of the DC semimicroelectrode within the cerebral cortex was determined by testing the field distribution of the antidromic response to a pyramidal tract volley (10). Intracellular recordings were taken by glass micropipettes filled with 3 mol·l^{-1} KCl or 2 mol·l^{-1} K-acetate using conventional amplification techniques. Intracellular stimulation was performed through the recording electrode by means of a bridge circuit. In order to reduce the pick-up of extracellular DC potentials during recording the membrane potential, either an AgAgCl electrode in the pressure foot on the surface of the gyrus or an additional microelectrode about 100 μm distant from the intracellular one served as a reference. Only, if the potential fluctuations during a seizure attack, recorded by the microelectrode for intracellular recordings in an extracellular position, were less than 1 mV in amplitude, the membrane potential changes determined by the actual electrode arrangement were evaluated further. Extracellular unit recordings were performed by glass micropipettes filled with 2.7 mol · l^{-1} NaCl.

Stimulation of the cortical surface was carried out by means of two electrodes mounted in the pressure foot. The pyramidal tract was stimulated bipolarly by aid of a comblike electrode which was positioned according to the stereotaxic atlas of Reinoso-Suarez (15). After the experiments the stimulation points were marked by coagulations and determined by histo-logical techniques.

The cells from which the recordings were taken have been classified as pyramidal tract cells and nonpyramidal tract cells (non-PT cells). A unit was assumed to be a PT cell if (a) a single stimulus applied to the ipsilateral pyramidal tract evoked action potentials at a constant latency and, in intra-cellular recordings, without preceding synaptic activity. It should be noted that antidromic spike invasion into soma regions was often blocked sub-sequent to seizure activity after repeated PTZ application and reappeared in the course of the interictal period. (b) The action potentials showed the ability to follow high-frequency stimulation at least up to 200 impulses/sec. (c) Collision of antidromic and orthodromic spikes was demonstrated (16). All neurons which did not show these criteria and were found in a depth of at maximum 1,000 μm below the cortical surface were considered to be non-PT cells (17). It is assumed that non-PT cells represent mainly cortical interneurons and afferent fibers (12). The present results are based on the analysis of 63 PT cells and of 43 non-PT cells.

Records were taken directly on an inkwriter and on film as well as on a FM tape. After the experiments, the bioelectric signals were evaluated as described by Knoll et. al. (11). This method makes it possible to recognize patterns in the DC potential occurring unpredictably and to relate mem-brane and action potentials of cortical neurons to the recognized waveform. The relation between these signals was examined by means of averaging and histogram techniques.

RESULTS

Relations of Cortical DC Shifts and Membrane Potential Changes of PT Cells

Repeated applications of PTZ in the anaesthetized animal finally evoke a seizure state characterized by periodically recurring convulsions (2). Both the duration of a single fit and the intervals between subsequent attacks are subject to considerable variations (19). In recordings from the surface of the cerebral cortex, this type of generalized seizure activity is always ac-companied by a prominent negative DC shift on which the spikes of the conventional EEG are superimposed. The relations between these DC dis-placements and membrane potential changes of PT cells were studied in a first series of experiments.

A representative example of curves traced by an oscilloscope is given in Fig. 1. The simultaneous recordings of the DC and MP potentials in A to D demonstrate that each surface-negative DC displacement associated with seizure discharges of increasing duration coincides with neuronal paroxys-mal depolarization shifts (PDS) in series of corresponding length. In Fig. 2

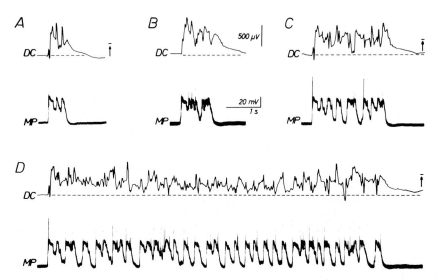

FIG. 1. A–D: Simultaneous recordings by an oscilloscope of the epicortical DC potential **(DC)** and of the membrane potential **(MP)** of a PT cell during seizure discharges of increasing duration.

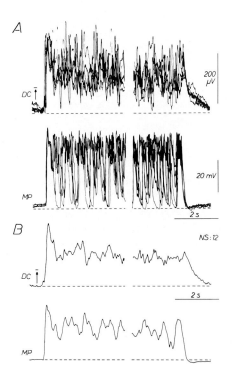

FIG. 2. Superimposition and averaging of simultaneous recordings of the epicortical DC potential **(DC)** and of the membrane potential changes of one PT cell **(MP)** during long-lasting seizure attacks. In the course of the seizure, the tracings are interrupted for about 1 min. **A:** Graphical superimposition of inkwriter tracings of five consecutive attacks. **B:** Average curves of 12 consecutive ictal DC and MP shifts calculated by a computer.

a number of such recordings obtained during consecutive attacks in the same experiment are superimposed graphically (A) and averaged by a computer (B). Both evaluations indicate that the mean surface-negative DC shift is closely related to the mean depolarization of PT cells in the course of a fit.

Besides this correspondence, the simultaneous DC and MP recordings also exhibit some essential differences concerning both the polarity and the time course of the potential fluctuations. Such differences are encountered both at the commencement and at the termination of seizure activity. In leads from the surface of the cerebral cortex the sustained negative DC shift is usually preceded by one or more rapid deflections, the direction of which may be negative, positive, or multiphasic. Independent of their actual polarity and time course, these prepotentials occur coincidently with the initial neuronal PDS which is very uniform in shape.

An example of this finding is illustrated in Fig. 3A and B. Such dissimilarities between DC reactions and MP changes of PT cells at the onset of seizure activity are always present provided that the DC component is led from the surface of the cerebral cortex. In DC recordings from deeper cortical layers the occurrence of fast prepotentials with varying polarity is regularly missing. The comparative measurements in Fig. 3C indicate that the depth response of the DC potential at the commencement of a

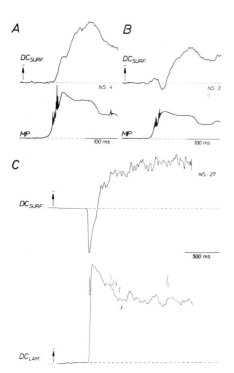

FIG. 3. **A, B:** Relations between epicortical DC shifts (**DC**$_{SURF}$) showing a different time course and paroxysmal depolarization shifts of PT cells (**MP**) at the onset of seizure activities. The tracings represent average curves. Number of sweeps (**NS**): four and three, respectively. **C:** Simultaneous recordings of DC shifts at the cortical surface (**DC**$_{SURF}$) and at a depth of 1700 μm below surface (**DC**$_{LAM}$) at the beginning of consecutive seizure attacks. The tracings represent average curves. NS: 27.

convulsive attack consists in an unidirectional and steep negative shift which shows an initial overshoot and then declines to a rather constant level. This finding is in accordance with earlier observations (7,19). In contrast to the DC deviations obtained in surface leads, the mean reaction of the DC component in deeper layers is almost congruent with the mean MP changes of PT cells.

Further differences between epicortical DC shifts and neuronal MP changes appear at the termination of a seizure attack. Consistent with previous investigations (3) the tracings in Fig. 1 show that the termination of convulsive activity is always accompanied by a steep re- and hyperpolarization of cortical neurons, whereas the negative DC shift returns slowly to the preictal level. Figure 4 demonstrates that the slope of the DC decay decreases with increasing duration of a convulsive fit. The slow return of the negative DC displacement to the preictal value is characteristic for surface leads. With progressive penetration of the cerebral cortex by the recording electrode the decay of the DC deviation increases in slope and finally turns to a transient positive shift. The results of a typical experiment are presented in Fig. 5. In Fig. 6B the mean DC deviations at the cortical surface and at a depth of 1,700 μm as well as the mean MP changes of a PT cell were calculated at 1-sec intervals from a number of repetitive seizure attacks in the same experiment as illustrated in Fig. 6A. It becomes evident that the depth response of the DC component at the termination of a convulsive fit is almost congruent with the neuronal MP shifts.

In summary, the results allow these conclusions: (a) During and after seizure activity the DC field potentials occurring in deeper cortical layers are closely related to MP fluctuations of PT cells. This finding suggests that these slow extracellular potential deviations are generated mainly by neuronal, especially somatic membranes. (b) The differences existing between

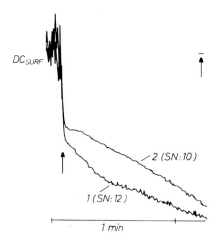

FIG. 4. Average curves of the decay of negative epicortical DC shifts (**DC**$_{SURF}$) at the termination of seizure attacks, which is marked by an arrow. Tracing 1 represents the average decay calculated from 12 consecutive seizures, each of which lasted about 2 min. Tracing 2 was calculated from 10 consecutive seizures, lasting about 20 sec longer than those in 1.

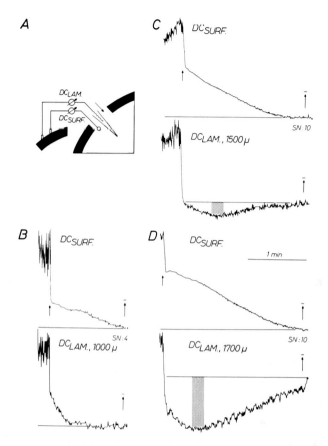

FIG. 5. Comparative DC recordings from the surface (**DC**$_{SURF}$) and at various depth (**DC**$_{LAM}$) of the cerebral cortex at the termination (arrows) of seizure attacks. **A:** Schematic drawing of the recording arrangement. **B–D:** With stepwise penetration of the cortex by the recording microelectrode, the slow decay of the negative DC shift found in the surface leads becomes accelerated and finally turns to a transient positive deflection (hatched columns). The preictal DC level is marked by horizontal lines. The tracings represent average curves (**SN** = number of sweeps).

DC field potentials at the cortical surface and MP changes of PT cells indicate that the epicortical DC shifts cannot, or only in part, be attributed to MP fluctuations of the cell soma in deeper cortical layers. Other generator structures such as dendrites and/or glial cells located more superficially in the cortex must be involved (18). (c) The close correspondence found between the mean epicortical DC shifts and the mean MP changes of PT cells *during* seizure activity can be explained by a parallel depolarization of the cell bodies in deeper layers and of the more superficially located generators by afferent impulses.

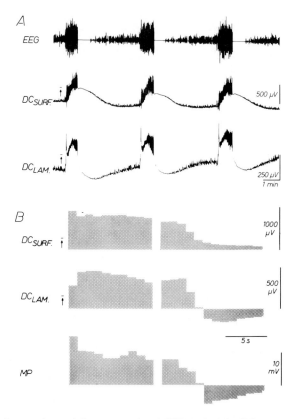

FIG. 6. A: Inkwriter tracings of the conventional EEG and of the DC potential led from the cortical surface (**DC**$_{SURF}$) and from a layer 1,700 μm below surface (**DC**$_{LAM}$) during repetitive seizure attacks. **B:** Calculations of mean epicortical DC shifts (**DC**$_{SURF}$), mean laminar DC shifts (**DC**$_{LAM}$), and of mean membrane potential changes of a PT cell (**MP**) at 1-sec intervals during and after several seizure attacks. The evaluation is interrupted for a period of about 1 min.

Relations of Seizure Discharges in the EEG and Membrane Potential Changes of PT Cells

The sustained negative DC shifts during seizure attacks described in the preceding chapter are superimposed with steep potential fluctuations which correspond to the well-known spike activity in the conventional EEG. A further aim of the present investigations was to examine whether these fast EEG transients are also related to changes in neuronal membrane potentials (Figs. 1 and 7). The tracings in Fig. 1 suggest that at least most of the sharp EEG waves recorded from the cortical surface coincide with a PDS of PT cells. Similar observations have been made by other investigators (9,14). However, polarity, time course, and amplitude of the EEG spikes vary to such an extent that definite conclusions as to the relationship between the fast EEG transients and neuronal events cannot be drawn from a mere visual evaluation of the curves. Therefore, a special method of pattern recognition was applied (11). The recordings in Fig. 7 demonstrate that certain patterns of potential fluctuations occur during seizure activity. They appear at irregular intervals and can easily be detected despite the variability of the ongoing trace. In Fig. 7B one example of such a waveform is marked by dotted lines. A superimposition of corresponding, subsequent patterns by means of an electronic display unit allows averaging of the curves. In the present study a total of six basic seizure patterns could be differentiated. They consist in unidirectional negative and positive waves, diphasic negative-positive or positive-negative deflections, and, finally, in multiphasic fluctuations (Fig. 7C).

To test the relations between the selected EEG patterns and the membrane potential changes of PT cells, the two bioelectric phenomena were recorded simultaneously and evaluated by averaging. With this procedure only the selected EEG pattern served as the technical trigger. Therefore, the correlation between the two signals is indicated by the amplitude as well as by the signal-to-background ratio in the MP recording. The results obtained with this method are summarized in Fig. 8. They show that each of the selected EEG patterns is closely related to a neuronal PDS. The finding implies that a rather uniform depolarization of PT cells may be accompanied by completely different seizure patterns in the EEG. This state-

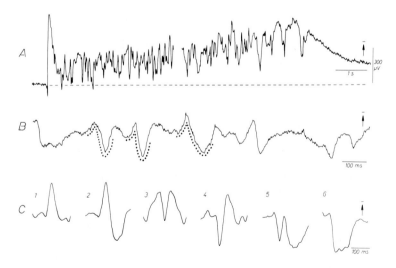

FIG. 7. A: Characteristic negative DC shift at the cortical surface during a seizure attack. The slow potential shift is superimposed with rapid deflections (EEG spikes). **B:** Recording as in **A** at a higher paper speed. The occurrence of a defined seizure pattern in this tracing is indicated by dotted lines. **C:** Basic seizure patterns in the EEG **(1–6)** isolated from a number of EEG recordings by means of pattern recognition. Average curves from 8 to 28 single potentials.

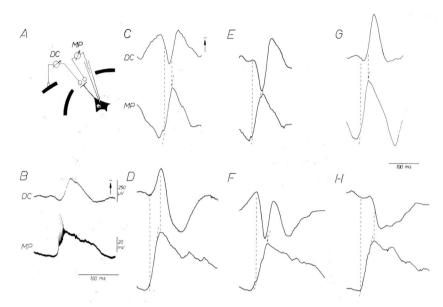

FIG. 8. Relations between various seizure patterns in the surface EEG **(DC)** and paroxysmal depolarization shifts of a PT cell **(MP). A:** Schematic presentation of the electrode arrangements for DC and MP recordings. **B:** Original simultaneous recordings of EEG and MP deflections during a single convulsive discharge. **C–H:** Average curves of EEG waves and related MP changes of a PT cell calculated from 8 to 28 single seizure discharges. The neuronal depolarizations are related to the EEG fluctuations by broken lines. The selected EEG patterns correspond to the six basic types presented in Fig. 7.

ment refers to recordings from the surface of the cerebral cortex. If the EEG spikes are led from deeper cortical layers, they appear as unidirectional negative deflections. A representative example of comparative recordings is given in Fig. 9. As a whole, these observations demonstrate that the fast EEG transients during seizure activity correspond very closely to membrane potential changes of PT cells, if the two bioelectric events are led from the same or at least immediately neighbouring layers of the cortex, whereas there are considerable differences both in polarity and time course, if the EEG potentials are recorded from the cortical surface. The same conclusion was drawn from the results of the DC measurements described in the preceding section.

The question is which mechanisms are responsible for the variability of seizure patterns in the surface EEG, while the reactions of PT cells consist in rather uniform depolarization shifts. At first sight it might be assumed that volume conduction plays an essential role in producing these differences. A more detailed analysis of the tracings, however, showed that this cannot account for the described variations of the epicortical field potentials. Therefore, another mechanism had to be considered. It is known from earlier investigations that polarity and time course of stimulus-related EEG poten-

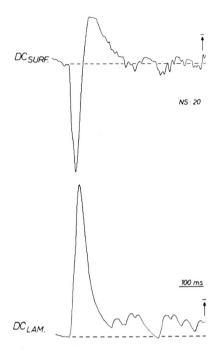

FIG. 9. Average curves of simultaneous recordings of convulsive discharges led from the surface **(DC$_{SURF}$)** and from a depth of 1,700 μm **(DC$_{LAM}$)** of the cerebral cortex. Number of sweeps **(NS):** 20.

tials depend on the level of the DC component on which they are super-imposed (1,8,13).

The existence of such a relationship in the present case was tested by a procedure illustrated in Fig. 10. At first, the actual DC level from which each single seizure pattern of the EEG arose was calculated using the method explained in Fig. 10A. Subsequently, the various selected EEG waves were displayed in relation to the different degrees of the negative DC shift encountered during a seizure attack. The results of such an evaluation are presented in the case of a typical experiment in Fig. 10B. It can be seen that the appearance of the EEG spike patterns in the course of the negative DC shift illustrated in Fig. 10C varies in a wide range. There is, however, a clear distribution of probability in the way that the EEG waves with a predominant negative component arise preferentially from low negative DC displacements, whereas monophasic positive spikes occur, exclusively, at high negative DC levels.

Such a relationship is demonstrable not only with single EEG transients as illustrated in Fig. 10, but also with longer sequences of seizure patterns. A typical experiment is presented in Fig. 11. The tracings show simultane-ous recordings of the membrane potential of a PT cells and of epicortical field potentials during a convulsive attack at different levels of the ongoing negative DC shift. At a comparatively low negative DC level, the sequences of the neuronal PDS are associated with EEG spikes that are mainly nega-

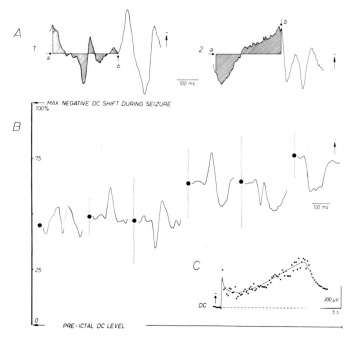

FIG. 10. Relation between basic EEG seizure patterns and level of negative DC shift at the cortical surface. **A1, A2:** At arrows **(b)** the seizure patterns concerned are defined to start. All potential fluctuations occurring in a period of 300 msec before these points are used for computation of the DC level at starting points **b.** The DC level is defined as the distance between the preictal level and the value at which the algebraic sum of negative and positive areas of EEG waves becomes zero. These actual levels are marked by arrows **(a). B:** Display of averaged EEG spike patterns in relation to DC level (ordinate) on which they occur. Dots and vertical bars: Mean ± SE. **C:** Time course of negative DC shift on which spike patterns in **B** are superimposed **(dots).**

tive in polarity. After the negative DC displacement has reached a higher level in the course of the same fit, the paroxysmal depolarizations of the neuron coincide with predominantly positive EEG deflections.

In summary, the results of this study show: (a) Each sharp EEG wave occurring within a series of seizure discharges is associated with a PDS at the soma membrane of PT cells. (b) Polarity and time course of the field potentials recorded from the surface of the cerebral cortex prove independent of the concomitant neuronal MP shifts. (c) The actual pattern of an epicortical seizure discharge is related to the local DC level. In accordance with previous investigations these findings suggest that both the DC shifts and the fast EEG transients appearing in surface recordings during seizure activity, can be attributed, if at all, only in part to a direct lead of somatic MP changes in deeper cortical layers (19). It must be assumed that the epicortical field potentials are produced mainly by other generators among

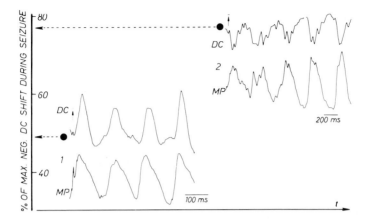

FIG. 11. Relation between trains of sharp EEG deflections **(DC)** and membrane potential changes of a PT cell **(MP)** during seizure activity with various amplitudes of the underlying negative DC shift (ordinate). The tracings represent average curves of eight single recordings each. In **1** and **2** the uniform neuronal depolarizations coincide with EEG deflections showing an opposite polarity.

which extrasomatic neuronal structures, such as dendrites and glial cells, may play a role.

The results obtained with surface recordings of the EEG and DC potentials can be explained by means of a hypothetical neuronal circuit drawn in Fig. 12. In Fig. 12A the upper tracings represent averaged DC reactions and MP changes of a PT cell during subsequent ictal discharges. In this case the epicortical field potential is mainly negative in polarity corresponding to a low negative DC level. The scheme in the lower part of Fig. 12A designs some kind of a flow chart of the neuronal processes supposed to underly the potential fluctuations. In this drawing, the light gray-tone arrow indicates the asynchronous afferent input to the cortex which determines the general DC level. The dark gray-tone arrows denote synchronized phasic volleys giving rise to a single convulsive discharge. In this case the cell soma and structures such as dendrites in the upper cortical layer are activated simultaneously. The depolarization of elements located near the cortical surface determines the potential fluctuation picked up by the epicortical recording electrode. Therefore, the neuronal PDS is associated with a monophasic negative field potential.

These conditions of potential generation change, however, if the asynchronous input to the cortex is enhanced. Such a situation is illustrated in Fig. 12B. In this case the general increase in background activity, which is reflected in a further rise of the negative DC shift, is indicated by a light, broad gray-tone arrow. On this condition, the relay cells to the upper cortical layers are highly active. An additional synchronized volley underlying a

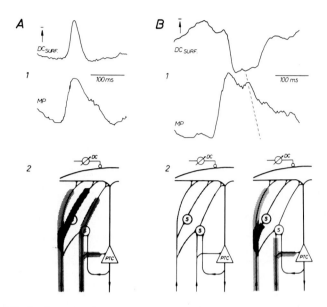

FIG. 12. Hypothetical neuronal processes responsible for the generation of different EEG spike patterns at the cortical surface (DC$_{SURF}$) with uniform depolarization shifts of PT cells **(MP). A1:** Example of a monophasic negative EEG spike pattern; average curves of 20 consecutive ictal discharges. **A2:** Schematic flow chart of neuronal excitation processes underlying the origination of tracings in **A1. PTC,** pyramidal tract cell; **S,** internuncial neuron, stellate cell. **Light gray-tone arrow:** Symbol for continuous asynchronous input to the cortex. **Dark gray-tone arrows:** Symbols for phasic volleys giving rise to single convulsive discharges. **B1:** Example of a monophasic positive sharp EEG wave pattern; average curves of 20 consecutive ictal discharges. **B2:** Schematic flow chart of neuronal excitation processes underlying the origination of tracings in **B1.** Symbols as in **A2.** Left scheme indicates state before positive EEG deflection. Right scheme shows changes of neuronal activity during positive deflection **(broken line).**

single convulsive discharge may cause excessive depolarizations of the internuncial elements and thus lead to a transient blockade of spike generation. Therefore, the phasic afferent volleys marked by dark gray-tone arrows in Fig. 12B2 cannot or only in part reach the upper cortical layer. Consequently, a disfacilitation of the superficial generator structures takes place resulting in a reduction of the asynchronous afferent input. This effect is illustrated by the smaller, light gray-tone arrow in the right scheme of Fig. 12B2. The disfacilitation is reflected in the monophasic positive EEG wave shown in the tracing in the upper part of Fig. 12B. As a whole, these mechanisms may explain why a rather uniform depolarization of PT cells can be associated with a variety of seizure patterns in the surface EEG.

The validity of the interpretation described above is greatly dependent on the actual activity changes of the relay cells during seizure discharges of various types. Therefore, this problem was studied in more detail by extracellular recordings from units identified as non-PT cells and, presumably, representing interneurons in the majority of leads. At first the discharge frequency of these elements was tested in relation to the local epicortical DC shifts in the course of convulsive fits. The results of such an experiment are displayed in Fig. 13. The average curves demonstrate that amplitude and time course of the negative DC displacements are clearly reflected in the discharge rates of the cells as far as the periods of ongoing seizure activity are concerned. It seems therefore justified to assume that a high negative DC level at the cortical surface is indeed accompanied by a high activity level of internuncial cells.

In a second step, the discharge rate of non-PT units was examined in relation to the various types of fast epicortical field potentials during seizure activity. Examples of predominantly negative waveforms in the surface EEG occurring at a low negative DC level are summarized in Fig. 14. The original tracings in A and B as well as the computed diagrams in C indicate that the negative field potentials in their rising phase are associated with high-frequency bursts of neuronal spikes. Figure 15 shows the relations between the activity of non-PT units and predominantly positive EEG deflections obtained in a seizure state with a significantly higher negative

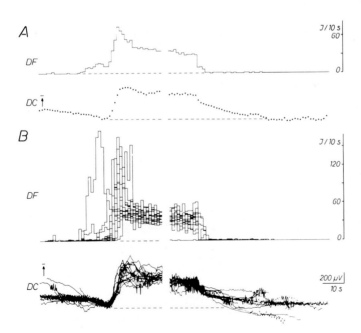

FIG. 13. Relations between negative DC shifts at the cortical surface **(DC)** and discharge frequency of non-PT cells in the cortex **(DF)** during seizure attacks. **A:** Average curves calculated from the tracings superimposed in **B.**

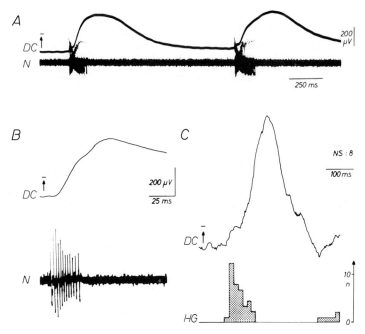

FIG. 14. Relations between monophasic negative sharp EEG waves **(DC)** and discharges of non-PT cells in the cortex **(N)** during seizure activity. **A, B:** Original recordings at different paper speeds. **C:** Average curve of sharp negative DC deflection calculated from eight single events **(NS). HG:** Corresponding average histogram of neuronal discharge rate.

DC level than the tracings displayed in Fig. 14. Both the original records in A and B and the average curves in C and D reveal that the positive EEG spikes run parallel with a transient decrease of the neuronal discharge frequency. This finding substantiates the basic assumption underlying the scheme in Fig. 12B that positive EEG deflections occurring in seizure states at a high negative DC level are due to a disfacilitation of generator structures in the upper cortical layer.

The type of positive EEG waves illustrated in Fig. 15 tends to be relatively slow and often shows a somewhat irregular time course. Besides this form, very steep positive deflections can be found which appear, preferentially, at low negative DC levels (Fig. 10). The comparative recordings in Fig. 16 demonstrate that the latter type of positive spikes is accompanied by an increase in discharge rate of non-PT elements. This finding, which is strictly contrasting to the neuronal silence during slow positive waves, corresponds with the results obtained in studies on sensory evoked potentials (6). Possibly, such fast positive spikes occurring in surface leads may be due to a synchronized, short-lasting depolarization of neuronal elements in deeper cortical layers.

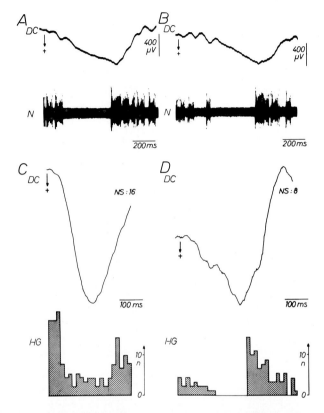

FIG. 15. Relations between monophasic positive EEG waves **(DC)** and discharges of non-PT cells in the cortex **(N)** associated with seizure activity. **A, B:** Original tracings. **C, D:** Average curves of positive EEG deflections calculated from 16 and 8 single events, respectively **(NS). HG:** Corresponding average histograms of neuronal discharge rates. The different discharge patterns in the two examples are reflected in different shapes of the epicortical EEG waves.

In summary, the present investigations suggest that field potentials recorded from the surface and from deeper layers of the cerebral cortex under seizure conditions are obviously generated by different structures. On the one hand, the EEG waves and DC shifts obtained in deeper cortical layers can be attributed to a summation of MP fluctuations at the cell soma, for instance of PT cells. On the other hand, slow waves occurring in surface leads are produced mainly by facilitation and disfacilitation processes on structures in the upper parts of the cortex. These structures may be dendrites, the potential generation of which may be modulated by surrounding glial elements.

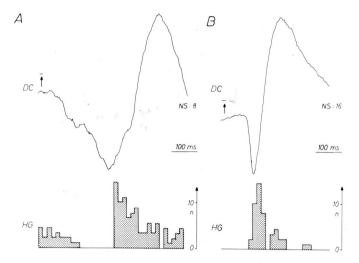

FIG. 16. Comparative recordings of two types of positive-negative EEG deflections and of corresponding histograms of the discharge rate of non-PT cells in the cortex occurring with seizure activity. The tracings represent average curves calculated from 8 and 16 single events, respectively **(NS)**. **A:** Relatively slow positive wave associated with a depression of neuronal activity. **B:** Sharp positive wave accompanied by a burst-like increase in neuronal activity.

REFERENCES

1. Caspers, H. (1959): Über die Beziehungen zwischen Dendritenpotential und Gleichspannung an der Hirnrinde. *Pfluegers Arch. Ges. Physiol.*, 269:157–181.
2. Caspers, H., and Speckmann, E.-J. (1969): DC potential shifts in paroxysmal states. In: *Basic Mechanisms of the Epilepsies*, edited by H. H. Jasper, A. A. Ward, and A. Pope. Little, Brown, Boston.
3. Caspers, H., and Speckmann, E.-J. (1972): Cerebral pO_2, pCO_2 and pH: Changes during convulsive activity and their significance for spontaneous arrest of seizures. *Epilepsia*, 13:699–725.
4. Caspers, H., and Speckmann, E.-J. (1974): Cortical DC shifts associated with changes of gas tensions in blood and tissue. In: *Handbook of Electroencephalography and Clinical Neurophysiology, Vol. 10, Part A: DC Potentials Recorded Directly from the Cortex*, edited by A. Rémond, pp. 10A–41, 10A–65. Elsevier, Amsterdam.
5. Creutzfeldt, O. D. (1969): Neuronal mechanisms underlying the EEG. In: *Basic Mechanisms of the Epilepsies*, edited by H. H. Jasper, A. A. Ward, and A. Pope. Little, Brown, Boston.
6. Creutzfeldt, O. D., and Houchin, J. (1974): Neuronal basis of EEG waves. In: *Handbook of Electroencephalography and Clinical Neurophysiology, Vol. 2, Part C: The Neuronal Generation of the EEG*, edited by A. Rémond. Elsevier, Amsterdam.
7. Ferguson, J. H., and Jasper, H. H. (1971): Laminar DC studies of acetylcholine-activated epileptiform discharge in cerebral cortex. *Electroenceph. Clin. Neurophysiol.*, 30:377–390.
8. Goldring, S., and O'Leary, J. L. (1954): Correlation between steady transcortical potential and evoked response. II. Effect of veratrine and strychnine upon the responsiveness of visual cortex. *Electroenceph. Clin. Neurophysiol.*, 6:201–212.
9. Gumnit, R. (1974): DC shifts accompanying seizure activity. In: *Handbook of Electroencephalography and Clinical Neurophysiology, Vol. 10, Part A: DC Potentials Recorded Directly from the Cortex*, edited by A. Rémond, pp. 10A–66, 10A–77. Elsevier, Amsterdam.

10. Humphrey, D. R. (1968): Re-analysis of the antidromic cortical response. I. Potential evoked by stimulation of the isolated pyramidal tract. *Electroenceph. Clin. Neurophysiol.*, 24:116–129.
11. Knoll, O., Speckmann, E.-J., and Caspers, H. (1974): Ein Verfahren zur Korrelierung verschiedener bioelektrischer Vorgänge mit definierten Potentialmustern im EEG. *Z. EEG-EMG*, 5:199–205.
12. Lance, J. W., and Manning, R. L. (1954): Origin of the pyramidal tract in the cat. *J. Physiol. (Lond.)*, 124:385–399.
13. O'Leary, J. L., and Goldring, S. (1964): DC potentials of the brain. *Physiol. Rev.*, 44: 91–125.
14. Prince, D. A. (1974): Neuronal correlation of epileptiform discharges and cortical DC potentials. In: *Handbook of Electroencephalography and Clinical Neurophysiology, Vol. 2, Part C: The Neuronal Generation of the EEG*, edited by A. Rémond. Elsevier, Amsterdam.
15. Reinoso-Suarez, F. (1961): *Topographischer Hirnatlas der Katze für experimentalphysiologische Untersuchungen*, 24 pp. (50 plates). Merck, Darmstadt.
16. Renaud, L. P., and Kelly, J. S. (1974): Identification of possible inhibitory neurons in the pericruciate cortex of the cat. *Brain Res.*, 79:9–28.
17. Renaud, L. P., and Kelly, J. S. (1974): Simultaneous recordings from pericruciate pyramidal tract and non-pyramidal tract neurons; response to stimulation of inhibitory pathways. *Brain Res.*, 79:29–44.
18. Somjen, G. G. (1973): Electrogenesis of sustained potentials. *Prog. Neurobiol.*, 1:199–237.
19. Speckmann, E.-J., Caspers, H., and Janzen, R. W. (1972): Relations between cortical DC shifts and membrane potential changes of cortical neurons associated with seizure activity. In: *Synchronization of EEG Activity in Epilepsies*, edited by H. Petsche and M. A. B. Brazier, pp. 93–111. Springer, New York.

Architectonics of the Cerebral Cortex,
edited by M. A. B. Brazier and H. Petsche.
Raven Press, New York © 1978.

Some Aspects of Plasticity in Parallel Visual Thalamocortical Pathways in the Cat

L. J. Garey

Institut d'Anatomie, University of Lausanne, Switzerland

Detailed architectonic study of the cerebral cortex has passed into and out of favour on many occasions, but it has reached the stage today of being firmly established as not only a morphological expression of cortical structure but also as a reflection of clear *functional* divisions within the cerebral cortex. Perhaps nowhere more clearly is this close anatomical and physiological relationship seen than in the mammalian visual system. It would seem likely that all mammals have secondary, tertiary, and even remoter cortical areas dealing with visual processes, innervated either directly from the primary visual thalamus or indirectly by cortical association pathways.

However, the structural and functional divisions at the cortical level must have a subcortical basis. This chapter will attempt to provide a brief review of the principal features of the organization of two parallel subsystems in the retinothalamocortical pathways of the cat and illustrate some recent findings on the differential reaction to sensory deprivation of two sets of neurons in the thalamic part of these pathways, each of which projects to an architectonically different cortical area.

VISUAL CORTICAL ARCHITECTURE AND ITS SUBCORTICAL BASIS

Physiological Evidence for Parallel Thalamocortical Pathways

In the cat, the visual cortex is divisible by its cyto- and myeloarchitectural features into three main areas: 17, 18, and 19 (1,40,43) (Fig. 1). In the present chapter area 19 and the other subsidiary visual areas now known to exist will not be considered. That there are also *functional* divisions in the cat's visual cortex was suggested by Talbot (56) who showed that there is a second representation of the visual field lateral to the primary visual cortex. Later Hubel and Wiesel (29) provided a clear description of the different physiological characteristics of these three major visual areas (17, 18, and 19). They proposed that the "complex" responses of neurons

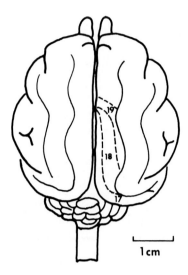

FIG. 1. Drawing of the dorsal surface of the brain of an adult cat to show, in the right hemisphere, the extent of the visual areas 17, 18, and 19. (Based on Otsuka and Hassler, ref. 40.)

in areas 18 and 19 depend essentially on intercortical transfer of information from "simple" cells in area 17, the primary visual cortex. However, much evidence has since been forthcoming that there are also important *parallel* subcortical inputs to the various visual areas which determine response characteristics in these areas. Axons from the retina relay in the lateral geniculate nucleus (LGN) of the thalamus. An anatomical basis for separate input from the LGN to areas 17 *and* 18 is well established (15, 16,18,39,42,60), and several lines of enquiry suggest that parallel pathways exist right through the visual system from retina to cortex (Fig. 2).

The retina of the cat contains various types and sizes of ganglion cells (32,36,49), and the optic nerve has axons of different diameters and conduction velocities (2,51,55). Enroth-Cugell and Robson (8) studied the physiological responses to stimulation of the ganglion cells of the cat's retina and were able to differentiate between "X cells" and "Y cells," as they termed them, on the basis of the degree of linearity of summation within their receptive fields. This classification was amplified and extended, also using physiological techniques, by Cleland et al. (6) and Ikeda and Wright (31), who accentuated the "sustained" and "transient" nature of the responses of the two respective cell types and, like Fukada (9), provided evidence that the axons of X cells conducted more slowly than those of Y cells. Hoffmann et al. (27,53) were able to trace two distinct pathways from the retina, through the LGN and on to the visual cortex, one having the characteristics of X cells and conducting relatively slowly, while the other was Y-like and conducted more rapidly. X afferents were, furthermore, found to project predominantly to the simple cells of area 17, and Y fibres to complex cells in area 18 (26,50,58) (Fig. 2). The division is not absolutely

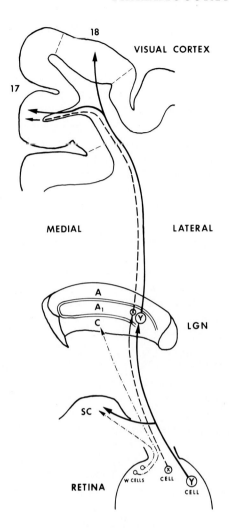

FIG. 2. Schematic drawing showing the projections of small W cells, medium X cells, and large Y cells from the retina of the cat to the lateral geniculate nucleus (LGN) and the superior colliculus (SC), and the onward projection of X and Y cells to areas 17 and 18 of the visual cortex.

strict, since both simple and complex cells exist in both areas 17 and 18, and cells with simple and complex characteristics can be driven by either X or Y afferents, at least in area 17 (28,47).

Anatomical Aspects of X and Y Cells

Naturally, in the light of such strong *physiological* evidence for a subcortical separation of inputs to architectonically and functionally different cortical areas, a *morphological* correlation was sought. Boycott and Wässle (4) have produced good anatomical evidence in the cat that retinal Y cells are the largest of the ganglion cells (the α cells), while the X cells are smaller (β cells). They also described very small γ cells, which probably represent the very slowly conducting "W cells" of Stone and Hoffmann (54), responsible for retinal input to the superior colliculus (11,25) (Fig. 2). Populations of neurons with different shapes and sizes also exist in the LGN of the cat (21,24,34). No *direct* correlation with their physiological activity has so far been possible, although Fukuda and Stone (12) have produced some preliminary indications that the medium-sized neurons are the equivalent of X cells and the large neurons the Y cells.

There is evidence from retrograde cell degeneration in the LGN after visual cortical lesions that distinct neuronal populations may project to the different cytoarchitectonic areas of the visual cortex. A lesion of area 17 in the cat caused shrinkage of the small and medium cell somata in the LGN, but when the lesion involved both areas 17 and 18 the large cells also underwent degenerative changes (15) (Fig. 3). These observations support the idea that the small and medium cells of the LGN send axons to area 17, while the largest cells send axonal collateral branches to areas 17 *and* 18. As the rapidly conducting axons of Y cells should be of relatively large diameter and, presumably, issue from large somata, there is, therefore, some indirect morphological evidence that X cells exert their main influence on area 17 and Y cells on 18 (Fig. 2). Garey and Powell (16) also noted that the degenerating axons entering area 18 from the thalamus after a lesion in the LGN had a much coarser appearance than those entering area 17.

Further morphological evidence that the neurons of the LGN projecting to area 18 are, at least in part, larger than those projecting to area 17 has come from studies involving the retrograde axonal transport of horseradish peroxidase (HRP). This enzyme, when injected into an area containing axonal ramifications, is absorbed and transported retrogradely along the axons to the parent cell bodies where its presence can be detected by a histochemical reaction (35). Maciewicz (37) injected HRP into the visual cortex of normal adult cats and studied the distribution of labelled cell bodies in the LGN. Gilbert and Kelly (17) and Garey and Blakemore (13) also used this technique, but measured the sizes of the labelled cells. When the injection was restricted to area 17, most of the thalamic neurons containing reaction product belonged to the small-cell population; when area 18 was injected selectively, a population of large cell bodies was labelled, although there was some overlap in the two cases. These results in the normal, mature cat, taken with the anatomical and physiological data concerning the distribution and features of X and Y cells discussed so far in this chapter, allow some confidence in equating the neurons labelled from area 18 with Y cells, and those labelled from area 17 with, predominantly, X cells; some Y cells will certainly be filled from area 17 also, owing to the branching of Y axons (15).

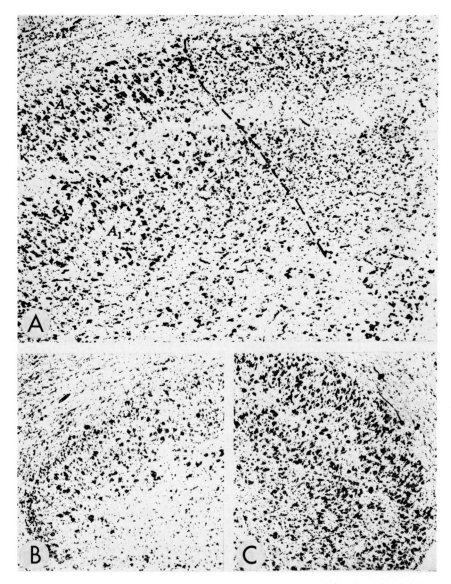

FIG. 3. A: Photomicrograph of part of the LGN of a cat showing the normal appearance of laminae A and A1 to the left of the dotted line; to the right of the line there is retrograde degeneration of large, medium, and small cells 37 days after a lesion in areas 17 *and* 18 of the ipsilateral visual cortex. **B:** The LGN of a cat which had a lesion confined to the ipsilateral area 17, 6 months previously. Even after this relatively long survival the largest cells of the nucleus have survived. **C:** The LGN of the opposite side to that in **B** to show its normal appearance. (From ref. 15.)

VISUAL DEPRIVATION

In order to take the line of correlative morphological and physiological experiments a step farther, a study has been made of the effects of visual deprivation on the parallel thalamocortical pathways in the cat (13). The experimental paradigm used monocular pattern deprivation by unilateral eyelid suture in young kittens combined with an attempt to identify X and Y cells in the LGN by injecting HRP into area 17 and 18 selectively some weeks later.

Effects of Visual Deprivation on the Lateral Geniculate Nucleus

The LGN of the cat is a laminated structure, with two main cellular strata, laminae A and A1, which receive, respectively, axons from the contralateral and the ipsilateral retina. There is also a complex of "C" laminae (22), similarly receiving segregated ipsi- and contralateral retinal inputs. In 1963 Wiesel and Hubel (59) reported that closure of one eye in a kitten resulted in a failure of normal growth of the neurons of the LGN laminae innervated by the closed eye. This effect was only obtainable during a sensitive period in the first 3 months of life (30) and was particularly marked if the deprivation was started at approximately 1 month of age. The original results have been widely confirmed (5,14,23,33). What one observes, if cell body sizes are measured in deprived LGN laminae and compared with those in normal laminae, is that the mean cell area is reduced by some 30% or more and that the largest cells observed in the normal laminae are not found in the deprived laminae (Figs. 4 and 5). Does this imply that these large cells, which by presumption could be the Y cells, *disappear* as a result of the monocular deprivation, or do they *specifically* fail to grow to full size, or do *all* cells fail to grow? Wiesel and Hubel (59) were, however, unable to detect any obvious change in the physiological responses of the LGN after monocular deprivation. But later Sherman et. al. (44) reported that they were unable to record the usual proportions of X and Y cells in the deprived laminae of the LGN of monocularly lid-sutured kittens: the percentage of Y cells that they found was drastically reduced. Perhaps, then, the Y cells *are* specifically affected by monocular deprivation.

---------------------------→

FIG. 4. Photomicrographs of the LGNs of a kitten after a left monocular deprivation from 1 to 8 weeks of age. **A:** The left LGN to show the lack of growth of neurons in lamina A1 ipsilateral to the deprived eye. **B:** The right LGN showing normal cells in lamina A1 and small cells in lamina A contralateral to the deprivation. **C:** A higher power view of the small neurons in lamina A of the right LGN compared with the normal ones in lamina A1; note the reduction of the largest cells in the deprived lamina. (From ref. 7.)

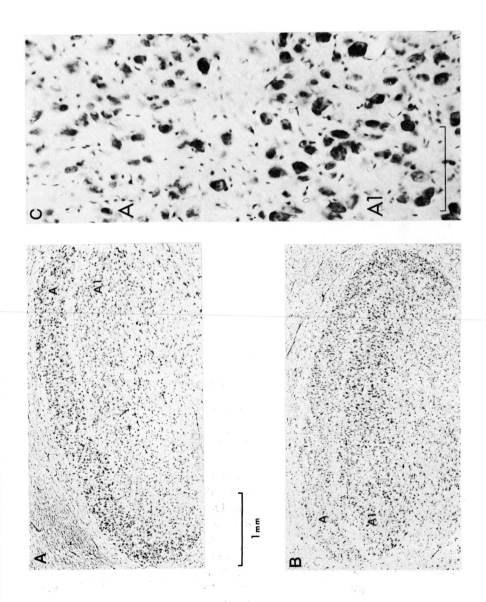

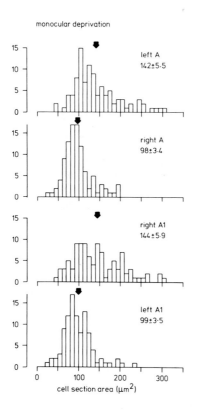

monocular deprivation

left A
142±5·5

right A
98±3·4

right A1
144±5·9

left A1
99±3·5

cell section area (μm²)

FIG. 5. Histograms showing the distribution of the cross-sectional areas of cells in laminae A and A1 of the LGNs of a monocularly deprived kitten (the same experiment as illustrated in Fig. 4). The arrows, and the figure to the right of each histogram, indicate the mean cell area (± SE). There is a reduction of some 30% in cell area in the deprived laminae, and the largest cells do not appear in them. (From ref. 7.)

Differential Effects of Visual Deprivation on X and Y Cells

In order to try to provide answers to the questions posed above, a series of kittens was reared with one eye closed by lid suture. Suturing was performed either at the age of 1 week or in the fifth or sixth week of life. At the age of approximately 3 months, a solution of 30% HRP was injected by pressure into the visual cortex using a microsyringe or a glass micropipette. One to three days later the animal was perfused with a buffered mixture of glutaraldehyde and paraformaldehyde. The injections of HRP were restricted either to area 17 or 18; in most cases area 17 was injected on one side and 18 on the other, but in some experiments the posterior part of 17 and the anterior part of 18 were injected on the same side. Coronal frozen sections of the brain were cut at 40 μm and incubated in diaminobenzidine containing hydrogen peroxide (19). This treatment causes the formation of a granular reaction product within the cells containing transported peroxidase (Fig. 6). A representative series of sections through the injection sites and the thalamus was mounted, and the Nissl substance of the neuronal somata lightly counterstained with cresyl violet. Neurons containing HRP reaction product were easily identified in the LGN after injection in either

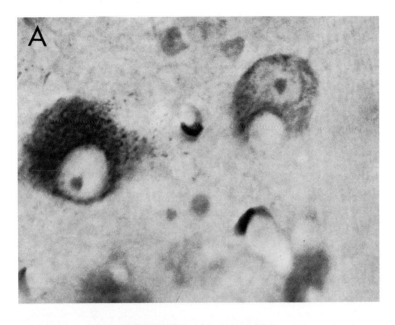

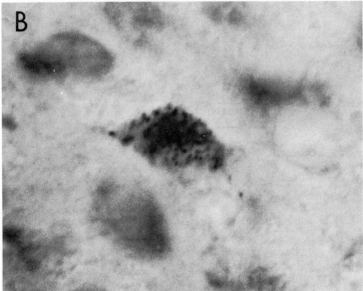

5μm

FIG. 6. A: Two cells in a nondeprived lamina of the LGN. The one on the left contains dark, granular reaction product after retrograde filling with HRP from area 18; it is representative of a normal Y cell. **B:** A labelled cell in a deprived lamina of the LGN, also filled from area 18, but belonging to the population of small neurons found after monocular deprivation. It is typical of the small, deprived Y cell described in the text.

area 17 or 18, using both light- and dark-field microscopy. With area 18 injections, marked cells also appeared in the pulvinar, the posterior nucleus and the nucleus lateralis posterior of the thalamus.

After defining the part of the LGN containing labelled neurons, sample fields were selected within which the HRP cells and the Nissl-stained, but unlabelled, cells were measured. Measurement was done by tracing the soma with the aid of a microscope drawing tube onto a digital graphics tablet (Tektronix 4953), the output of which was interfaced to a Nova 2 computer. In this way the cross-sectional area of sampled cells was calculated, and data stored for subsequent statistical analysis and display. Cells were measured only from laminae A and A1; the extreme lateral part of lamina A, projecting to the monocular part of the visual cortex and receiving its afferents from the monocular nasal portion of the retina, was avoided, as it is known that morphological (23) and physiological (44) changes after monocu-

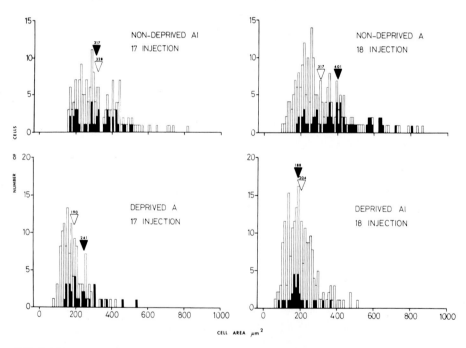

FIG. 7. Histograms of the distribution of the cross-sectional area of cells in laminae A and A1 of the LGN of a kitten monocularly deprived from the age of 1 week to 3 months. Open columns represent measurements of *all* cells sampled, and the black columns the cells which were marked by retrograde transport of HRP. The *open* and *filled* arrows indicate, respectively, the mean cell area of the *total* cells and the *HRP* cells. Note that there is a difference in overall cell size between normal and deprived laminae of some 30%. Cells filled by area 17 injection are of the same size as the total mean in the nondeprived lamina A1, and these cells (mainly X cells) are about 20% smaller in the deprived lamina A. After area 18 injection, marked Y cells are larger than the total population in the nondeprived lamina A, and are *50% smaller than normal Y cells* in the deprived lamina A1. The distribution of these very small deprived Y cells is also much more restricted than the normal distribution of Y cells. A schematic summary of these results is given in Fig. 8.

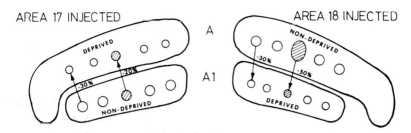

FIG. 8. Summary diagram of the findings of the experiments described here. Laminae A and A1 of the LGN are shown: open and hatched circles represent, respectively, neurons unlabelled and labelled with HRP reaction product. It can be seen that the left lamina A and the right lamina A1 (deprived laminae) contain total cell populations which are 30% smaller than in the other lamina of the same side. The cells marked on the left (after area 17 injection) are presumably mainly X cells, and are only 20% smaller in the deprived lamina than in the nondeprived. Marked cells on the right (after area 18 injection: proposed Y cells) are very large in the nondeprived lamina; they are 50% smaller in the deprived lamina, where they are even smaller than the deprived X cells demonstrated in the opposite thalamus.

lar deprivation do not occur in these sites. The C complex was also avoided because of the possibility of input from the third group of retinal ganglion cells, the W cells (54) which perhaps innervate the C laminae (61) and were not the object of the present analysis. Samples were taken from lamina A1 and the binocular part of lamina A, and, as far as possible, the samples were similar between laminae as to the part of the visual field they represented. However, the samples could not always be exactly similar because the number of labelled neurons in a deprived lamina was generally considerably less than in the nondeprived lamina adjacent to it, an effect previously described by Thorpe and Blakemore (57). This phenomenon resulted in the proportion of labelled to unlabelled cells in any sample to vary, and therefore no conclusions can be drawn from this work as to the ratios of various cell types.

By comparing the areas of the cells, both labelled and unlabelled, measured in deprived and nondeprived laminae of the LGN, the efficacy of the monocular deprivation was ascertained: the deprived laminae contained neurons whose mean size was some 25 to 50% less than in the "normal" laminae (Figs. 7 and 8). When the cells filled from the injection in area 17 (probably, therefore, mainly X cells) were studied, it was seen that the mean size of the marked somata was similar to that of the unmarked ones (or, equally, of the total population of marked and unmarked cells). However, the mean size of cells filled from area 18 (the proposed Y cells) was significantly greater than that of the total population (Fig. 7). In the deprived laminae, after area 17 injection, labelled cells were larger than the overall population, but, after area 18 injection, were of similar size or slightly smaller than the total mean. A comparison of the sizes of the labelled cells revealed that deprived X cells filled from area 17 were significantly smaller than their nondeprived counterparts, but that the Y cells labelled by area

18 injection were *even smaller,* both compared with cells in the correspond-ing nondeprived laminae and, furthermore, with the deprived X cells filled by area 17 injection (Figs. 7 and 8). It can be seen from the histograms (Fig. 7) that the distribution of marked cells on the side of the injection in area 17 was not grossly different in the deprived lamina A from that in the normal lamina A1, although there was a slight fall in the mean and a tendency for the peak in the small cell population to be more marked. However, the histo-grams after area 18 injection (Y cells) reveal a dramatic change from a broad, fairly flat distribution in the *nondeprived* lamina A to a sharply peaked distribution restricted to the small cells in the *deprived* lamina A1 (Fig. 7).

CONCLUSIONS

In summary, in nondeprived laminae, the postulated X cells, or rather those somata labelled from area 17, which should include some Y cells also, were roughly of the same mean size as the overall LGN population, whereas the supposed Y cells were much larger. In deprived laminae, X cells *do* exhibit a failure to grow normally, but much less so than the Y cells, with the ultimate result that the Y cells become smaller than the X cells (Fig. 8). These results, then, support the findings of Sherman et. al. (44) that the Y cells of the LGN are more affected by monocular deprivation than the X cells. No evidence was found of cell *loss* in the deprived laminae.

It remains for the significance of the two parallel inputs to the visual cortex in the cat to be determined. That X and Y systems can also exist in animals with an LGN whose principal cells probably project *only* to area 17 has recently been shown in the rat (10), the monkey (38,46) and the tree shrew (45); this would suggest that the division of functional properties over more than one visual area by direct afferents from the LGN is not a prerequisite for the development of X and Y systems.

It is unclear why, in the cat, a separate branch of the Y system should project to area 18 and be probably its major subcortical afferent. An im-portant function of the Y input to the visual cortex is probably concerned with visuomotor coordination. Y cells have been implicated in motion detec-tion (31,52) and may innervate monosynaptically those complex cells in the cortex which send efferents to the superior colliculus (41), which, in turn, has an important role in visually guided behaviour (48). Area 18 also receives afferents from the nucleus lateralis posterior of the thalamus, itself in-nervated from the superior colliculus (20). Perhaps, therefore, area 18 is more suited to the gross detection of objects in the visual field, whereas area 17 is equipped for fine-grain analysis of the detected objects (58). Further, if, as seems likely from the results of the experiments described here, Y cells are more susceptible to deprivation than X cells, it could be that the Y system provides a more modifiable input from the visual world to the visual cortex than that derived from a relatively "hard-wired" X system (3): it may be that the main functional significance of Y cells is in their adaptive role.

ACKNOWLEDGMENT

This work was carried out in collaboration with Dr. Colin Blakemore of the Physiological Laboratory, University of Cambridge, and was supported by the Swiss National Science Foundation (3/2460/74) and the Medical Research Council of Great Britain (G/972/463/B). Exchange visits were made possible by grants from the European Training Programme in Brain and Behaviour Research and the Roche Research Foundation. M. Gissler and M. Dürsteler were responsible for computer programming and M. C. Cruz, R. M. Cummings, and B. Rhodes for technical help.

REFERENCES

1. Bilge, M., Bingle, A., Seneviratne, K. N., and Whitteridge, D. (1967): A map of the visual cortex in the cat. *J. Physiol. (Lond.)*, 191:116–118P.
2. Bishop, G. H., and Clare, M. H. (1955): Organization and distribution of fibers in the optic tract of the cat. *J. Comp. Neurol.*, 103:269–304.
3. Blakemore, C., and van Sluyters, R. C. (1975): Innate and environmental factors in the development of the kitten's visual cortex. *J. Physiol. (Lond.)*, 248:663–716.
4. Boycott, B. B., and Wässle, H. (1974): The morphological types of ganglion cells of the domestic cat's retina. *J. Physiol. (Lond.)*, 240:397–419.
5. Chow, K. L., and Stewart, D. L. (1972): Reversal of structural and functional effects of long-term visual deprivation in cats. *Exp. Neurol.*, 34:409–433.
6. Cleland, B. G., Dubin, M. W., and Levick, W. R. (1971): Sustained and transient neurones in the cat's retina and lateral geniculate nucleus. *J. Physiol. (Lond.)*, 217:473–496.
7. Dürsteler, M. R., Garey, L. J., and Movshon, J. A. (1976): Reversal of the morphological effects of monocular deprivation in the kitten's lateral geniculate nucleus. *J. Physiol. (Lond.)*, 189–210.
8. Enroth-Cugell, C., and Robson, J. G. (1966): The contrast sensitivity of retinal ganglion cells of the cat. *J. Physiol. (Lond.)*, 187:517–552.
9. Fukuda, Y. (1971): Receptive field organization of cat optic nerve fibers with special reference to conduction velocity. *Vision Res.*, 11:209–226.
10. Fukuda, Y. (1973): Differentiation of principal cells of the rat lateral geniculate body into two groups: Fast and slow cells. *Exp. Brain Res.*, 17:242–260.
11. Fukuda, Y., and Stone, J. (1974): Retinal distribution and central projections of Y-, X-, and W-cells of the cat's retina. *J. Neurophysiol.*, 37:749–772.
12. Fukuda, Y., and Stone, J. (1976): Evidence of differential inhibitory influences on X- and Y-type relay cells in the cat's lateral geniculate nucleus. *Brain Res.*, 113:188–196.
13. Garey, L. J., and Blakemore, C. (1977): Monocular deprivation: Morphological effects on different classes of neurons in the lateral geniculate nucleus. *Science*, 195:414–416.
14. Garey, L. J., Fisken, R. A., and Powell, T. P. S. (1973): Effects of experimental deafferentation on cells in the lateral geniculate nucleus of the cat. *Brain Res.*, 52:363–369.
15. Garey, L. J., and Powell, T. P. S. (1967): The projection of the lateral geniculate nucleus upon the cortex in the cat. *Proc. Roy. Soc. Lond. [Biol.]*, 169:107–126.
16. Garey, L. J., and Powell, T. P. S. (1971): An experimental study of the termination of the lateral geniculo-cortical pathway in the cat and monkey. *Proc. Roy. Soc. Lond. [Biol.]*, 179:41–63.
17. Gilbert, C. D., and Kelly, J. P. (1975): The projections of cells in different layers of the cat's visual cortex. *J. Comp. Neurol.*, 163:81–106.
18. Glickstein, M., King, R. A., Miller, J., and Berkley, M. (1967): Cortical projections from the dorsal lateral geniculate nucleus of cats. *J. Comp. Neurol.*, 130:55–76.

19. Graham, R. C., and Karnovsky, M. J. (1966): The early stages of absorption of injected horseradish peroxidase in the proximal tubules of mouse kidney: Ultrastructural cytochemistry by a new technique. *J. Histochem. Cytochem.*, 14:291–302.
20. Graybiel, A. (1972): Some extrageniculate visual pathways in the cat. *Invest. Ophthalmol.*, 11:322–332.
21. Guillery, R. W. (1966): A study of Golgi preparations from the dorsal lateral geniculate nucleus of the adult cat. *J. Comp. Neurol.*, 128:21–50.
22. Guillery, R. W. (1970): The laminar distribution of retinal fibers in the dorsal lateral geniculate nucleus of the cat: A new interpretation. *J. Comp. Neurol.*, 138:339–368.
23. Guillery, R. W., and Stelzner, D. J. (1970): The differential effects of unilateral lid closure upon the monocular and binocular segments of the dorsal lateral geniculate nucleus in the cat. *J. Comp. Neurol.*, 139:413–422.
24. Hayhow, W. R. (1958): The cytoarchitecture of the lateral geniculate body in the cat in relation to the distribution of crossed and uncrossed optic fibers. *J. Comp. Neurol.*, 110: 1–64.
25. Hoffmann, K. P. (1973): Conduction velocity in pathways from retina to superior colliculus in the cat; a correlation with receptive-field properties. *J. Neurophysiol.*, 36:409–424.
26. Hoffmann, K. P., and Stone, J. (1971): Conduction velocity of afferents to cat visual cortex: A correlation with cortical receptive field properties. *Brain Res.*, 32:460–466.
27. Hoffmann, K. P., Stone, J., and Sherman, S. M. (1972): Relay of receptive-field properties in dorsal lateral geniculate nucleus of the cat. *J. Neurophysiol.*, 35:518–531.
28. Hubel, D. H., and Wiesel, T. N. (1962): Receptive fields, binocular interaction and functional architecture in the cat's visual cortex. *J. Physiol. (Lond.)*, 160:106–154.
29. Hubel, D. H., and Wiesel, T. N. (1965): Receptive fields and functional architecture in two non-striate visual areas (18 and 19) of the cat. *J. Neurophysiol.*, 28:229–289.
30. Hubel, D. H., and Wiesel, T. N. (1970): The period of susceptibility to the physiological effects of unilateral eye closure in kittens. *J. Physiol. (Lond.)*, 206:419–436.
31. Ikeda, H., and Wright, M. J. (1972): Receptive field organization of "sustained" and "transient" retinal ganglion cells which subserve different functional roles. *J. Physiol. (Lond.)*, 227:769–800.
32. Kelly, J. P., and Gilbert, C. D. (1975): The projections of different morphological types of ganglion cells in the cat retina. *J. Comp. Neurol.*, 163:65–80.
33. Kupfer, C., and Palmer, P. (1965): Lateral geniculate nucleus: Histological and cytochemical changes following afferent denervation and visual deprivation. *Exp. Neurol.*, 9:400–409.
34. Laemle, L. K. (1975): Cell populations of the lateral geniculate nucleus of the cat as determined with horseradish peroxidase. *Brain Res.*, 100:650–656.
35. LaVail, J. H., and LaVail, M. M. (1972): Retrograde axonal transport in the central nervous system. *Science*, 176:1416–1417.
36. Leicester, J., and Stone, J. (1967): Ganglion, amacrine and horizontal cells of the cat's retina. *Vision Res.*, 7:695–705.
37. Maciewicz, R. J. (1975): Thalamic afferents to areas 17, 18 and 19 of cat cortex traced with horseradish peroxidase. *Brain Res.*, 84:308–312.
38. Marrocco, R. T. (1976): Sustained and transient cells in monkey lateral geniculate nucleus: Conduction velocities and response properties. *J. Neurophysiol.*, 39:340–353.
39. Niimi, K., and Sprague, J. M. (1970): Thalamo-cortical organization of the visual system in the cat. *J. Comp. Neurol.*, 138:219–250.
40. Otsuka, R., and Hassler, R. (1962): Über Aufbau und Gliederung der corticalen Sehsphäre bei der Katze. *Arch. Psychiatr. Neurol.*, 203:212–234.
41. Palmer, L. A., and Rosenquist, A. C. (1974): Visual receptive fields of single striate cortical units projecting to the superior colliculus in the cat. *Brain Res.*, 67:27–42.
42. Rossignol, S., and Colonnier, M. (1971): A light microscope study of degeneration patterns in cat cortex after lesions of the lateral geniculate nucleus. *Vision Res.*, Suppl 3: 329–338.
43. Sanides, F., and Hoffmann, J. (1969): Cyto- and myeloarchitecture of the visual cortex of the cat and of surrounding integration cortices. *J. Hirnforsch.*, 11:79–104.
44. Sherman, S. M., Hoffmann, K. P., and Stone, J. (1972): Loss of a specific cell type from dorsal lateral geniculate nucleus in visually deprived cats. *J. Neurophysiol.*, 35:532–541.

45. Sherman, S. M., Norton, T. T., and Casagrande, V. A. (1975): X- and Y- cells in the dorsal lateral geniculate nucleus of the tree shrew (Tupaia glis). *Brain Res.*, 93:152–157.
46. Sherman, S. M., Wilson, J. R., Kaas, J. H., and Webbe, S. V. (1976): X- and Y- cells in the dorsal lateral geniculate nucleus of the owl monkey (Aotus trivirgatus). *Science*, 192:475–477.
47. Singer, W., Tretter, F., and Cynader, M. (1975): Organization of cat striate cortex: A correlation of receptive-field properties with afferent and efferent connections. *J. Neurophysiol.*, 38:1080–1098.
48. Sprague, J. M., and Meikle, T. H. (1965): The role of the superior colliculus in visually guided behavior. *Exp. Neurol.*, 11:115–146.
49. Stone, J. (1965): A quantitative analysis of the distribution of ganglion cells in the cat's retina. *J. Comp. Neurol.*, 124:337–352.
50. Stone, J., and Dreher, B. (1973): Projection of X- and Y- cells of the cat's lateral geniculate nucleus to areas 17 and 18 of visual cortex. *J. Neurophysiol.*, 36:551–567.
51. Stone, J., and Freeman, R. B. (1971): Conduction velocity groups in the cat's optic nerve classified according to their retinal origin. *Exp. Brain Res.*, 13:489–497.
52. Stone, J., and Fukuda, Y. (1974): Properties of cat retinal ganglion cells: A comparison of W- cells with X- and Y- cells. *J. Neurophysiol.*, 37:722–748.
53. Stone, J., and Hoffmann, K. P. (1971): Conduction velocity as a parameter in the organisation of the afferent relay in the cat's lateral geniculate nucleus. *Brain Res.*, 32:454–459.
54. Stone, J., and Hoffmann, K. P. (1972): Very slow-conducting ganglion cells in the cat's retina: a major, new functional type? *Brain Res.*, 43:610–616.
55. Stone, J., and Holländer, H. (1971): Optic nerve axon diameters measured in the cat retina: some functional considerations. *Exp. Brain Res.*, 13:498–503.
56. Talbot, S. A. (1942): A lateral localization in the cat's visual cortex. *Fed. Proc.*, 1:84.
57. Thorpe, P. A., and Blakemore, C. (1975): Evidence for a loss of afferent axons in the visual cortex of monocularly deprived cats. *Neurosci. Lett.*, 1:271–276.
58. Tretter, F., Cynader, M., and Singer, W. (1975): Cat parastriate cortex: A primary or secondary area? *J. Neurophysiol.*, 38:1099–1113.
59. Wiesel, T. N., and Hubel, D. H. (1963): Effects of visual deprivation on morphology and physiology in the cat's lateral geniculate body. *J. Neurophysiol.*, 26:978–993.
60. Wilson, M. E., and Cragg, B. G. (1967): Projections from the lateral geniculate nucleus in the cat and monkey. *J. Anat.*, 101:677–692.
61. Wilson, P. D., and Stone, J. (1975): Evidence of W- cell input to the cat's visual cortex via the C laminae of the lateral geniculate nucleus. *Brain Res.*, 92:472–478.

Architectonics of the Cerebral Cortex,
edited by M. A. B. Brazier and H. Petsche.
Raven Press, New York © 1978.

Identification and Localisation of Some Relay Cells in Cat Visual Cortex

D. Sanides and *F. Donate-Oliver

Abteilung für Neurobiologie, Max Planck-Institut für Biophysikalische Chemie, D-3400 Göttingen, Federal Republic of Germany

In recent years injection of horseradish peroxidase (HRP) has been successfully employed for retrograde labelling of cell bodies of relay cells with axonal terminations in the site of injection. It thus was possible to identify in monkey striate cortex type and location of cell bodies of neurons with different corticocortical or subcortical projections (6,15,16). Neurons with a common axonal projection were shown to be localized in the same cytoarchitectonic layer(s) or even sublayer(s) and to have similarly shaped cell bodies and dendritic fields. The question arises whether a similar kind of specialization is found in surrounding visual areas and in visual areas of other species.

In cat visual cortex, Maciewicz (7) and Gilbert and Kelly (1) have demonstrated that some pyramidal cells in layers (L) II and III project to surrounding visual areas. The target of the majority of L II–III cells, however, is still unknown. Medium to large pyramidal cells in L V have been found to project to the superior colliculus (1,2,8), and a few may also project to the dorsal lateral geniculate nucleus (LGNd) (3). More than 50% of the neurons in L VI of areas 17, 18, and 19 appear to project to the LGNd (1,3,12). L VI neurons in the Clare-Bishop area, however, may also have axonal endings in areas 17 and 18 (1).

PONTINE PROJECTION

Following HRP injections into the pontine nuclei of cats, we found cells containing fine dark HRP granules, typical for retrograde labelling, exclusively in L V (Fig. 1). They were extremely rare in the lateral gyrus (areas 17 and 18), but more common in the lateral wall of the lateral sulcus (area 19), the suprasylvian gyrus and sulcus (including the Clare-Bishop area). Another accumulation of HRP-labelled cells was found in the splenial gyrus.[1]

---

* *Present address: Departamento c. Morfologicas, C.U. Soria, Soria, Spain.*
[1] See Sanides et al. (11) for detailed descriptions of experiments with HRP injections in the pontine nuclei.

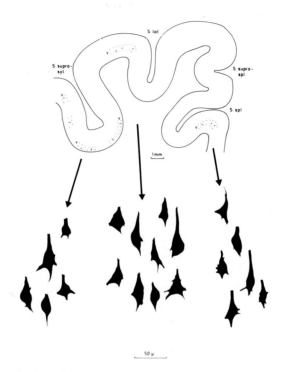

FIG. 1. Drawing of a frontal 60-μm section through cat visual regions with peroxidase-containing cells following pons injection represented by dots. Layer V is indicated by broken lines. Below are camera lucida drawings of the peroxidase-labelled cells from this and one adjacent section. **S. supra-syl.,** suprasylvian sulcus; **S. lat.,** lateral sulcus; **S. supra-spl.,** suprasplenial sulcus; **S. spl.,** splenial sulcus.

All of these cells belonged to the pyramidal type with thick apical dendrite. Their cell body was medium sized or large (relative to surrounding Nissl-stained perikarya) and often quite slender, almost spindle-shaped. The density of labelled cells was very low. We never found more than a dozen cells in a single 60 μm section in this region.

GENICULATE PROJECTION

In contrast to the pontine projection, cells projecting to the LGNd are very numerous and extremely densely clustered in areas 17, 18, and 19 as shown by some large test injections in the LGNd (Fig. 2). Our results agree with previous findings (see above) that the majority of L VI cells have axon terminals in the LGNd. Most of them could be classified as pyramidal by their conspicuous apical dendrite. Their perikarya usually were small round, pear-shaped, or triangular. In addition we found some larger pyramidal cells with perioxidase in L V, similar to Holländer (3). One reason for the inconsistent findings concerning involvement of L V pyramids in the genicu-

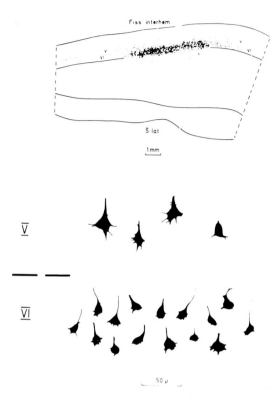

FIG. 2. Drawing of a horizontal 60-μm section through the lateral gyrus of the cat with peroxidase-containing cells following injection of the lateral geniculate body represented by dots. The L V to L VI boundary is indicated by the broken line. Below are camera lucida drawings of a few peroxidase-labelled cells of L V and VI of this region. **Fiss. interhem.,** interhemispheric fissure; **S. lat.,** lateral sulcus.

late projection may be differences in size and differences in location of the HRP injections within the lateral geniculate. Possibly these cells project only to a subnucleus of the LGN or to a neighbouring region such as the pulvinar as in the monkey (6). This question has to be settled by further investigations with small HRP injections.

COMMISSURAL PROJECTION

In another series of experiments we studied cells with commissural projections in cat visual cortex. In order to get a rough picture of this projection, we made large unilateral HRP injections into the visual cortex. The injection extended from the top of the lateral gyrus down to the bottom of the splenial sulcus. The enzyme had diffused through most parts of areas 17, 18, and somewhat into area 19 as well as the cortex in the splenial sulcus. As other authors have pointed out, however, the peripheral zone of dif-

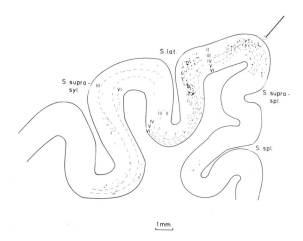

FIG. 3. Drawing of a frontal 60-μm section through cat visual regions with peroxidase-containing cells following contralateral lateral gyrus injection represented by dots. Some of the layers are indicated by broken lines. See Fig. 1 for abbreviations. The arrow points to the areal limit between areas 17 and 18.

fusion is probably not significant for retrograde labelling, rather the zone immediately surrounding the track of the injection needle [for an extensive discussion of these technical problems see Lund et al. (6)].

Figure 3 shows the outlines of a typical 60-μm section contralateral to the site of injection[2] with all HRP-labelled cells represented by dots and the laminar boundaries, as seen after Nissl counterstaining, indicated by broken lines. Two large dense clusters of cells were labelled, on top of the lateral gyrus (around the limit between areas 17 and 18) and on the medial bank of the lateral sulcus (in area 19). Besides, numerous labelled cells were located on the medial bank of the suprasylvian sulcus (Clare-Bishop area). A few labelled cells were scattered throughout the suprasylvian gyrus. In addition, a small group of cells in the bottom of the splenial sulcus contained peroxidase.

Most HRP-labelled cells lay in the lower part of L III. However, a few cells were found more superficially and some in the deeper layers as well. The laminar distribution and typology of cells differed somewhat between the three main cell foci: In the lateral gyrus on both sides of the 17–18 areal boundary, labelled cells were encountered from the upper part of L III through L VI (Fig. 4). Most of them lay in L III close to L IV, were typical pyramidal cells, and were usually quite large. More superficial and deeper pyramids usually were smaller. In L VI some cells with rather small round cell bodies were labelled which appear to represent the typical L VI pyramidal and spindle cells as seen in Golgi-stained material (9,12).

The most remarkable feature of this region, however, were neurons in

---

[2] The level of the section corresponds approximately to Horsley Clarke Anterior 7.

L III and IV with rounded perikarya without a conspicuous apical dendrite and numerous, usually very fine dendrites radiating in all directions (Fig. 4). Their size relative to the surrounding pyramidal perikarya was small to medium. All these features would characterize typical stellate cells (4,9,10). Unfortunately, the HRP labelling was not sufficient to distinguish dendritic spines. Thus, a distinction between "spiny" and "nonspiny stellates" was not possible. However, only "spiny stellate" cells have been found to send their axon toward the white matter (4,5). Thus, these cells probably belong to the "spiny stellate" type.

On the medial bank of the lateral sulcus (area 19) the distribution of cells was similar as at the area 17–18 boundary (Fig. 3). Here, however, almost exclusively pyramidal cells contained enzyme granules (Fig. 5). No cells were encountered which would appear definitely as stellate type cells. In addition to the small pyramidal and spindle cells, L VI here contained some horizontal cells, similar to those which Tömböl et al. (12) found in this layer in Golgi-impregnated material.

On the medial bank of the suprasylvian sulcus, HRP-labelled cells were

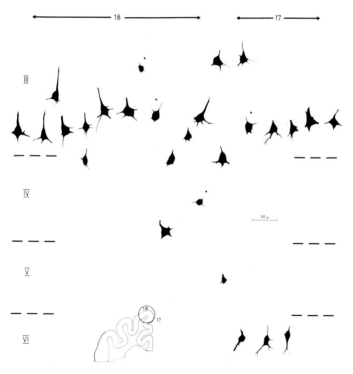

FIG. 4. Camera lucida drawings of representative HRP-labelled cells of Fig. 3 in the lateral gyrus (areas 17 and 18; see inset). The extent of the two areas is indicated by the arrows on the top. Cortical layers are indicated by broken lines and roman numerals on the sides. Stellate-type cells are marked by small stars.

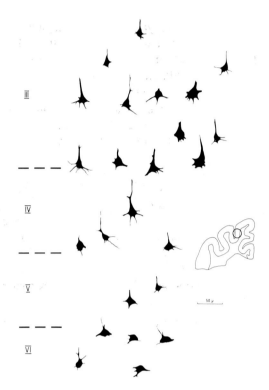

FIG. 5. Camera lucida drawings of representative HRP-labelled cells of Fig. 3 in the medial bank of the lateral sulcus (area 19; see inset). Cortical layers are indicated by broken lines and roman numerals on the side.

less numerous than in the other regions (Fig. 3). Besides, their laminar distribution was different since they occurred mainly in two layers, III and VI, in the latter frequently at the L V boundary (Fig. 6). In L III only pyramidal cells contained HRP granules. Their size varied from medium to large, the large ones being restricted to the deep part of L III. In L VI several HRP-labelled cell types were encountered: (a) pyramidal cells, mainly at the L V boundary, (b) a few spindle cells, and (c) a few horizontal cells. The most distinctive features of this region, however, are the large number of labelled (d) *inverted pyramids* with a thick apical dendrite descending toward the white matter, whereas thin dendrites extend upward from the base of the cell body. Similar cells were described by Tunturi (13) as "special auditory cells" in the dog and by van der Loos (14) as "improperly oriented" pyramidal cells in visual cortex of several mammals.

These preliminary results on commissural projections indicate that cortical relay cells with commissural projections may be located in different layers and may belong to different cell types in different cortical areas.

The observed HRP-labelled stellate-type cells contralateral to the site of

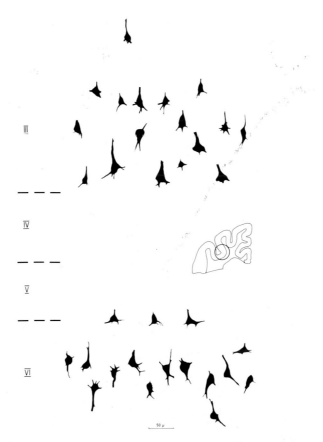

FIG. 6. Camera lucida drawings of representative HRP-labelled cells of Fig. 3 in the medial bank and bottom of the suprasylvian sulcus (Clare-Bishop area; see inset). Cortical layers are indicated by broken lines and roman numerals on the sides.

injection indicate that stellate cells may have a commissural projection. Hitherto stellate cells have always been considered to be short axon cells (Golgi II) with solely local intracortical axonal ramification. Only for the so-called "spiny stellates" the full extent of the axon has never been shown. In view of the present results one should look if some "spiny stellates" really are long axon cells. An alternative explanation for the HRP content of these cells is that they received the enzyme transsynaptically from neighbouring pyramidal cells. However, so far a transsynaptic transport of HRP has not been demonstrated.

ACKNOWLEDGMENT

We would like to thank Mrs. E. Hoeps for her technical assistance and Mrs. C. Rauschenbach for her help in preparing the figures.

REFERENCES

1. Gilbert, C. D., and Kelly, J. P. (1975): The projections of cells in different layers of the cat's visual cortex. *J. Comp. Neurol.*, 163:81–105.
2. Holländer, H. (1974): On the origin of the corticotectal projections in the cat. *Exp. Brain Res.*, 21:433–439.
3. Holländer, H. (1976): On the origin of corticofugal projections in the visual system. In: *Afferent and Intrinsic Organization of Laminated Structures in the Brain*, edited by O. Creutzfeldt. Springer Verlag, Berlin.
4. LeVay, S. (1973): Synaptic patterns in the visual cortex of the cat and monkey. Electron microscopy of Golgi preparations. *J. Comp. Neurol.*, 150:53–86.
5. Lund, J. S., and Boothe, R. G. (1975): Interlaminar connections and pyramidal neuron organization in the visual cortex, area 17, of the macaque monkey. *J. Comp. Neurol.*, 159:305–334.
6. Lund, J. S., Lund, R. D., Hendrickson, A. E., Bunt, A. H., and Fuchs, A. F. (1975): The origin of efferent pathways from primary visual cortex area 17, of the macaque monkey as shown by retrograde transport of horseradish peroxidase. *J. Comp. Neurol.*, 164:287–303.
7. Maciewicz, R. J. (1974): Afferents to the lateral suprasylvian gyrus of the cat traced with horseradish peroxidase. *Brain Res.*, 78:139–143.
8. Magalhães-Castro, H. H., Saraiva, P. E. S., and Magalhães-Castro, B. (1975): Identification of corticotectal cells of the visual cortex of cats by means of horseradish peroxidase. *Brain Res.*, 83:474–479.
9. O'Leary, J. L. (1941): Structure of the area striata of the cat. *J. Comp. Neurol.*, 75:131–164.
10. Sanides, D., and Sanides, F. (1974): A comparative Golgi study of the neocortex in insectivores and rodents. *Z. Mikrosk. Anat. Forsch.*, 88:957–977.
11. Sanides, D., Albus, K., and Donate-Oliver, F. (1977): Cells of origin of the visual cortico-pontine projection in the cat. *Pflugers Arch. [Suppl.]*, Vol. 368 (R 43):171.
12. Tömböl, T., Hajdu, F., and Somogyi, Gy. (1975): Identification of the Golgi picture of the layer VI cortico-geniculate projection neurons. *Exp. Brain Res.*, 24:107–110.
13. Tunturi, A. R. (1971): Classification of neurons in the ectosylvian auditory cortex of the dog. *J. Comp. Neurol.*, 142:153–166.
14. van der Loos, H. (1965): The "improperly" oriented pyramidal cell in the cerebral cortex and its possible bearing on problems of neuronal growth and cell orientation. *Bull. Johns Hopkins Hosp.*, 177:228–250.
15. Wong-Riley, M. T. T. (1974): Demonstration of geniculocortical and callosal projection neurons in the squirrel monkey by means of retrograde axonal transport of horseradish peroxidase. *Brain Res.*, 79:267–272.
16. Zeki, S. M. (1974): Functional organization of a visual area in the posterior bank of the superior temporal sulcus of the rhesus monkey. *J. Physiol. (Lond.)*, 236:549–573.

Architectonics of the Cerebral Cortex,
edited by M. A. B. Brazier and H. Petsche.
Raven Press, New York © 1978.

Localisation of Cortical Functions by Multiregional Measurements of the Cerebral Blood Flow

David H. Ingvar

Department of Clinical Neurophysiology, University Hospital, Lund, Sweden

The cerebral blood flow is normally controlled by the oxidative metabolism of the nervous tissue ("metabolic regulation of CBF") (12). Hence, measurements of the regional cerebral blood flow (rCBF) mirror regional functional changes in the brain. By means of multidetector devices and isotope techniques based upon residue detection (16), functional "landscapes" in the brain (7), or cerebral "ideograms" (8), can be recorded at rest and during different forms of sensory-motor and mental activity.

METABOLIC REGULATION OF THE CEREBRAL BLOOD FLOW

A comprehensive survey of all factors involved in the metabolic regulation of rCBF cannot yet be made. Some factors appear normally to play subordinate roles, such as the cerebral vasomotor innervation. Potassium, and possibly also calcium ions, may influence the caliber of the brain vessels by their effects on the smooth muscle cells. However, it still appears that CO_2, generated by the active nerve cells and the main determinant of the extracellular pH, is the most important regulatory factor. An augmented neuronal activity increases the output of CO_2. This lowers the tissue pH, and vasodilatation is induced. Reduced activity gives a higher pH with vasoconstriction.

TECHNICAL CONSIDERATIONS

This chapter is based upon rCBF studies with the intraarterial ^{133}Xe clearance technique which has a high reproducibility (12). From regional clearance curves, different rCBF parameters can be calculated including the flow in grey matter compartments. It is this variable especially that demonstrates distinctly different regional patterns during various forms of brain activity in neurologically normal patients, as well as in patients with brain disorders (16). Recently, colour display systems have been devised with which cerebral ideograms based on regional flow measurements can be recorded (13,22).

THE NORMAL RESTING CEREBRAL IDEOGRAM

At rest, in undisturbed neurologically normal subjects awake, the ideogram of the dominant hemisphere shows typical features. The flow (activity level) is about 10 to 30% higher in premotor and frontal regions as compared to the hemisphere mean, and correspondingly lower in postcentral structures, especially temporally. This *hyperfrontal* pattern is highly reproducible, provided measuring conditions of rest are rigidly observed (15). It is easily changed by procedures that alter the sensory-motor situation or the mental activity of the subject studied (see below) (5).

Using concepts mainly developed by Luria (17), the cerebral ideogram of resting consciousness signals a high activity in efferent parts of the hemisphere, situated anterior to the sylvian-rolandic fissures. These regions are responsible for programming and synthesis of behaviour in its widest sense. Apparently, even when one is awake, there is a high activity in these parts of the brain, a finding which indicates that resting wakefulness may imply "simulation" of behaviour. The low activity level in postcentral efferent structures may imply that normally, at rest, these parts of the brain are exposed to inhibition (21).

SENSORY-MOTOR AND SPEECH IDEOGRAMS

An increased sensory input, up to levels of slight pain (without overt behavioural or motor responses), augments the mean hemisphere flow level, but the hyperfrontal flow distribution of resting awareness is retained (14) (Fig. 1).

In contrast, voluntary motor activity, such as rhythmic clenching of the fist, augments the rCBF over the contralateral rolandic field (Fig. 2). At the same time the activity may fall somewhat in frontal structures. Distinct local activations of other parts within the cortical homunculus chart can also be recorded (18,20).

During speech, a more widespread activation of the dominant hemisphere takes place, involving the upper, anterior, and posterior speech cortices, as well as motor structures for face–tongue–larynx (Fig. 3). During reading there is, in addition, an occipital activation (15).

MENTAL ACTIVITY

Problem solving, reasoning, and motor ideation, all constituting various types of abstract mentation, not accompanied by any, or at least very limited behavioural changes and motor events, induce an activation especially of premotor and frontal regions. If the mentation is of the verbal type it appears that temporal and sylvian regions are also activated (7,8).

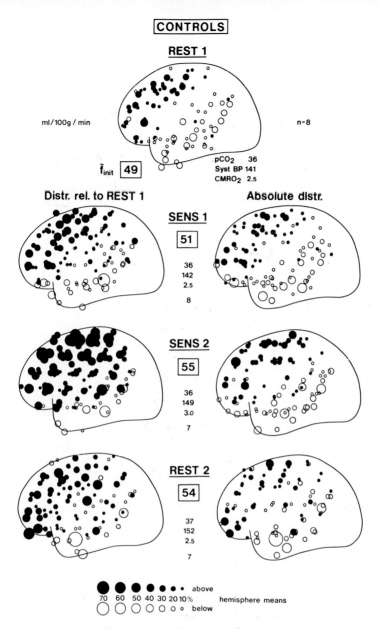

FIG. 1. Sensory ideograms. Diagrams of the distribution of the blood flow in the left hemisphere in eight neurologically normal subjects at rest, during weak electrical stimulation of the right frontal area **(SENS 1),** and during a stronger stimulation of the same region with an intensity giving discomfort and/or slight pain **(SENS 2).** It is seen that weak stimulation ("touch") of the contralateral thumb gave a small increase of the mean flow, while pain gave a significant increase ($p < 0.05$). During pain, the $CMRO_2$ also increased from 2.5 to 3.0 ml/100 g/min, a significant change ($p < 0.05$). Two sets of diagrams are shown. **To the left:** The flow distributions have been plotted, using the resting mean (49 ml/100 g/min) as a reference. It is seen that this type of plot shows the generalized aspects of the flow increase during touch and slight pain. **To the right:** The flow distributions have been plotted in relation to the new higher levels. It is then seen that the resting "hyperfrontal" flow distribution is retained in the two situations with weak and strong cutaneous stimulation (14). See Fig. 2.

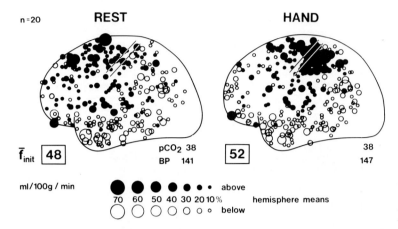

FIG. 2. Example of cerebral motor ideogram. Superimposed diagrams of rCBF measurements in 20 subjects at rest **(left)** and during voluntary clenching of the right hand **(right).** The mean flow in the two situations is given in boxes (48 and 52 ml/100 g/min calculated as f_{init} values from the initial part of the clearance curves). In the diagram, flows above the individual hemisphere mean flows have been denoted in black circles and flows below the mean in open circles, in accordance with the scale given at the bottom of the diagram. Note that at rest there is a clear-cut predominance of higher flows in structures situated anterior to the sylvian-rolandic fissure. The lowest flows were recorded in temporal regions as well as parietooccipitally. During voluntary hand movements the resting ideogram changed dramatically and a clear-cut flow peak was seen over the hand area in the rolandic region and also in postcentral and parietal areas. At the same time there was a moderate flow decrease in frontal structures (5).

ABNORMAL PATTERNS

Organic brain disorders alter the normal cerebral ideograms described above. On the whole, brain lesions, not only diffuse ones, reduce the mean hemisphere flow (activity) level. In addition, regional flow (activity) reductions are recorded in regions where focal lesions have occurred. Multiregional rCBF measurements can thus be used to quantify the functional state of telencephalic structures, e.g., in patients with *chronic traumatic brain lesions* (10).

A number of clinical studies with the rCBF technique have been devoted to *cerebrovascular lesions* caused by hemorrhage or thrombosis. The acute phase is often characterized by a vasoparalysis with cerebral hyperemia at the site of the lesion where the normal autoregulation of the cerebrovascular resistance is lost (19). In chronic patients, the low level of hemisphere flow often parallels in a striking fashion the loss of higher functions, and regional flow reductions can often be clearly related to focal neurological symptoms.

In *focal cortical epilepsy* rCBF studies have revealed regions of hyperemia within the epileptogenic focus (4,6). Such findings have been made also in cases with normal neurological findings and without abnormalities in neuroradiological and brain-scanning investigations, as well as—in some cases—with a normal EEG. These studies indicate that the rCBF technique

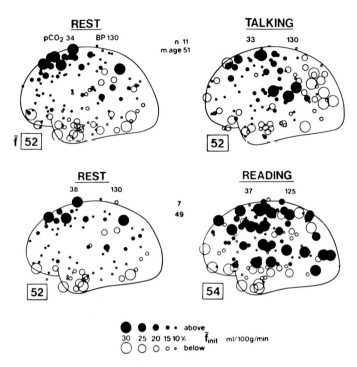

FIG. 3. Two series of cerebral speech ideograms are shown. **a:** Eleven normal subjects measured at rest and during "automatic speech" (enumeration of weekdays or months). **b:** Seven subjects measured at rest and during reading of a neutral text. The ideograms of talking and reading differed substantially from those at rest (plotted in absolute terms in relation to the actual means during talking and reading, respectively). In both situations, the highest flows were recorded over the premotor, the middle rolandic, and the posterior sylvian regions. Note that during talking (with closed eyes) the flow in occipital parts decreased, while it was higher in this region during reading. Symbols as in Fig. 2. (Replotted from ref. 15.)

may be used with great advantage even for diagnostic purposes in focal cortical epilepsy. Possibly also flow measurements during induction of focal seizures may reveal new aspects of the spread of epileptic discharge in the cerebral cortex.

In *organic dementia* (Fig. 4) with loss of neurons due to primary degenerative disorders or disseminated cerebrovascular lesions, the cerebral oxygen uptake, and secondarily the cerebral blood flow, is reduced. The distribution of the flow decrease also correlates in a meaningful way with the subsymptoms of dementia. Memory deficits are accompanied by a temporal decrease, agnostic symptoms by a flow reduction in occipitoparietotemporal regions, etc. (11). Regions with the lowest flows show the most marked loss of neurons (1).

Chronic schizophrenia with its well-known perceptual and behavioural symptoms differs from organic mental disorders by its lack of cerebral morphological changes. In addition, the *mean* brain metabolism and blood

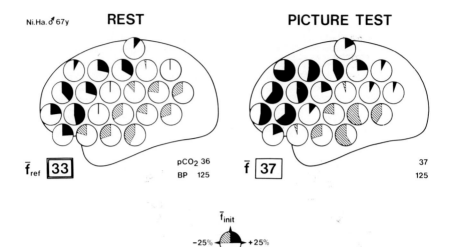

FIG. 4. Organic dementia. Cerebral ideograms obtained from a 67-year-old man who had suffered from increasing memory disturbances and confusion for the last 3 years. At the time of the rCBF study he had great difficulties in recognizing people and he could not read. At rest **(left diagram)** the flow distribution showed a decrease of the mean flow (33 ml/100 g/min; normal value 55). The distribution was in principle normal ("hyperfrontal"). However, the difference between the high-flow region in anterior parts of the brain and in posterior parts was more marked than normally (normally about 20%, here about 40 to 60%), indicating an ischemic region in the temporooccipital part. During a picture test **(right diagram)** an activation was seen in frontal part, but the flow in temporal occipital decreased even further. The patient could only recognize a few of the pictures shown, with great difficulty. At the bottom of the figure, the symbols used are explained. In every detector field 12 o'clock denotes the hemisphere mean flow. Values *above* the mean are shown in *black;* 25% above equal to 3 o'clock. Flow values *below* the mean are shown as *hatched* sectors; 25% below the mean equal to 9 o'clock.

flow remain normal even in deteriorated cases. However, the flow (activity) distribution in the dominant hemisphere measured with the rCBF technique is "reversed," showing a (*hypofrontal*) pattern with low frontal, and high postcentral flows, correlating to autism/inactivity and to cognitive disturbances, respectively (2,3,9). Both in organic dementia and in schizophrenia there are, furthermore, deviations from the normal rCBF changes during mental activation.

These findings indicate that rCBF measurements—at rest and during activation procedures—may be used to study the pathophysiological background of mental disorders even of those lacking a specific morphological substrate.

CONCLUDING REMARKS

The studies summarized above have conclusively demonstrated that the cerebral blood flow is not constant. Although the mean hemisphere flow level may only change to a limited extent, important regional alterations take place, often amounting to 50% or more, as related to the resting level during *physiological* changes of brain functions accompanying sensory-motor and mental activity. Such changes lead to a redistribution of flow from inactive to active regions. This takes place by means of inherent tissue mechanisms responsible for the metabolic regulation of the cerebral blood flow.

In general, the observations made in neurologically normal patients who have undergone routine measurements of rCBF have confirmed many classic concepts on the functions of the cerebral cortex. Here one may first mention the clear-cut and regional activation of rolandic structures during voluntary motor activity. With the aid of rCBF measurements, one can say that the homunculus chart has been confirmed with physiological methods. Also the observations during speech should be mentioned. In principle they have confirmed that automatic uncomplicated formulation of repetitive well-known words activates in the dominant hemisphere the speech cortices as well as sensory-motor centres within the face–mouth–larynx region.

However, the regional blood flow studies have revealed several new and interesting details of the dynamic interaction between larger cortical fields during various forms of brain activity. Here one may first recall the unex-pected observation that the resting cerebral ideogram in a conscious awake subject shows such a typical distribution of flow/activity. Elsewhere (5,7,8), the functional implications of this pattern have been discussed. Apparently, resting consciousness implies a high activity in efferent-motor parts of the cerebral cortex, responsible for programming behaviour in its widest sense. This might indicate that resting consciousness constitutes some type of "simulation" of behaviour. Evidence has also been summarized above that this pattern is amplified, i.e., the general activity level of the hemisphere is increased and with a retention of the hyperfrontal distribution of activity, in situations characterized by increased consciousness — awareness — during sensory stimulation and various forms of ideation.

Another aspect that as yet has not been fully elucidated is the finding that an increased sensory input appears in general to augment the activity more in efferent-motor structures precentrally than postcentrally. This again ap-pears paradoxical and so does the fact that voluntary motor activity pro-vokes a substantial activation of postcentral-parietal regions. This finding (the "sensory-motor paradox"; Ingvar, 1975) indicates that methods which measure mass activity in the brain ("brain work") may reveal a new aspect of the cortical functions. The observations mentioned indicate, for example, that it is not the reception of sensory stimulation which requires an increased brain work but the perceptual consequences and that these in their turn re-quire activation of centres which synthesize the behavioural response to the stimulation in question. Similarly, it appears as if the feedback sensory con-trol of voluntary motor activity may require a much larger metabolic brain work than the mere execution of the motor act via the precentral motor cortex.

It should be stressed that the results summarized here are few and should be looked upon as preliminary in several ways. The rCBF technique has, however, opened up a great new possibility for systematic studies of the functions of the cerebral cortex including its highest functions pertaining to mentation. However, present rCBF techniques yielding adequate and reproducible values are hampered by the fact that they require intracarotid injections of isotopes. Several attempts to substitute the isotope labelling of the brain with inhalation have been tried with some success. However, there are limitations caused by isotope contamination of extracerebral structures, and, in addition, the spatial resolution is also smaller than with the intraarterial technique.

At present, several attempts are being made to develop three-dimensional atraumatic techniques by means of which isotope clearance can be studied in all parts of the brain following inhalation of a suitable tracer. These techniques are principally related to computer tomography, which in recent years has come to dominate the neuroradiological field. Although there are no three-dimensional techniques for flow measurements available today for clinical routine studies, one can already envisage that techniques will be developed within a not-too-distant future. Then it will be possible to study in quantitative terms the interaction between superficial cortical structures and subcortical nuclei in the brainstem and spinal cord.

ACKNOWLEDGMENT

This work was supported by the Swedish Medical Research Council (Project No. B75-14X-00084-12A) and by the Wallenberg and Thuring Foundations, Stockholm.

REFERENCES

1. Brun, A., Gustafson, L., and Ingvar, D. H. (1976): Clinical symptoms, neuropathological findings and regional cerebral blood flow in Alzheimer's disease. *Acta. Neurol. Scand.* (*submitted for publication*).
2. Franzén, G., and Ingvar, D. H. (1975): Abnormal distribution of cerebral activity in chronic schizophrenia. *J. Psychiatr. Res.,* 12:199–214.
3. Franzén, G., and Ingvar, D. H. (1975): Absence of activation in frontal structures during psychological testing of chronic schizophrenics. *J. Neurol. Neurosurg. Psychiatry,* 38:1027–1032.
4. Hougaard, K., Oikawa, T., Sveinsdottir, E., Skinhøj, E., Ingvar, D. H., and Lassen, N. A. (1976): Regional cerebral blood flow in focal cortical epilepsy. *Arch. Neurol.,* 33:527–535.
5. Ingvar, D. H. (1975): Patterns of brain activity revealed by measurements of regional cerebral blood flow. In: *Brain Work,* edited by D. H. Ingvar, and N. A. Lassen, pp. 397–413. Munksgaared, Copenhagen.
6. Ingvar, D. H. (1975): rCBF in focal cortical epilepsy. In: *Cerebral Circulation and Metabolism,* edited by T. W. Langfitt, L. C. McHenry, Jr., M. Reivich, and H. Wollman, pp. 361–364. Springer-Verlag, New York.

7. Ingvar, D. H. (1976): Functional landscapes of the dominant hemisphere. *Brain Res.*, 107:181–197.
8. Ingvar, D. H. (1977): L'ideogramme cérébrale. *Encéphale,* 3:5–33.
9. Ingvar, D. H., and Franzén, G. (1974): Cerebral activity in chronic schizophrenia. *Lancet,* 2:1484–1485.
10. Ingvar, D. H., and Gadea Ciria, M. (1975): Assessment of severe damage to the brain by multi-regional measurements of cerebral blood flow. In: *Outcome of Severe Damage to the Central Nervous System.* CIBA Foundation Symposium 34, pp. 97–120. Elsevier, Amsterdam.
11. Ingvar, D. H., and Hagberg, B. (1976): Cognitive reduction in presenile dementia related to regional abnormalities of the cerebral blood flow. *Br. J. Psychiatry,* 128:209–222.
12. Ingvar, D. H., and Lassen, N. A. (Eds.) (1975): *Brain Work.* Munksgaard, Copenhagen.
13. Ingvar, D. H., and Philipson, L. (1977): Distribution of cerebral blood flow in the dominant hemisphere during motor ideation and motor performance. *Annals Neurol.,* 1 (*in press*).
14. Ingvar, D. H., Rosén, I., Elmqvist, D., and Eriksson, M. (1976): Activation patterns induced in the dominant hemisphere by skin stimulation. In: *Sensory Functions of the Skin,* edited by Y. Zotterman. Pergamon Press, London (*in press*).
15. Ingvar, D. H., and Schwartz, M. (1974): Blood flow patterns induced in the dominant hemisphere by speech and reading. *Brain,* 97:273–288.
16. Lassen, N. A., and Ingvar, D. H. (1972): Radioisotopic assessment of regional cerebral blood flow. In: *Progress in Nuclear Medicine,* edited by J. Potchen, and V. R. McCready, pp. 1/376–409. Karger, New York.
17. Luria, A. R. (1966): *Higher Cortical Functions in Man.* London, Tavistock Publications.
18. Olesen, J. (1971): Contralateral focal increase of cerebral blood flow in man during arm work. *Brain,* 94:635–646.
19. Paulson, O. B. (1971): Cerebral apoplexy (stroke): Pathogenesis, pathophysiology and therapy as illustrated by regional blood flow measurements in the brain. *Stroke,* 2:327–360.
20. Roland, P. E., and Larsen, B. (1976): Focal increase of cerebral blood flow during stereognostic testing in man. *Arch. Neurol.,* 33:551–558.
21. Skinner, J. E., and Lindsley, D. B. (1973): The non-specific mediothalamic frontocortical system: Its influence on electro-cortical activity and behaviour. In: *Psychophysiology of the Frontal Lobes,* edited by K. H. Pribram, and A. R. Luria, pp. 185–234. Academic Press, New York.
22. Sveinsdottir, E., Torlof, P., Risberg, J., Ingvar, D. H., and Lassen, N. A. (1971/72): Monitoring regional cerebral blood flow in normal man with a computer-controlled 32-detector system. *Eur. Neurol.,* 6:228–233.

Architectonics of the Cerebral Cortex,
edited by M. A. B. Brazier and H. Petsche.
Raven Press, New York © 1978.

EEG Coherence as a Measure of Cerebral Functional Organisation

J. C. Shaw, K. O'Connor, and C. Ongley

*M.R.C. Clinical Psychiatry Unit, Graylingwell Hospital,
Chichester, Sussex PO 19 4 PQ, England*

This paper presents some experimental results which replicate work that we have already published (20). The experiments are representative of our attempts to find a relationship between the electroencephalogram (EEG) and functional organisation in the brain. This work differs from almost all other presentations in this volume in that it uses human subjects and a noninvasive technique. Its relevance to these other contributions is to indicate one way in which their findings may come to be used in a practical way with clinical problems. Since our interest is in clinical psychiatry, it is appropriate to explain its relationship to the theme of this symposium.

CENTRAL FUNCTIONAL ORGANISATION AND PSYCHIATRIC DISORDER

There is accumulating evidence from several sources that in some psychiatric disorders there are anomalies of cerebral functional organisation. This is particularly so in the case of the psychoses, especially schizophrenia. The description "anomalies" rather than "abnormalities" is used for two reasons. First, there can be gross disturbances of behaviour in these cases without any signs of organic cerebral pathology. Second, the anomalies may be related to the type of functional organisation found in other individuals who show no signs of abnormal behaviour, but who have characteristics with lower than average incidence. An example is left-handedness.

Evidence for such functional anomalies have been discussed elsewhere (19,20), but some pertinent examples follow. The considerable evidence for a pathological involvement of the limbic system in schizophrenia has been reviewed by Torrey and Peterson (22), and Taylor's (21) finding of a specific class of lesion in patients with temporal lobe epilepsy who also develop psychosis is relevant. There is increasing evidence that such functional pathology may be lateralised to the left (dominant) hemisphere. Thus, Flor-Henry (9) discusses evidence that psychosis involves a dysfunction of the dominant hemisphere, while in neurosis the nondominant hemisphere is implicated. Lishman and McMeekan (14) found evidence for a less specific left hemisphere dominance in patients with a functional psychiatric disorder, and increased sinistrality in their patients appeared to be acquired rather than inherited. Using a variety of psychophysiological measures, Gruzelier and Hammond (11) conclude that "the dominant hemisphere of schizophrenics displays 'weak' nervous system dynamics." Beaumont and Dimond (3) have found that interhemisphere integration is impaired in schizophrenic patients. The significance for psychiatry of functional differences between the cerebral hemispheres has been fully reviewed by Galin (10). He showed how such differences may influence behaviour, give rise to abnormal behaviour, and also result in psychodynamic conflicts of behaviour.

It follows that the measurement of the characteristics of cerebral functional organisation may be of considerable importance for a biological development of psychiatry. It is our belief that the EEG may help with this measurement.

The conventional visual interpretation of clinical EEG records shows no specific difference between the records of psychiatric patients and those of normal individuals when patients with obviously organic or epileptic causes for their illnesses are excluded. Nevertheless, power spectral analysis can demonstrate group differences between the EEGs of psychiatric patients and normal control subjects. These differences are usually explained in terms of differing levels of activation or arousal. One of us has proposed an alternative explanation, namely that the differences are due to the anomalies of cerebral functional organisation in psychiatric patients suggested by the above evidence (19).

In summary, the presence of anomalies of cerebral functional organisation is a factor in psychiatric disorders and the EEG may be one way of detecting this in groups of individuals. The aim of our work is, therefore, to examine the relationships between the EEG and cerebral functional organisation more closely to see if it may be possible to use the EEG to make clinically useful inferences about the individual patient.

THE RELATION OF THE EEG TO ELECTROCORTICAL ACTIVITY

The EEG recorded from the scalp arises from electrical activity in the neurones of the cortex (6,8), although this may in turn be under the influence of the activity of deeper structures (16). The physical relationship between the scalp EEG and the electrocortical activity is such that only its gross features can be measured. This is in such contrast to the results obtained with histological or invasive techniques described in the other papers in this volume that it must be emphasised.

To detect significant EEG activity on the scalp, the underlying electrocortical activity must be synchronised over a wide area—about 6 sq cm according to Cooper et al. (4). In addition, the tissue between scalp surface and cortex is a sufficiently good volume conductor for the fields from different cortical areas to summate so that at best the scalp record is a rather gross average of the activity (4,7). Attempts to improve the resolution of scalp EEG measurement by spectral analysis shows even further sources of error. Thus, Pfurtscheller and Cooper (18) have shown that the amplitude of a particular frequency component on the scalp may also depend on its phase relationship at different parts of the cortex. Some propagated activity may not be visible at all on the scalp for this reason.

These physical aspects of the relationship of the scalp EEG to electro-cortical activity are in marked contrast to other electrophysiological studies in this volume. Lopes da Silva (15), for example, is able to examine the association between electrocortical activity from electrodes a few millimeters apart. Scalp EEG electrodes are invariably several centimeters apart and detect activity arising over a wide area.

A MODEL FOR THE STUDY OF EEG FUNCTIONAL ORGANISATION RELATIONSHIPS

The above considerations make it necessary to use a conceptual model for the study of EEG-cerebral functional organisation relationships, which is quite crude compared with those used for the similar study of cortico-cortical or thalamocortical associations. At present we use the classic model that the EEG arises from areas of cortex that are involved in synchronous electrical activity when they are at rest. Any area that is active because it is processing information becomes desynchronised. The regions involved in this functional aspect of EEG generation are probably limited to the second functional unit of Luria (17). A further characteristic is that there are areas of relatively independent synchrony so that the EEG is not composed of activity attributable to a single source of synchronisation, but to a topographic distribution of such sources. Thus, the common alpha rhythm activity of the EEG is not necessarily present as a unitary activity (5).

This model is in agreement with the compatible models of Elul (8) and Lopes da Silva (15), although they use much finer measurement resolution and relate to smaller cortical areas.

One inference made from this model is that an analysis of the topography of the EEG using the coherence function may be more valuable than an analysis by autospectra alone. It was postulated that the correlation between EEG activities from two areas at rest would change if one of these areas became active and therefore desynchronised. This is schematised in Fig. 1, which represents a section through a cortical slab and overlaying scalp. In Fig. 1a, the slab abc is at rest and giving rise to synchronous activity. The activity from the overlying electrode derivations will have contributions from the coherent activity in this slab, and from neighbouring regions whose activity is not coherent with it. If now the portion ab becomes

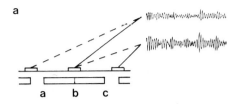

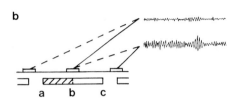

FIG. 1. Classic model of EEG generation. **a:** Cortical slab **abc** is at rest and generates synchronous activity. **b:** Part **ab** of cortex is active and desynchronised.

active and desynchronised, as in Fig. 1b, then the relative proportion of its contribution to the EEG signals in the two channels will change and so the correlation between the two signals will also change.

In practice, the correlation between pairs of signals is measured by the coherence function that computes correlation as a function of frequency. Coherence analysis is illustrated in Fig. 2. In Fig. 2a, a single noise generator N (t) is applied to two identical selective filters. The outputs of the filters are two identical narrow band noise signals and so the coherence between them is unity. If now the output from another noise generator n (t) is added in to one channel as in Fig. 2b, n (t) being independent of N (t), the coherence between the filter outputs is reduced. The model of Fig. 1

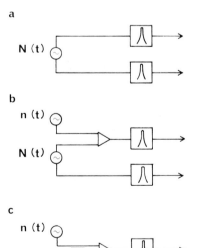

FIG. 2. Model for signal coherence. **n(t), N(t), and m(t)** are independent noise generators. The filters have identical characteristics. **a:** Output of filters has unity coherence for the filter pass band. **b:** Coherence of filter output is reduced because of independent noise **n(t)** added to one filter input. **c:** Generator model for EEG model of Fig. 1. **R** is an attenuator.

could then be represented by Fig. 2c in which N (t), n (t), and m (t) are independent noise generators and R is an attenuator. The output from filter 1 represents the activity of the electrodes overlying ab of Fig. 1 and the output of filter 2 that from the electrodes above bc. Desynchronisation of ab would be represented by an increase in the attenuation of R.

A comprehensive frequency analysis system for the PDP 12 computer has been developed by one of us (C.O.) to compute power spectra and coherence functions using the Fast Fourier Transform. Coherence as computed has the dimensions of a correlation coefficient squared. Both power spectra and coherence functions are derived as 15 term spectra from 2 to 30 Hz, each term with a bandwidth of nearly 2 Hz. The spectra may be appropriately averaged over any required number of EEG epochs. The validity of our use of this system has been tested empirically and will be described elsewhere (*in preparation*).

EXPERIMENTAL INVESTIGATION OF EEG-FUNCTIONAL ORGANISATION RELATIONSHIP

Introduction

The relationship between the EEG and cerebral function organisation has been investigated by studying subjects with differing hand preference. There is evidence that right-handed and left-handed individuals differ in this organisation (2,13). In the right-preferent individual, the left hemisphere is concerned with verbal activity and other serial forms of information processing, the right hemisphere with visuospatial activity and parallel processing generally. In left-preferent individuals, this lateralisation of function appears to be less specific. Beaumont (2) has suggested a model in which right preference is associated with a few large functional units of high specificity, whereas in left preference there are many smaller units of lower specificity.

Groups of right- and left-preferent individuals are thus representative of differing forms of cerebral functional organisation. It was hypothesized that the change in the topography of the EEG when the subjects carried out mental tasks would be different for the two groups. Two quite independent experiments to examine this hypothesis in such groups have now been carried out.

Method

Different subjects were used for the two experiments. In each experiment the subjects attended the laboratory on two occasions. Only for the second occasion were results of experiment I analysed; the first occasion was regarded as a laboratory acclimatisation session and it had a differing procedure. In experiment II, essentially the same procedure was used on both occasions so that reliability could be measured.

Subjects were selected for the right- and left-preferent groups on the basis of their scores on laterality questionnaires. In the first experiment this was Humphrey's questionnaire (12). For the second, a more detailed procedure was used and was composed of Annett's questionnaire (1), with additional questions designed by one of us (K.O.) to obtain a wider range of scores, and some manual performance tasks. These were Crawford's manual dexterity test, and tests that compared both hands for writing, grip strength, and finger-tapping speed. The manual tests were presented on both occasions, and all but the tapping test scores were found to be significantly reliable ($p \leq 0.05$).

EEGs were recorded with the subject sitting comfortably in a darkened room with eyes shut under three conditions presented in random order over subjects. (A further condition was included in the second occasion of experiment II but is not considered here.) The conditions were rest and mental arithmetic and spatial imagery tasks. The tasks were intended to involve the left and right hemispheres, respectively, in right-preferent subjects in accordance with the laterality model referred to above. They were presented in 5-sec trials with random intervals between, similar trials being marked during the rest condition.

The EEG was recorded with a common reference montage from FZ to C4, P4, O2, T4, and T6 on the right hemisphere and to C3, P3, O1, T3, and T5 on the left side (10–20 International System). The 10 channels and a trial marker signal were recorded on paper and on an analogue magnetic tape system. Subsequently, eight trials for each condition and eight channels of EEG were transferred to digital tape for analysis.

Further details of these and other aspects of the methodology have been published (20).

Results

When experiment I was carried out, it was anticipated that the intra-hemisphere coherence spectra would be the most interesting of the results and would enable us to test the model referred to above. However, Mr. O'Connor observed that the interhemisphere coherence in the alpha band changed from the rest to the task condition in a way that discriminated the right- and left-preferent groups, particularly for the parietal channels. It was primarily to test the reliability of this finding that experiment II was undertaken. The following results are, therefore, restricted to (a) the FZ-P4 and FZ-P3 EEG channels, and (b) alpha band measures obtained by appropriately combining the 8-, 10-, and 12-Hz frequency bands of our 15-term spectra. Power was summed over these spectral bands. Coherence values were found by taking the Z-transform of the square root of the computed coherence values and averaging these over the same spectral bands. The interhemisphere coherence change score referred to below is the task minus rest value of this transformed coherence. The results presented here are summarised in Tables 1 and 2.

TABLE 1. *Differences between right-preferent (R) and left-preferent (L) groups*

Experiment occasion group			Spatial imagery task				Mental arithmetic			
			Mean	SE	U	p	Mean	SE	U	p
Coherence change score										
I	2	R	0.082	0.030			0.040	0.043		
		L	−0.062	0.027	16	0.004	−0.069	0.041	21	0.01
II	1	R	0.035	0.023			0.037	0.030		
		L	−0.021	0.033	48	0.09	−0.002	0.045	76	0.37
II	2	R	0.052	0.038			0.058	0.024		
		L	−0.035	0.027	40	0.03	−0.069	0.037	24	0.003
Power change score										
I	2	R	0.017	0.089			−0.113	0.109		
		L	−0.040	0.076	46	0.17	−0.075	0.071	57	0.41
II	1	R	0.081	0.108			0.183	0.072		
		L	−0.015	0.048	63	0.30	0.078	0.058	56	0.12
II	2	R	0.034	0.098			0.015	0.121		
		L	−0.084	0.106	60	0.25	−0.036	0.149	75	0.43

Experiment I, N = 11 per group; II, N = 12 per group.
SE, standard error of mean.
U, Mann-Whitney U for test of difference between groups.
p, chance probability of the obtained value of U.

TABLE 2. *Correlation between EEG scores and laterality scores for right- (R) and left-preferent (L) groups, and for combined (R + L) groups*

Experiment occasion group			Coherence change score		Power change score	
			r_s	p	r_s	p
Laterality questionnaire						
I	2	R	0.691	0.014	−0.025	0.47
		L	−0.263	0.210	−0.200	0.26
		R + L	0.755	0.0005	0.102	0.32
II	2	R	0.474	0.05	0.007	0.49
		L	−0.242	0.22	0.156	0.30
		R + L	0.677	0.0007	−0.153	0.23
Manual dexterity score						
		R	0.753	0.006	−0.019	0.47
		L	0.587	0.025	−0.343	0.13
		R + L	0.561	0.004	0.142	0.25

Experiment I, N = 11 per group; II, N = 12 per group.
r_s, Spearman rank correlation coefficient.
p, chance probability of obtained value of r_s.

Experiment I

Each group contained 11 subjects and there are two main findings from this experiment (20). The first was that the change in interhemisphere coherence from rest to task (FZ-P2/FZ-P3) discriminated the two groups. Not only was the difference between the two groups statistically significant (Mann-Whitney $U = 16$, $p = 0.004$ for spatial imagery; $U = 21$, $p = 0.01$ for mental arithmetic), but the direction of change tended to be different for the two groups. Thus, in the case of the spatial imagery task, 8 of the 11 right-preferent subjects showed an increase in interhemisphere alpha coherence and 8 of the 11 left-preferent showed a decrease. Of the six individuals who did not fit this pattern of sign of change, all but one had relatively lower scores on the laterality questionnaire than the remaining subjects. This led to the second main finding. Within each group, subjects were divided into two classes determined by the score on the Humphrey questionnaire. We found that the higher laterality scores were associated with a positive interhemisphere change in the right-preferent and with a negative change in the left-preferent subjects. (Fisher exact probability test, $p = 0.011$.)

Further evidence for such an association in the data of experiment I has been found since the above results were published. Within each group, the correlation between the coherence change scores and the laterality scores was only significant for the right-preferent group (right-preferent group, $p = 0.014$; left-preferent group, $p \leqslant 0.2$). However, the groups were combined in the following way. The sinistrality scores were considered to be on the same continuum as the dexterity scores, but having a negative sign. This is valid because a dextral or sinistral score is the number of questions scoring "right" or "left" divided by the total number. Thus, the sinistrals could have a dextral score of unity minus their sinistrality score. It does not change the rank order of the laterality scores but may change the rank order of the EEG scores and also increases the number of degrees of freedom. Spearman's rank-order correlation coefficient for this combined group was highly significant ($r_s = 0.759$, $p \leqslant 0.0005$).

The above results relate to the spatial imagery task. Similar, but statistically less significant results, were obtained for the mental arithmetic task.

Power spectral measures were compared with the coherence measures by calculating the difference in alpha band power between the parietal electrodes and measuring how this changed during the task conditions. This power change score did not discriminate between the groups, or relate to the laterality scores.

Thus, our main finding of experiment I was an association between an EEG measure (the change in interhemisphere coherence from task to rest), and a behavioral measure (a laterality score), related to functional organisation in the brain.

Experiment II

Experiment II was a replication to test the reliability of the above findings. There were 12 subjects in each group. The design and method were essentially the same as experiment I except as indicated in the method section above. The results are presented for the first time here and are again restricted to those from the parietal channels, FZ-P4, FZ-P3, and the alpha frequency band.

There were two main comparisons that could be made between experiments I and II to test the reliability of the results of experiment I. The first of these was to see if the interhemisphere coherence change scores obtained on the second occasion of experiment II discriminate between the groups as was the case in experiment I. Considering only the spatial task, we found that the score was again positive in 8 of the 12 right-preferent and negative in 8 of the 12 left-preferent subjects. The scores differed significantly between the two groups (Mann-Whitney $U = 40, p = 0.032$).

In the second comparison, the association between the laterality scores and the coherence change scores was examined. Taking the questionnaire scores alone (i.e., excluding the manual dexterity scores) the association within groups was again only significant for the right-preferent group. But combining the groups as before resulted in a significant association (Spearman's rank-order correlation coefficient $r_s = 0.677, p \leq 0.0007$). In the case of the manual dexterity scores, there was a clear association with the coherence change scores within the groups when these scores were combined, excluding the finger-tapping test (right-preferent group, $r_s = 0.753$, $p = 0.006$; left-preferent group, $r_s = 0.587, p = 0.025$).

The subjects in experiment II experienced the same conditions on two occasions. The reliability of their scores could therefore be determined. On the first occasion 9 of the 12 right-preferent subjects had a positive interhemisphere change score and in 8 of the 12 left-preferent subjects it was negative. Thus, the score of one right-preferent subject changed from positive to negative from the first to the second occasion, but his first occasion score was quite low. In five of the left-preferent group, the score changed sign between occasions, and again these were the subjects with the relatively lower scores. The difference between groups on the first occasion was not significant, but was in the expected direction (Mann-Whitney $U = 48, p = 0.09$).

The consistency over the two occasions of subjects' coherence change scores was determined, again using Spearman's rank correlation coefficient. There was a significant correlation between occasions (right-preferent group, $r_s = 0.66, p = 0.014$; left-preferent group, $r_s = 0.53, p = 0.04$; combined groups $r_s = 0.623, p = 0.0014$).

The above results describe the change from rest produced by the spatial imagery task. The mental arithmetic task resulted in similar changes on the second occasion, but the difference between groups was not significant on the first occasion (first occasion $U = 76$, $p = 0.37$; second occasion $U = 24$, $p - 0.0028$). On the second occasion, 9 of the 12 right-preferent group had a positive coherence change score and in 10 of the left-preferent subjects it was negative. The correlation between occasions of the change produced by this task was not significant.

The relative efficiency of coherence measures and power spectral measures was investigated for the results of experiment II. In experiment I, a hemisphere difference in power score was used, but, in experiment II, the ratio of the right hemisphere power to the left hemisphere power was determined because this is commonly used to measure the effect of tasks on the EEG. This ratio was calculated for the alpha band by combining the 8-, 10-, and 12-Hz spectral bands as before, and the change in the ratio from rest to task investigated. On both occasions, the difference between groups was not significant for either task. The correlation between occasions within groups was not significant and there was no correlation between the power ratio change score and laterality scores.

Discussion

The measure we have used in the work described in this paper is an interhemisphere coherence change score. The change is a change from a rest state produced by carrying out a task. Only FZ-P4 and FZ-P3 electrode derivations and the alpha band have been considered here.

This interhemisphere coherence change score discriminated the right- and left-preferent groups in two experiments using different subjects when the task required spatial imagery. A mental arithmetic task gave similar but less significant results. These findings were consistent over the two occasions of the second experiment. In both experiments, a correlation between the coherence change score and a score of the laterality of cerebral function was obtained. This relationship was stronger with the right- than the left-preferent subjects and this would seem to fit the model for a more diffuse organisation of function in the latter (2). No significant relationship between these factors and power change scores was found.

We interpret these findings as showing an association between an EEG coherence measure and a behavioural measure which is determined by functional organisation in the brain.

The model of Fig. 1 that led us to use coherence analysis is clearly inadequate. It is obvious from Fig. 2 that a change in coherence could arise from several factors, for example, an increase in uncorrelated activity as well as a topographical change in correlated activity. However, only one (common reference) scalp derivation in each hemisphere and the alpha band have been considered in this paper. We have data from four channels in each hemisphere and frequencies from 2 to 30 Hz. In addition, our common reference montage was chosen so that the tape-recorded data could be transformed to an equivalent bipolar montage. This further data will be examined to see if a more appropriate model can be derived, and to see if it reinforces the above relationship.

If a satisfactory model of the relationship between the EEG and cerebral functional organisation can be derived in this way, the value of the EEG for investigating the significance of anomalies of functional organisation in psychiatric disorders may be enhanced.

REFERENCES

1. Annett, M. (1970): A classification of hand preferences by association analysis. *Br. J. Psychol.,* 61:303–321.
2. Beaumont, J. G. (1974): Handedness and hemisphere function. In: *Hemisphere Function in the Human Brain,* edited by S. J. Dimond and J. G. Beaumont, pp. 89–120. Elek Science, London.
3. Beaumont, J. G., and Dimond, S. J. (1973): Brain disconnection and schizophrenia. *Br. J. Psychiatry,* 123:661–662.
4. Cooper, R., Winter, A. L., Crow, H. J., and Walter, W. G. (1965): Comparison of subcortical, cortical and scalp activity using chronically indwelling electrodes in man. *Electroencephalogr. Clin. Neurophysiol.,* 18:217–228.
5. Cooper, R., and Mundy-Castle, A. C. (1960): Spatial and temporal characteristics of the alpha rhythm: A toposcopic analysis. *Electroencephalogr. Clin. Neurophysiol.,* 12:153–165.
6. Creutzfeldt, O., and Houchin, J. (1974): Neuronal basis of EEG waves. In: *Handbook of Electroencephalography and Clinical Neurophysiology, Vol. 2, Part C,* edited by O. Creutzfeldt, pp. 4–55. Elsevier, Amsterdam.
7. de Lucchi, M. R., Garoutte, B., and Aird, R. B. (1962): The scalp as an electroencephalographic averager. *Electroencephalogr. Clin. Neurophysiol.,* 14:191–196.
8. Elul, R. (1972): The genesis of the EEG. In: *Int. Rev. Neurobiol., Vol. 15,* edited by C. C. Pfeiffer and J. R. Smythies, pp. 227–272. Academic Press, New York.
9. Flor-Henry, P. (1974): Psychosis, neurosis and epilepsy. *Br. J. Psychiatry,* 124:144–150.
10. Galin, D. (1974): Implications for Psychiatry of left and right cerebral specialisation. *Arch. Gen. Psychiatry,* 31:572–583.
11. Gruzelier, J., and Hammond, N. (1976): Schizophrenia: A dominant hemisphere temporal-limbic disorder? *Res. Comm. Psychol., Psychiatr. Behav.,* 1:33–72.
12. Humphrey, M. E. (1951): Consistency of hand usage. A preliminary enquiry. *Br. J. Educ. Psychol.,* 21:214–224.
13. Levey, J. (1974): Psychobiological implications of bilateral asymmetry. In: *Hemisphere Function in the Human Brain,* edited by S. J. Dimond and J. G. Beaumont, pp. 121–183. Elek Science, London.
14. Lishman, W. A., and McMeekan, E. R. L. (1976): Hand preference patterns in psychiatric patients. *Br. J. Psychiatry,* 129:158–166.
15. Lopes da Silva, F. H. (1976): The cortical sources of alpha rhythms analysed by depth profiles (*this volume*).
16. Lopes da Silva, F. H., Van Lierop, T. H. M. T., Schrijer, C. F., and Storm Van Leeuwen, W. (1973): Organisation of thalamic and cortical alpha rhythms: Spectra and coherences. *Electroencephalogr. Clin. Neurophysiol.,* 35:627–639.
17. Luria, A. R. (1973): *The Working Brain.* Allen Lane, London.
18. Pfurtscheller, G., and Cooper, R. (1975): Frequency dependence of the transmission of the EEG from cortex to scalp. *Electroencephalogr. Clin. Neurophysiol.,* 38:93–182.
19. Shaw, J. C. (1976): Cerebral function and the EEG in psychiatric disorder: A hypothesis. *Psychol. Med.,* 6:307–311.
20. Shaw, J. C., O'Connor, K., and Ongley, C. (1976): The EEG as a measure of cerebral functional organisation. *Br. J. Psychiatry,* 130:260–264.
21. Taylor, D. C. (1975): Factors influencing the occurrence of schizophrenia-like psychosis in patients with temporal lobe epilepsy. *Psychol. Med.,* 5:249–254.
22. Torrey, E. F., and Peterson, M. R. (1974): Schizophrenia and the limbic system. *Lancet,* 2:942–946.

Architectonics of the Cerebral Cortex,
edited by M. A. B. Brazier and H. Petsche.
Raven Press, New York © 1978.

Depth Profiles of Electrocortical Activities and Cortical Architectonics

*H. Petsche, *I. B. Müller-Paschinger, **H. Pockberger,
**O. Prohaska, **,*P. Rappelsberger, and *R. Vollmer

* Neurophysiological Institute of the University of Vienna, and ** Brain Research Institute of the Austrian Academy of Sciences, Vienna, Austria

The question as to what degree the histological structure of the cortex is reflected by its electrical behaviour has been studied by our group by two different approaches: (a) by analysis of the spatiotemporal behaviour of surface events (this volume, p. 281) and (b) by analysis of intracortical events in histologically verified regions. Because of the great variability of electrical patterns observed, statistical methods had to be applied, above all the estimates of power, coherence, and phase spectrum. These studies were performed almost exclusively on seizures hoping that, by initiating seizures under equivalent conditions, the afterdischarges would present fairly standardized patterns, as opposed to the continually changing spontaneous EEG. This expectation, however, often proved to be delusive, even if in many cases characteristic patterns for certain regions were found.

But for still another reason, seizures were chosen as the main subject of our studies: in surface recordings, seizures frequently present themselves as very regular patterns which, at first sight, seem to offer better conditions for their analysis than spontaneous activities. However, this assumption also turned out to be erroneous as soon as these patterns were investigated with multiple intracortical electrodes: in most cases they turned out to be composed of different oscillations in a very complex manner. For the same reason activities from only two regions, the A. striata and the A. praecentralis granularis, are dealt with in this chapter.

This report, based on studies of cortical activities by means of a multiple depth electrode, demonstrates that the epicortically recorded activities reflect only in an infinitely small degree the electrical processes taking place in deeper cortical levels. This proves once more that the electrical conductivity of the grey matter is relatively small. Moreover, the studies shed new light on the phenomenon of the phase reversal often found between surface and deep cortical layers, which has caused some authors to postulate vertical dipoles within the cortex. Finally, particular attention is paid to the nature of regular, "tonic" seizure patterns, the analysis of which has largely contributed to an understanding of intracortical mechanisms and their histological background.

Most of the previous examinations in this field were restricted by the small number of electrodes and by the difficulty in attaining enough exactness of their dimensions in manufacturing them. This was the reason why one of us (14) undertook to develop a multielectrode on a common carrier needle, based on thin-film technology.

METHODS

These experiments were carried out on 12 unanesthetized and artificially respirated rabbits under Alloferrin, a synthetic, curare-like drug. Both ossa jugularia were fixed by curved metal bars. The animals were repeatedly infiltrated locally with a 3% procaine solution. It is very unlikely that the animals felt pain during the recording, since rabbits are generally very sensitive to any kind of arousal, yet these experimental animals presented a normal EEG at rest, without a continuous arousal reaction.

After removal of the scalp, small trephine holes (less than 3 mm Ø) were made over the areas to be studied. The dura was removed. Immediately the trephine hole filled with cerebrospinal fluid so that no other procedure was required to prevent the cortex from drying out. Seizures were produced either by N-penicillin-g, topically applied or intracortically injected (5 μl of a 1 M solution) at least 10 mm distant from the site of recording, or by bifrontal application of electrical current (200 Hz, 2 ms, up to 30 mA).

Recordings were made by means of the multielectrode (Fig. 1) (14). This electrode has, on a small needle as a carrier (0.3 mm wide), 8 Ag-AgCl contacts of 50 × 50 μm at 300 μm distances vertically arranged. One millimeter below contact 8 (c.8), a ninth contact was applied for measuring the contribution of electrically active regions underlying the cortex (particularly the hippocampus). The impedance of the contacts measured on the average 0.5 MΩ at 10 Hz. The Ag-AgCl contacts were chlorided before each experiment. This multielectrode was introduced into the cortical region to be studied by a microdrive (DKI) under microscopic control until the uppermost contact just disappeared under the cortical surface.

The electrode contacts were connected to the inputs of impedance transformers, the outputs of which led to a Schwarzer EEG machine (32 channels). The recordings were made simultaneously with common reference (nasal bone) and in bipolar linkages. Moreover, the activities were monitored on an eight-channel Omniscope (Siemens) and a selection of them was stored on tape (Ampex FR 1300, seven channels). Power spectra, coherence, and phase functions were computed by an IBM 370/145 programmed by P. Rappelsberger.

After each experiment, a microelectrode filled with Alcian blue in 3 M potassium citrate was immediately lowered close to the multielectrode by a

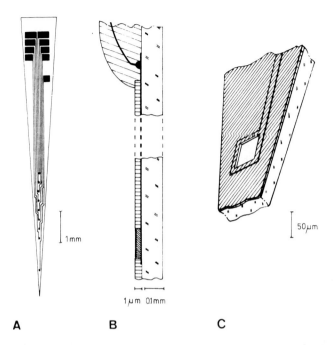

A   B   C

FIG. 1. The multielectrode and its dimensions. Eight contacts of Ag-AgCl 50 × 50 μm in size at distances of 300 μm are adhered to a plane glass carrier of 0.1 mm diameter. Contact 9, 1 mm below c.8, is used for recording the activities of structures immediately subjacent to the neocortex. **A:** Layout of the contacts and their connections. **B:** Cross section through the multielectrode demonstrating the carrier, one contact, its conducting line and the insulation layer. **C:** Oblique view of a free contact.

hydraulic microdrive (DKI) down to a target level where the activity recorded by this multielectrode was identical with a certain characteristic activity of one of the contacts of the multielectrode. Here, the dyestuff was electrophoretically expelled. After the experiment, the animals were killed by thiopental and perfused with Boin's solution for histological processing.

In order to quantify the data obtained by this multielectrode, the following calculations were performed: simultaneous power spectra of seven of the eight traces, squared coherence, and transformed coherence estimates between adjacent recordings and the phase spectra. The phase differences were used to calculate the delays in milliseconds and sometimes the speed in centimeters per second.

Note: In the present context the word "spike" has to be understood as used in electroencephalography to designate the fast transients in the upper part of the frequency range as found mostly during seizures. It is never used here for cellular discharges that are out of the scope of this paper. In the same sense, "wave" is generally used for field potentials in the lower frequency range of the EEG spectrum.

RESULTS

Spontaneous Activities

In contrast to the human EEG, the rabbit's activity at rest varies considerably. An organized alpha rhythm is missing. The striate area is characterized by groups of irregular slow waves several hundreds of microvolts in amplitude with frequencies in the delta range (Fig. 2). These groups usually last only up to a few seconds and alternate with periods of low activity in the alpha and theta range, indicating an arousal reaction. That this latter activity is not produced by the neocortex but by the underlying hippocampus and is projected to the neocortex by volume conduction, was proved by three observations: (a) the theta voltage is highest at contact 9 (c.9), just above the hippocampus, (b) its amplitude decreases toward the superficial recording sites, and (c), in contrast to endogeneous cortical activities,

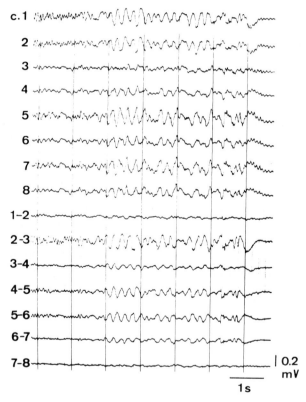

FIG. 2. Spontaneous activity in A. striata. Common reference and bipolar recordings. Two generators are present (c.1 and c.2, and c.4 to c.7), separated by a zone of minimal activity (zero zone) in c.3. These two generators are often linked together and oscillate in reverse phase.

its coherence is high throughout the cortical profile, its phase being zero, (d) it is missed in bipolar recordings. Obviously, the striate area is most likely to exhibit volume-conducted theta activity as the dorsal hippocampus is here immediately below the cortex.

These slow-wave groups, usually best seen in the two uppermost contacts, are reflected, in the deeper layers, by similarly shaped groups of waves which, however, at first sight never represent a true mirror image in spite of the fact that they appear phase-reversed on closer examination. However, these wave groups in the deeper layers usually have more of higher frequency components (as is best seen in the power spectrum) and are usually of higher amplitude than the waves close to the surface. The first impression is that both these events are generated by a single generator, a dipole extending through nearly the total width of the cortex. This is further supported by the observation that very little activity is found in the zone between these two seemingly phase-reversed activities. This holds true also for other activities, such as visually evoked potentials, sleep, and for most seizure patterns; this zone is called "zero zone" in the following description.

In addition, however, to the abovementioned differences in shape between these two activities above and below the zero zone, there are yet other signs indicating that they come from different sources. One is the frequent autonomy of either the upper or the lower activity: both are sometimes present without being reflected beyond the zero zone (Fig. 2). Moreover, coherence estimates are not consistent with the assumption of a single generator underlying these activities. By this finding, earlier observations are confirmed (10,12), according to which a low coherence was ascertained for the slow components of seizure patterns in the vertical dimension of the cortex.

The spontaneous activity of the precentral area is quite different from the one observed in the striate area. Characteristic for the precentral region is an alternation between groups of faster waves (preponderantly 12 to 15 Hz), often appearing in the form of spindles, with groups of slow waves in the delta range (Fig. 3). The fast waves are most variable in amplitude and usually do not exceed the delta waves that attain voltages of up to 800 μV. Figure 3 offers several sections of spontaneous activity from one experiment in order to demonstrate the high variability of these events. The fast activity has its zero zone in c.3. Even with the naked eye it can be seen that these fast waves, although occurring on both sides of the zero zone and mostly simultaneously, come from different generators, since there are considerable differences in shape. In spite of this, there are many potentials among them showing a phase reversal when recorded under the usual EEG conditions. A more careful analysis of the intracortical recordings, however, demonstrates that the shape of the potentials in many cases changes considerably from one trace to the adjacent one. This observation suggests

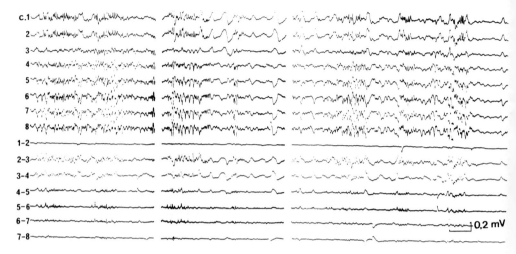

FIG. 3. Spontaneous activity in A. praecentralis granularis. Groups of delta waves alternate with spindle-like activity. The groups of delta waves also appear to be due to two generators separated by a zero zone. With regard to the periods of spindle activity, several additional generators below the zero zone contribute to the formation of this pattern.

the presence of several electrical sources (at different distances from the surface and of different vertical extension) underlying this complex pattern. A closer examination of the simultaneously recorded bipolar traces gives some evidence of this variability even at the standard recording speed.

As in the case of the delta groups in both regions, the spindles, too, may occur isolated above and below the zero zone.

The delta groups of the precentral area are usually higher in amplitude in the layers close to the surface than in the deeper cortical layers. Their zero zone is not identical with the zero zone of the spindles but is usually somewhat deeper (Fig. 3 shows the zero zone for spindles at c.3, for delta waves between c.3 and c.4). Otherwise, what has been said for the spindles was also found for delta groups (apparent phase reversal, difference in shape on each side of the zero zone, occasional autonomy on both sides). These findings lead to the conclusion that both activities on this side and beyond the zero zone, although caused by different generators, are often linked together.

Activity Evoked by Intermittent Light Stimulation (ILS)

A behaviour similar to the spontaneous activity was found for photically evoked activities in the striate area (Fig. 4). In each of the three samples taken from different experiments, the photically evoked potentials were distinct in the uppermost and the deeper cortical layers, separated by a zero zone, the extension of which differed but little. In Fig. 4, B1, the zero zone

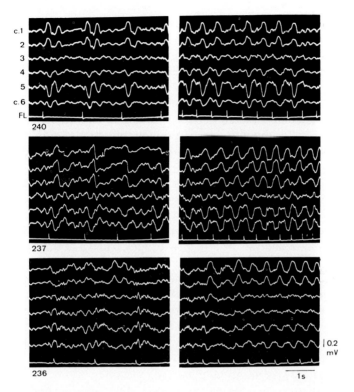

FIG. 4. Visually evoked activity recorded from A. striata at low and higher flicker rates from three experiments. In experiment 236, the recording electrode was close to A. retrosplenialis granularis beta. Common reference recordings. The evoked potentials in the upper and the lower cortical layers are closely related to each other and are also separated by a zero zone (c.3 in 240). The position of this zero zone may shift on changing the flicker frequency (right part of the sample from 237). The potentials are suppressed by arousal stimuli (last second of the right part of 240). In this figure, as in Figs. 5 and 7, the common reference recordings were photographed from the omniscope.

seems to be 300 μm deeper than in the other two samples. This is due to the multielectrode having been less deeply introduced into the cortex. Again the two evoked potentials in the two levels of the cortex are related to each other and seem to be phase-reversed without, however, presenting true mirror images. There is also no significant coherence between these two activities.

The right column of records of Fig. 4 demonstrates the oscillations produced by ILS at approximately 2 Hz. The evoked potentials are easily suppressed by noise (see last second of the record A2 in Fig. 4). The relatively great variety of the shape of the evoked potentials depends on the place within the striate area from which they were recorded: the record 236 was taken from a site located more medially than in the other two experiments, closer to the A. retrospinalis granularis beta (16). Its flicker responses are less distinct than the responses in the other two experiments. This may also account for the evoked potentials in depth which, in this experiment, are considerably smaller than in the other two samples.

There is still another fact deserving attention, namely the change of the position of the zero zone in Fig. 4, B2: this record shows a sudden change of the FL frequency from 1.9 Hz to 2.6 Hz after the fifth flash. Up to this flash, c.4 participates in the activity below and c.3 in the activity above, the zero zone thus being situated between these two contacts. But, beginning with flash 6, c.4, for the duration of a few waves, participates in neither of these activities: this indicates that the zero zone has shifted down by 150 μm.

The problem of time relationships between the evoked potentials produced in these different cortical layers has not been thoroughly studied as yet. The spectral estimates of the few samples investigated thus far result in an equal distribution of the power peaks of evoked activity and activity at rest. The phase analysis of a regular driving pattern of the experiment in which Fig. 4, B2, was recorded, yields, for the main frequency, a delay line from c.1 downward with the following phase differences between adjacent contacts: 17, 42, 51, 17, and 9 degrees. These data, however, do not permit any conclusive statements concerning the temporal organization of the evoked potentials, since they only relate to the slow waves. The (probably more essential) fast events produced by each flash are inconsistent and have to be studied with averaging techniques if data on temporal relationships are to be collected.

The responses to light flashes may also occur only on one side of the zero zone.

Thiopental Narcosis

In order to seek possible characteristic differences between seizure patterns and the activities observed intracortically after application of a narcotic drug, thiopental was administered gradually within a period of 3 min at a dosage high enough to produce the well-known alternating sleep pattern (Fig. 5, left column, third trace from top). The figure shows recordings c.1 through c.7 from the multielectrode situated in the striate area at different time intervals after the beginning of the administration. During thiopental administration, too, the intracortically recorded patterns also mostly differed from the surface recording.

At the beginning of the thiopental effect, a rather uniform, low-voltage slow activity is seen throughout the cortex, superimposed by yet lower fast waves. Very soon (second section from top) an irregular activity up to 500 μV develops and is clearly different in c.1 and c.2 as compared with the recordings from about c.4 downward. The deeper traces are characterized by the presence of more higher frequency components. In section 3 from top, the stage of the alternating pattern is attained. The pattern

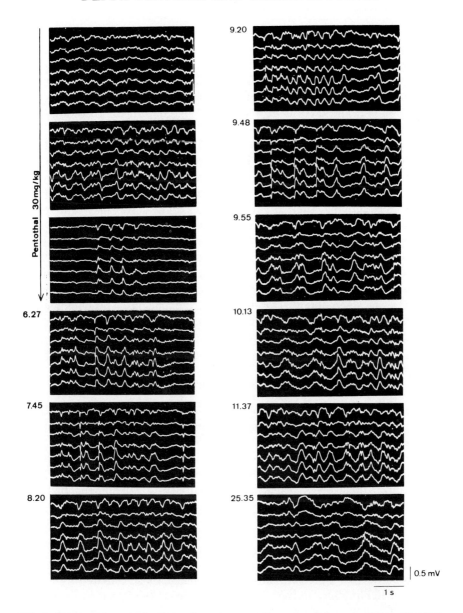

FIG. 5. Thiopental narcosis. Recordings from c.1 through c.7 from A. striata after fractionated application of thiopental (10 mg/kg/min). The numbers indicate time in minutes and seconds after the beginning of the application. Both the extension and position of the zero zone change (compare 9.48 with 25.35); the activities of the layers below the zero zone are more complex than those of the more superficial layers; in the deep layers, sharp waves that are not often seen near the surface (at 7.45 and 9.48) occur; regular periods of waves at this depth often have no correspondence superficially (at 9.20).

now consists of groups of fairly regularly repeating transients that are indistinguishable from epileptic discharges. The phase reversal is here particularly marked in the delta waves, the zero zone of which seems to extend over more than 300 μm, which is the distance between the contacts. The vertical extension of the zero zone, however, changes, as does also its position (see the records at 9.48 as compared with the record at 25.35 and others). It is further to be noted that the frequently occurring sharp waves in the deep layers (particularly at 7.45 and at 9.48) are not always reflected by the cortical activity. In the depth, there are also complex potentials (at 9.55 and at 11.37) without any corresponding activity at the surface. Moreover, upon closer examination of these records, different generators occupying different vertical ranges of the cortex may be detected. One particularly convincing example is the activity at 8.20 when the regularly repeating transients at 1.45 Hz are replaced by a 2.9-Hz activity; for the slow activity, there is a clear-cut zero zone at c.3 with a comparatively steep potential gradient toward c.1 and c.2. But the subsequent activity of 2.9 Hz has a zero zone extending further down, sometimes as far down as c.4, where the steep potential gradient toward c.5 begins. This demonstrates once more that both the sites and vertical ranges of the generators giving rise to distinct features in the EEG are variable.

Seizure Patterns

Because of the extreme variability of intracortically recorded seizure patterns, the results obtained from the A. striata and from A. praecentralis granularis will be dealt with in separate sections. Although the patterns observed in these two areas are so characteristic that anybody acquainted with this domain is able to define their origin merely by looking at them, the patterns themselves display such a variety of phenomena that they deserve to be dealt with in a separate section.

Area Striata

Seizures elicited by electrical stimulation and those initiated by locally applied penicillin differ in this area only insofar as the first kind commonly begins with an irregular activity, whereas the beginning of the second kind consists of a regular fast activity developing from a penicillin spike, the afterdischarges of which go over into a self-sustained activity. However, the later stages of the seizure fail to show any significant differences. Most characteristic for striate seizures are long-lasting periods of tonic activity, presenting an almost sinusoidal pattern of usually 8 to 10 Hz.

In the following figures, a few of the most frequently occurring patterns are presented.

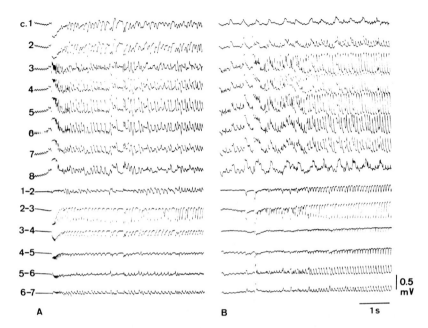

FIG. 6. Two typical sections from seizures recorded from A. striata. **A:** After electrical stimulation. **B.** Initiated by an intracortical penicillin focus 12 mm rostrally from the multi-electrode. A typical feature is the appearance of electronegative spikes, most prominently in the layers below the zero zone (c.4 and c.5 in **A**), accompanied by arcade-like waves of the same frequency near the surface (c.1 and c.2). In penicillin-induced seizures, the involvement of the total width of the cortex occurs within a few seconds when the seizure has been elicited by a distant focus, in contrast to the sudden and simultaneous onset in all layers after local application of the drug. The in-phase delta transients in the common-reference recordings of **B** are volume-conducted from the underlying hippocampus.

The salient features of striate seizures are shown in Fig. 6A and B from two different experiments. The seizure of Fig. 6A was produced by electrical stimulation. The section of the seizure starts with a large electronegative shift most distinctly expressed in the layers from c.3 downward, covered with high-frequency discharges, the maximum of which coincides with the maximum of the negative shift (at c.5). This burst is followed by irregularly discharging negative transients, with maximum amplitude also in c.5. In the upper two contacts, there is, instead, a positive shift free from any burst. Only the electronegative irregular transients (c.4 to c.8) are reflected by arcade-like waves of the same frequency. This can best be seen in the bipolar linkages. It often happens that the fast transients appear at a lower repetition rate: in this case, the arcade-like waves recorded from near the surface have the appearance of a more or less regular spike-and-wave pattern (9).

Figure 6B, elicited by intracortical application of penicillin 12 mm rostrally, shows the same development of fast negative transients within the lowest two-thirds of the cortex, but this time without being accompanied by phase-reversed waves in the topmost layers. Figure 6B demonstrates, in addition, two other frequently seen features, namely a distinct vertical spreading of the seizure from its maximum (c.3 to c.5) down as far as c.6 and up to c.2. This is a common finding when the seizure is triggered from a distant penicillin focus in the same hemisphere.

Moreover, there are, in all common-reference recordings, high-amplitude electronegative delta transients with a slight decrease in amplitude toward the surface that are not seen in the bipolar records. These are remnants of a hippocampal seizure: the hippocampus, having the lowest seizure threshold, in most cases produces an afterdischarge which, however, is by far shorter in duration than cortical afterdischarges.

Regular tonic seizure patterns, sometimes of a duration of up to 15 sec, are frequently observed in the striate area. Even if these patterns, when seen merely in surface recordings, appear to be easily interpretable, their intracortical organization poses problems that are treated in detail by Rappelsberger, *this volume*. Here, only some of the intricate electrographic features are to be presented in one sample of a seizure of 3 min duration following intermittent light stimulation (ILS) after topical application of penicillin (Fig. 7). This seizure is characterized by the presence of several, fairly long-lasting tonic periods of quite different organization. A short description is given to underscore its salient features.

The seizure starts from the burst of a penicillin spike. The penicillin spikes themselves are also different between the uppermost and the lower levels of the cortex, the record of c.3 representing a superimposition of these two types of discharges. The seizure first shows a tonic pattern of roughly 25 Hz composed of all cortical levels with an amplitude maximum at c.3. A few seconds after its beginning (Fig. 7, second sample), this pattern is suddenly replaced by activity of much higher voltage composed of arcade-like 14-Hz waves (best visible at c.5 and c.6) interlocked with electronegative spikes on their peaks. The spikes themselves are most marked in c.3. C.1 seems, for this part of the seizure, to represent the zero zone. This form of arcade-like regular waves in the deeper layers of the cortex, each superimposed by a spike and best seen in the middle layers, is often encountered in tonic seizures.

In the next sample, recorded 15 sec after the beginning of the seizure the same phenomenon occurs, but at a lower frequency and often alternating with blunter-shaped waves that have a double peak (best visible in c.4 to c.6): 35 sec after the beginning, the pattern becomes more irregular and the superimposition of waves and spikes in c.4 to c.7 and the preponderant presence of spikes in c.4 to c.7 become more definite. After 65 sec the pattern shows, in the 2nd and 3rd sec, an example of the abovementioned irregular spike-and-wave pattern in surface recordings accompanied, in the depth, chiefly by spikes. This pattern occurs again, but even less regu-

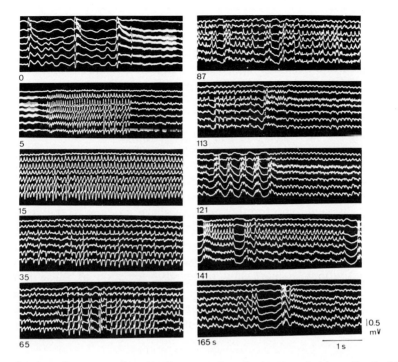

FIG. 7. Sections from one seizure lasting more than 2 min, recorded from the A. striata after local application of penicillin. Common reference recordings from c.1 to c.7 at different intervals from the start of the seizure (the numbers indicate seconds). Note the great variability of shape, frequency, and amplitude distribution of the different tonic episodes within the cortical width.

larly, after 87 sec. Now, in contrast to the first minute of the seizure, c.1 also shows wave activity, the zero zone for delta having shifted downward.

An entirely new tonic pattern appears after 113 sec with a regular 9.5-Hz activity in c.1, c.7, and c.8 (out-of-phase with respect to c.1) accompanied by its double frequency, 19 Hz, with maximum voltage in c.3. Almost the same pattern occurs once more after 121 sec after a few groups of clonic discharges that are only poorly reflected in the surface recordings. After 141 sec another new type of tonic pattern appears, again at 9.5 Hz, but this time with the waves (with double spikes) in the same region where, just previously, the 19-Hz component prevailed. These latter, on the contrary, are now best marked in c.7 and c.8 where immediately before the basal frequency was prominent. The last portion of this seizure (after 165 sec) finally shows, after a clonic group, a tonic pattern in which the upper harmonics are barely visible.

It is obvious that these so extremely different tonic patterns are caused by the presence of several generators that are interlocked at different phases. Special attention should be paid to a phenomenon shown in Fig. 7 at 5 sec, where the total width of the cortex seems to be switched on and off to give rise, for a couple of seconds, to an entirely different pattern. This phenomenon of switching on and off has also been observed with topographical recordings from extended areas of the cortex and has turned out to be accompanied by a sudden change of the entire spatiotemporal organization in the horizontal plane too (8,21).

Area Praecentralis Granularis

Seizures in this area elicited either by electrical stimulation or by application of penicillin show an even more complicated intracortical organization than seizures in the striate area. Patterns as demonstrated in Figs. 8 and 9 are fairly characteristic for this area. In sharp contrast to the striate area where seizures, initiated by whatever kind of stimulus, begin abruptly, they slowly develop in the precentral area, usually with the deep layers leading (Fig. 8A). Subsequently, the layers close to the surface start with an irregular spiking activity with increasing frequency. As soon as these transients appear, the deep areas produce slower and higher amplitude activities with intermingled spikes. The fully developed seizure (Fig. 8B, recorded at different speeds) shows two levels of mostly interlocked activities with

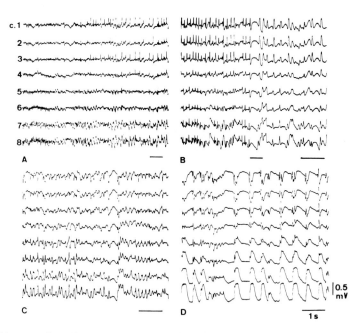

FIG. 8. Four sections from one seizure elicited by electrical stimulation and recorded from the A. praecentralis granularis. In contrast to the striate area, precentral seizures differ mainly by their gradual onset, by their lesser connectivity between deep and superficial layers and by the comparatively rare finding of a zero zone.

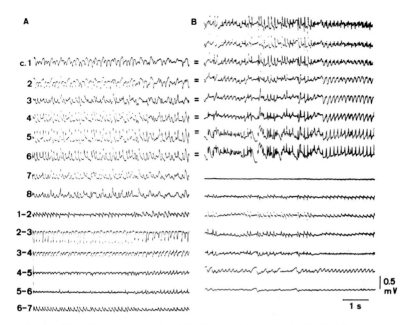

FIG. 9. Two sections from two seizures initiated electrically and recorded from A. praecentralis granularis. In **A,** the electrode was protruded by the distance of two contacts (i.e., 600 μm) in order to explore the activity of the deepest cortical regions. For a short while, a zero zone appears between c.2 and c.3. **B:** Tonic seizures appear in the precentral area more rarely and with shorter duration than in the striate area. They are superimposed by waves and spikes having their generator zones at different positions but largely superimposed on each other. This section corresponds to an early stage of the seizure (compare the end of Fig. 8A).

maxima in c.1 and c.8 and decreasing in amplitude to c.4 and c.5, respectively, where they superimpose. However, as the next part of the seizure (Fig. 8C) shows, the activity of the deep layers increases and extends further upward at the expense of the activity near the surface that now shows electropositive spikes. The seizure ends with an irregular spike-and-wave pattern (Fig. 8D) which, in contrast to that seen in the striate area, displays the spikes most markedly in the upper half of the cortex, the waves being most prominent in the deep cortical regions.

With regard to this region, the question of the existence of a phase reversal and a zero zone is difficult to answer. In any case both are inconstant in seizures. In the spike-and-wave-groups of Fig. 8D, it is true that the waves near the surface appear as a somewhat distorted mirror image of the waves observed in the deepest cortical layers, but there is no such phase reversal for the spikes. At some instances, however, a clear phase reversal with a zero zone is found (Fig. 9A, recorded during another seizure after the multi-electrode had been protruded by 600 μm, i.e., the distance of two contacts), easily recognizable by the high bipolar amplitude c.2 to c.3. The instability of both the presence and the position of a zero zone is a characteristic finding in this region.

Tonic patterns occur similarly in the precentral area but they are less frequent and of shorter duration than in the striate area. One pattern is shown in Fig. 9B. It starts shortly after the irregular transients in the upper layers have fully developed. Its main frequency is 7.5 Hz. As in the striate area, it seems to be composed of a wave component, best visible in c.4 to c.6, bearing a spike near its top. Another often-observed phenomenon (12) is distinctly visible in this record: in following the shape of the tonic potentials from c.5 upward, one notes that the depression between the negative peak of the wave and the spike becomes deeper, i.e., the spike moves away from the peak of the wave. This was shown to be caused by an upward spreading of the spike with respect to the wave.

Histological Correlations

The greatest difficulty in studying the intracortical phenomena of synchronization and in finding their histological correlates has been an exact marking of the position of the contacts. It would be possible to deposit silver electrolytically, but the risk of damaging the multielectrode by this procedure is too great. Therefore, an indirect method was chosen using a dye-filled microelectrode that was introduced near the multielectrode to a depth where characteristic electrographic features had been observed. But although an attempt was made to define, as exactly as possible, the position of the zero zone and of maximal amplitude by marking these zones by means of the microelectrode filled with Alcian blue, this procedure has not yielded fully satisfying results.

The difficulties are not solely due to the manipulation, but also in many cases to defining these zones in the often *Proteus*-like seizure patterns observed on the screen of the oscilloscope. The attempted electrohistological correlations, presented in the following pages, therefore, can give only a rough approximation.

The possibility of correlating physiological and histological data is still further limited by the recording device. For many cases, the 50×50 μm measuring contact surfaces have turned out to be still too large and the 300-μm distances too great to define possible histological substrates with sufficient exactitude. The following considerations, therefore, are mainly based on the fact that the location of the electrode was histologically verified and the multielectrode was introduced in such a way that the uppermost contact just disappeared below the cortical surface.

Figure 10 shows profiles through the two cortical regions that were studied, together with a schema of the multielectrode on the same scale.

One of the most constant findings in the striate area was the presence of two activities separated by a zero zone. This holds true for spontaneous

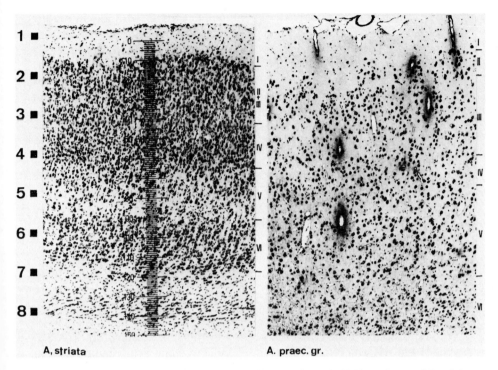

FIG. 10. Profiles through the two cortical regions investigated with the scheme of the eight contacts of the multielectrode true to scale. Lamination according to Rose (16). Gomory 1 scale mark = 10 μm.

activities, for photically evoked potentials and for the greater part of seizure activities. If one takes into account the cortical profile, it is most likely that the nerve cells of layers II and III and V are involved in producing these two activities. This assumption is corroborated by the fact that the power spectra of these patterns usually have maxima in these regions. The zero zone coincides with a level where the apical dendrites bifurcate. Considering the high significance of these dendrites for conducting the fast seizure components corticopetally (10), and the observation that there is a steep gradient of the fast electronegative transients at this level, the assumption of the distribution pattern of apical dendrites being involved in the phenomenon of the zero zone becomes still more probable.

With regard to the high-amplitude, negative fast transients below the zero zone (Fig. 7), the nerve cells of layers IV and V seem to yield the most important contribution.

There are, however, many phenomena that cannot yet be referred to any histological basis. This holds true for the change of the zero level in visually evoked potentials with changing ILS frequency and also for various seizure patterns and particularly for thiopental narcosis.

In the precentral area, only the spontaneous activity with its alternating spindle and delta pattern shows a clear-cut zero zone. According to the profiles of power spectra, the zero zone is wider than in the striate area. Its position corresponds approximately to the lower part of layer III. If, as was presumed for the striate area, here too, the splitting up of apical dendrites may be connected to this phenomenon, it would be tempting to find out whether the special type of bifurcation, as described by Fleischhauer and Detzer (3) might be the reason for the larger vertical extent of the zero zone. These authors found strikingly different formations of dendritic bundles in these two regions.

In all likelihood, the formation of the delta groups of spontaneous activity also takes place mainly in layers II and III and layer V. No morphological substrate whatsoever can be presumed for the potentials composing the spindles. They are probably produced by cell populations of various vertical extension with different degrees of mutual interlocking.

The precentral seizure patterns deserve special consideration. Since, as emphasized above, these patterns are more intricate than in the striate area, attempts at coordinating them with morphological features are even more difficult. One characteristic finding in this region, the irregular spiking at the early stage of a seizure (see Fig. 8A), seems to be caused by nerve cells of layer III, probably also II. In the section of the seizure shown in Fig. 8B, layers II and III and V and VI seem to be active and firmly interlocked in phase. A similar phase locking seems to be present in the stage of irregular spike and waves toward the end of the seizure (Fig. 8D), the only difference being that layer VI seems to produce mainly slow waves, whereas the spikes are most visible from layer IV to V upward where they propagate corticopetally. (It is, however, possible that the spikes, too, originate in the deepest layer but are hidden in the steep rising phase of the locally present large waves.) There are sometimes indications of the presence of a zero zone (Fig. 8E) roughly corresponding to layer IV.

Concerning the tonic pattern represented in Fig. 9, one may claim that the largest spikes are found in layers VI, V, and perhaps also IV, being characterized by the production of slowly rising 7.5-Hz waves, whereas the upper cortical layers are mainly characterized by the presence of spikes propagating toward the uppermost layers.

This is only a preliminary attempt at coordinating physiological and histological facts. A verification of these findings has to be left to further studies with an improved system both of histological marking and of recording by manufacturing multielectrodes of smaller dimensions.

DISCUSSION

These studies aimed at an elucidation of the intracortical spatiotemporal behaviour of normal and seizure activities in the vertical dimension of the cortex. They are a continuation of previous reports (10,13) in which different cortical activities were studied by means of equidistant semimicroelectrodes in different depths, their activities having been compared with the simultaneous epicortical events. These examinations resulted in the finding of an electrical anisotropy of the cortex and finally gave rise to the discovery of the apical dendritic bundles by Fleischhauer et. al. (4), a structure probably engaged in conducting the fast electrical events (called "spikes" in the EEG jargon) from the deep pyramidal layer antidromically to more superficial layers. Arguments for such an assumption have been presented previously (11,13). Further evidence for such a mechanism is supplied by this chapter. In the present context, it appears not unlikely that the relatively long-extended zones of closest apposition of the apical dendrites, which take about 20% of their total surface[1] are involved in the synchronization of discharges. Further investigations (15) brought some evidence that the greater part of the waves occurring during regular tonic seizure patterns may also be conducted along the apical dendrites.

One of the main reasons for starting this project was the search for the generators of the different EEG events. Since there is overwhelming evidence that the cortical nerve cells play a leading role in the generation of the electrical activity of the cortex, great emphasis was laid upon possible histological correlations between electrical and histological features. The concept "generator zone," coined by us in 1974, is to be understood in a merely descriptive sense and does not involve any physiological meaning whatsoever. By "generator zone" we imply only the volume of cortical tissue where a field potential of a distinct shape may be recorded. The results presented have contributed to the definition of the vertical dimension only of this volume, since the multielectrode was used only for vertical penetrations of the cortex.

Evidently, these generator zones have no strict limits but continually merge with adjacent zones where the field potentials in question continually diminish. Hence, it would be preferable to define their size in terms of the space constant. But at present the data that can be given concerning the sizes of the generator zones are only approximations; the main limiting factor is the fact that as a rule the EEG waves are compound events made up of at least two individual field potentials with a different size and position of their generator zones.

It is our intention not to focus our attention on the possible nature of field potentials, since the experiments discussed in this paper do not contribute to this question. Nevertheless, we ought to present, without any further comment, our hypothetical view concerning the origin of these field potentials seen as characteristic graphoelements in our recordings. We think that they are the outcome of an interaction of a limited population of neurons and interneurons, mainly reflecting the summation of the entirety

---

[1] Latz, H. (1975): Quantitative Messungen an Dendritenbündeln in der Hirnrinde des Kaninchens. Thesis, Bonn, 97 pp.

of EPSPs and IPSPs evoked by this system. The evidence for seizure patterns consisting of a great number of such small populations being linked together and acting in a temporal sequence was underscored in the above-mentioned papers. With regard to the phenomenon of synchronization in seizures, therefore, these generator zones may be conceived as representing a kind of elementary events.

In addition to a thorough study of seizure patterns, main emphasis was laid on the exploration of activity at rest in the two regions studied. In either instance, evidence was found for the existence of two main generators, one situated close to the surface and approximately corresponding to layers II and III, the other in the depth of the cortex. Although these two generators seem upon crude examination to be phase-reversed at many moments, the assumption of a single vertical dipole is not in accordance with the facts, since the coherence between these activities is low and they may also occur independently from one another. The two activities are usually separated from each other by a zone of minimal activity, called zero zone by us, which does not seem to contribute to electrogenesis. The small activity here encountered has turned out to be a mixture of the activities seen in the adjacent layers.

There are several reasons for assuming that different generators participate in the formation of the intracortical electrical activity. One of the most thorough studies of this question was performed by Calvet et. al. (1) and by Scherrer and Calvet (17) who, in chronically prepared cats, described three different generators of EEG wave activity: type A, reaching down to about 500 μm and having no temporal counterpart in the frequency of cellular discharges; type B, with good time relation to pyramidal cell discharges and which the authors considered as composed of two dipoles, the one reaching down to approximately 1,000 μm, the other, with the opposite sign, found between 1,000 μm and 2,000 μm below the surface; and finally type C, also considered to be composed of two partial dipoles, at about the same position as B and only observed during slow wave sleep.

The histological interpretation of the zero zone where minimal electrogenesis was found is at present impossible. The width of this zone, in the striate area, is less than the distance between adjacent contacts, i.e., than 300 μm. In the precentral area, it may be somewhat larger than 300 μm. It is tempting to ask whether there is some likelihood of a connection between the position of the zero zone and the bifurcation of the apical dendrites of layer V pyramidal cells, which takes place somewhat below zero zone. But in the absence of further data to be obtained with more closely spaced electrode contacts and smaller contact surfaces, any further conjectures are unjustified. It is worthy of note, however, that, during spontaneous activity, the position of the zero zone remains relatively unaltered, in contrast to seizures, in which zero zones quite different from those found in spontaneous activity seem to be present.

This applies also to the spontaneous spindle activity in the precentral area. Its intricate pattern is a good example of the merging of several generator zones of different position and vertical extension. Almost the same holds true for the intracortical sleep pattern produced by thiopental. Its variability, which is even higher than the one observed in seizures, deserves special study.

In seizures, the situation is somewhat more complicated. There is no doubt that, in seizures, in addition to the generator zone in the deep layers, layers close to the surface may also become autonomously active. This is also stressed by Speckmann et al. (18), who, although finding very stable relationships between membrane potential of deep pyramidal neurons and cortical DC shifts (and also sometimes field potentials), arrive at the conclusion that additional superficial structures mediate the DC displacements at the surface of the cortex, whereas in the layer of the large pyramidal cells, the DC shifts could be explained by the summation of slow membrane transients of the cortical neurons. Further evidence for the existence of generator structures beneath the cortical surface has been supplied by Creutzfeldt et al. (2) who found that the amplitude of the epicortical positive wave is related to the slope of the neuronal depolarization shift and increases with the steepness of PDS. Another previous observation (13) underscores this assumption of two main generators in seizures: when amplitude histograms of seizure patterns were made at different levels of the cortex, the skewness had, in the uppermost levels, a reversed sign as compared with the histograms from deep cortical activities; zero skewness was found in the zero zone.

As for the penicillin-induced seizures, and according to the studies of Matsumoto and Ajmone Marsan (6,7), it seems most likely that the cellular discharges during the paroxysmal depolarization shift (PDS), representing the synchronized activation of a large number of excitatory synapses on the same neuron (5), are the triggering mechanisms for inducing other cells to fire in synchrony with the PDS. Attention has therefore to be focused on the beginning of penicillin-induced seizures. They start in the striate area after local application of the drug in a most constant manner: a burst of spikes (electronegative beneath the zero zone) appears in all cortical layers simultaneously and develops into a regular self-sustained activity, being most prominent in layers IV and V (Fig. 8A). However, as may be seen in Fig. 8, the amplitude profile through the cortex does not remain stable during the seizure. It is, however, beyond the scope of this chapter to discuss in any detail the problems of the variability of the power profiles. Suffice it to mention that, in becoming involved in electrogenesis, the zero zone may undergo considerable alterations. These samples show that the basic concept of two cortical generators as being mainly involved in the spontaneous activity of the striate area is insufficient to explain the variety of electrical events in seizures.

There is, in striate area seizures, one striking difference in the onset of seizures according to the kind of application of penicillin: when locally applied, the seizures start as described above, with a sudden involvement of all layers by a burst of spikes. However, when the seizures were initiated by an intracortical injection of penicillin several millimeters distant in the same hemisphere, they usually start from layers IV and V, where they increase in amplitude and slowly include layers VI and I to III. It may take several seconds before the seizure attains its full amplitude throughout the cortex. Considering that the callosal and corticocortical afferents terminate mainly in the three first layers, the specific afferents from the thalamus predominantly in layer IV and to a lesser extent also in layer II (19), it is most likely that these striate seizures are initiated from the precentral area (where penicillin was injected intracortically) via the thalamus.

Phase and coherence analyses were made on a few seizure episodes. The general tendency of the fast components to spread in an epicortical direction as described previously was confirmed. The same holds true for a detailed analysis of the tonic seizure patterns, which are a common feature in the striate area. Figure 8 demonstrates their intricate structure. This finding renders almost hopeless any attempt to understand the mechanisms underlying these patterns. Studies of the cellular counterpart also yield no further information. Scherrer and Calvet (17) only mention that, during tonic stages, cells tend to discharge at a very high but almost constant rate. There is no indication, however, of the layer these cells were recorded from.

The seizures recorded from the precentral area are distinguished from the striate seizures by several characteristic features, among which the following are the most important: the rare appearance of a zero zone, the tendency of layers I to III to develop a seizure from transient negative spikes, delayed by several seconds with respect to a slowly recruiting seizure pattern in the deepest layers, and, finally, the occurrence of spike-and-wave patterns, in which the waves are most prominent in the deepest layers, the spikes being most easily observable in the upper half of the cortex. Finally, only rare and short periods of tonic patterns occur in this area.

In the precentral area, layers II and III seem to have generally a stronger tendency to develop self-sustained activities than in the striate area, where these layers depend mostly on deeper activities. This is to be expected, since the width of layers II and III is, in the precentral area, almost twice as large as in the striate area. The same holds true for the ratio of layers V and VI. To explore the depth of the cortex, the multielectrode proved to be too short so that it had to be further protruded to study the activities in the deepest cortical levels that often turned out to accommodate several generators. The local tonic patterns encountered, however, are generally composed of the same arcade-like waves of the basal frequency, firmly interlocked with spikes, as commonly seen in the striate area. In the same way, the spike components follow the general tendency to spread corticopetally.

Just a few words about the cortical interconnections possibly involved in forming these different generator zones and interlocking them. A discussion of this point is, however, limited by the fact that this study concerns the spatiotemporal relationships in one dimension only, namely in the Z axis of the cortex.

It seems not unlikely that interactions between nerve cells of the pyramidal type and of the Golgi type II play the most important role in the origin of self-sustained activities. There are enough candidates in each layer of the cortex, except layer I, to meet these conditions. Evidently, a conclusive answer to the question of the nature of the generators themselves can only be given after extensive studies at the cellular level. As far as the spatiotemporal organization in the vertical extension of the cortex is concerned, the role of dendritic bundles in maintaining synchronization by connecting layer-V discharges with the generator layers II and III has been discussed in previous papers (4,10). In addition, in this context the system of initial collaterals, recently studied by Tömböl (20) in the visual cortex of the cat, is considered to be of the utmost importance. This system, that Tömböl considers "the most general and widely distributed, as well as quantitatively the most important," creates widespread mutual connections in the vertical and horizontal directions. Briefly stated, its vertical connections are arranged as follows: layer-V pyramidal cells give off, within 100 to 150 μm distance from the parent cell, long vertically ascending side branches with short side branches terminating in small bulbs, which probably contact the apical dendrites of these cells. Possibly, this system is involved in the spreading and synchronization of the cellular bombardment during a seizure. The same is true for the initial collaterals of the cells of layer VI. Moreover, the Meynert cells in layer V contact the dendrites and the somata of pyramidal cells of layers III and II.

These findings, obtained from Golgi material, however, should not create the impression that the circuitries underlying the continually changing generators and their mutual connections are rigid systems. These are only a few of certainly far more pathways that may be taken by the neuronal events in producing the fascinating event of a seizure.

ACKNOWLEDGMENT

This research was supported by the Fonds zur Förderung der wissenschaftlichen Forschung (Nr. 2186 and M 3/1726) and by the European Training Programme in Brain and Behaviour Research (ETPBBR). The calculations were performed in the Rechenzentrum der Medizinischen Fakultät der Universität Wien.

REFERENCES

1. Calvet, J., Calvet, M. C., and Scherrer, J. (1964): Etude stratigraphique corticale de l'activité électroencéphalographique spontanée. *Electroenceph. Clin. Neurophysiol.,* 17:109–125.

2. Creutzfeldt, O., Watanabe, S., and Lux, D. H. (1966): Relations between EEG phenomena and potentials of single cortical cells. II. Spontaneous and convulsoid activity. *Electroenceph. Clin. Neurophysiol.,* 20:19–37.
3. Fleischhauer, K., and Detzer, K. (1975): Dendritic bundling in the cerebral cortex. In: *Advances in Neurology, Vol. 12: Physiology and Pathology of Dendrites,* edited by G. W. Kreutzberg, pp. 71–77. Raven Press, New York.
4. Fleischhauer, K., Petsche, H., and Wittkowski, W. (1972): Vertical bundles of dendrites in the neocortex. *Z. Anat. Entwicklungsgesch.,* 136:213–223.
5. Matsumoto, H., Ayala, G. F., and Ajmone Marsan, C. (1969): Neuronal behavior and triggering mechanism in cortical epileptic focus. *J. Neurophysiol.,* 5:688–704.
6. Matsumoto, H., and Ajmone Marsan, C. (1964): Cortical cellular phenomena in experimental epilepsy: Interictal manifestations. *Exp. Neurol.,* 9:286–304.
7. Matsumoto, H., and Ajmone Marsan, C. (1964): Cortical cellular phenomena in experimental epilepsy: Ictal manifestations. *Exp. Neurol.,* 9:305–326.
8. Petsche, H. Nágypal, T., Prohaska, O., Rappelsberger, P., and Vollmer, R. (1975): Approaches to the spatio-temporal analysis of seizure patterns. In: *CEAN—Computerized EEG Analysis,* edited by G. Dolce, and H. Künkel, pp. 111, 127. Fischer, Stuttgart.
9. Petsche, H., Pockberger, H., Prohaska, O., Rappelsberger, P., and Vollmer, R. (1977): Simultaneous laminar intracortical recordings in seizures. *Electroenceph. Clin. Neurophysiol.,* 42:414–416.
10. Petsche, H., Prohaska, O., Rappelsberger, P., and Vollmer, R. (1975): The possible role of dendrites in EEG synchronization. In: *Advances in Neurology, Vol. 12: Physiology and Pathology of Dendrites,* edited by G. W. Kreutzberg, pp. 53–70. Raven Press, New York.
11. Petsche, H., and Rappelsberger, P. (1971): Spatio-temporal and laminar analysis of self-sustained cortical activity. *Riv. Patol. Nerv. Ment.,* 93:16–44.
12. Petsche, H., and Rappelsberger, P. (1973): The problem of synchronization in the spread of epileptic discharges leading to seizures in man. In: *Epilepsy—Its Phenomenon in Man,* edited by M. A. B. Brazier, pp. 121–151. Academic Press, New York.
13. Petsche, H., Rappelsberger, P., and Frey, Z. (1972): Intracortical aspects of the synchronization of self-sustained bioelectrical activities. In: *Synchronization of EEG Activities,* edited by H. Petsche, and M. A. B. Brazier, pp. 263–284. Springer-Verlag, Wien.
14. Prohaska, O., Olcaytug, F., Womastek, K., and Petsche, H. (1977): A multielectrode for intracortical recordings produced by thin-film technology. *Electroenceph. Clin. Neurophysiol.,* 42:421–422.
15. Rappelsberger, P., Prohaska, O., Petsche, H., and Vollmer, R. (1975): Application of a special time domain technique to epi- and intracortically recorded epileptic seizures. In: *Quantitative Analysis of the EEG,* edited by M. Matejcek, and G. K. Schenk, pp. 297–308. AEG-Telefunken, Konstanz.
16. Rose, M. (1931): Cytoarchitektonischer Atlas der Großhirnrinde des Kaninchens. *J. Psychol. Neurol. (Leipzig),* 43:353–440.
17. Scherrer, J., and Calvet, J. (1972): Normal and epileptic synchronization at the cortical level in the animal. In: *Synchronization of EEG Activities in Epilepsies,* edited by H. Petsche, and M. A. B. Brazier, pp. 112–132. Springer-Verlag, Wien.
18. Speckmann, E. J., Caspers, H., and Janzen, R. W. (1972): Relations between cortical DC-shifts and membrane potential changes of cortical neurons associated with seizure activity. In: *Synchronization of EEG Activities in Epilepsies,* edited by H. Petsche, and M. A. B. Brazier, pp. 93–111. Springer-Verlag, Wien.
19. Tömböl, T. (1972): Golgi analysis of the sensory-motor cortex of the rabbit. In: *Synchronization of EEG Activities in Epilepsies,* edited by H. Petsche, and M. A. B. Brazier, pp. 25–36. Springer-Verlag, Wien-New York.
20. Tömböl, T. (1975): Collateral axonal arborizations. In: *Golgi Centennial Symposium: Perspectives in Neurobiology,* edited by M. Santini, pp. 133–141. Raven Press, New York.
21. Vollmer, R., Petsche, H., Pockberger, H., Prohaska, O., and Rappelsberger, P. (1977): Spatiotemporal analysis of cortical seizure activities in a homogeneous cytoarchitectonical region *(this volume).*

Architectonics of the Cerebral Cortex,
edited by M. A. B. Brazier and H. Petsche.
Raven Press, New York © 1978.

Spatiotemporal Analysis of Cortical Seizure Activities in a Homogeneous Cytoarchitectonic Region

*R. Vollmer, *H. Petsche, **H. Pockberger, **O. Prohaska, and *,**P. Rappelsberger

*Neurophysiological Institute of the University of Vienna, and **Brain Research Institute of the Austrian Academy of Sciences, Vienna, Austria

The most interesting feature of the cerebral cortex and still its greatest enigma is its electrical activity. Although it has been shown that cellular activity increases during certain surface phenomena and decreases during others (1–3), no general conclusions can be drawn as far as the steadily changing electrocorticogram (ECoG) is concerned. It has been shown by statistical analysis that only a time-limited correlation exists between cellular behaviour and the ECoG (4). This led to the conclusion that "the ECoG is produced by intermittent synchronization of selected groups of nerve cells" (5). Hence, it follows that a one-dimensional analysis of the ECoG seems to be insufficient to yield all the information that is probably included in the ECoG. Therefore, it seems reasonable to study the cerebral activity topographically.

Spatiotemporal analysis is occasionally used in clinical neurophysiology, especially for evoked potentials and for the analysis of epileptic seizures (for reference see ref. 15). It was reported that, during epileptic seizures, cortical equipotential maps — representing the ECoG — obey certain rules that suggest a connection between electrical behavior and cortical morphology (14). This line of research was pursued in the following years (9,10). The main results were as follows:

1. The conventional ECoG can be expressed in terms of positive and negative parts of potential fields (P-fields) which need not behave in the same way.
2. Special pathological situations exist in which these fields seem to change their places ("propagation").
3. This propagation may take place in a very regular manner.
4. Cytoarchitectonic borderlines influence the propagation of these P-fields.
5. Propagation can be prevented by vertical incisions down to the layer VI.

Since these findings seem to indicate that certain fundamental structural properties of the cortex may be reflected by its electrical activity, a more thorough study of the surface activity during epileptic seizures was undertaken.

MATERIALS AND METHODS

Experiments were carried out on 16 adult rabbits of both sexes with an average weight of 2.5 kg. The choice of this animal was prompted by several considerations: the rabbit is the animal with the largest uncurved cortex and therefore most suitable for topographical studies with multiple electrodes. Moreover, theoretical considerations have shown that the convolution of the cortex, which may be found in other animals, is the main source of distortion of common reference recordings (8).

After light anesthesia with a short-time barbiturate (thiopental) tracheotomy was performed under local anesthesia with 2% procaine. The animals were immobilized by d-tubocurarine and artificially respirated with room air. Body temperature was maintained with a heating device between 37 and 39°C. The head was fixed in a stereotactic frame and the skull was opened. Pressure points and open wounds were heavily infiltrated with repeated infiltrations of 2% procaine. The dura was removed and recordings were carried out directly from the cortical surface. Different cortical areas were studied: the parietal region, the striatal area, and the area retrosplenogranularis beta (17), but of primary interest was the electrical activity of the striatal cortex.

Recordings were made with 7×7 Ag-AgCl electrodes with a diameter of 0.3 mm and an interelectrode distance of 1 or 2 mm. These electrodes were arranged in a square of 6 mm length and fixed together with synthetic resin. The whole arrangement was placed stereotactically on the cortex under microscopical control. Recordings were made against a remote electrode on the nasal bone. From these 49 electrodes, 16 leads, forming a square, were deliberately chosen and registered on a 16-channel EEG machine. As the criterion for the selection of the derivations, the choice in most cases was that cortical site where the highest spontaneous or evoked activity was recorded. Seizures were elicited by epi- or intracortical application of 1 M Na-penicillin G solution (PNC), in some cases also by intravenous application of pentylenetetrazol (Cardiazol®). The electrical activity of the 16 electrodes was stored on a magnetic tape, which was connected to a multiplexer, for later calculations. In all cases the chosen electrodes formed a square, covering a surface of 9 or 36 mm² of the cortex.

MATHEMATICAL TREATMENT OF THE DATA

Isopotential lines were calculated according to the method given by Trappl (19), which has been modified by Rappelsberger and Prohaska. Calculations were performed by a 370/145 IBM computer at the Medizinisches Rechenzentrum der Universität Wien. Equipotential maps were calculated every 2, 4, and 8 msec, depending on the nature of the electrical activity, i.e., high-frequency events needed closer time intervals than ECoG curves containing lower frequencies. The data presented here are based on more than 10,000 equipotential maps of several minutes of ECoG activity. Such an enormous amount of data makes reduction necessary. Therefore, major attention was given to the behaviour of the positive or negative potential fields (Fig. 1). After visual inspection of the equipotential maps, the place of the maximum of the P-field was marked and followed through successive equipotential maps, thus analyzing its behaviour in time and space. With this procedure the emergence and decay of P-fields of different polarity and size can be followed over time. To do this, the points of maxima of subsequent P-fields were connected by lines. These lines are thus speed vectors representing the change of position of the fields at equal time intervals, usually every 8 msec. This method has its limits, however, since it is only feasible if P-fields of more or less circular circumference are present on the equipotential maps, where the position of the maximum is representative for the position of the whole field. Actually, however, particularly during irregular ECoG patterns, this does not occur so that a visual examination of the maps is indispensable. Some of the material that has been gained with this method has been published recently elsewhere (10).

RESULTS

Among the countless electrical phenomena the cerebral cortex is capable of producing, there are some that are characteristic for epileptic events: (a) the "spike," (b) the beginning of a seizure, (c) the tonic activity, (d) the clonic activity, and (e) irregular self-sustained activities that are difficult to classify.

An epileptic focus is characterized by "spike" activity. Repeated spikes are the first sign of a penicillin-induced seizure, which starts with tonic activity, then undergoes a sudden change and the pattern (c), (d), and (e) alternate in an unforeseeable manner.

Spikes

A description of the spatiotemporal features of ECoG spikes by topographical methods was given in a previous paper (10). These results are corroborated by the present findings and may be briefly summarized as follows.

These spikes usually start with a positivity somewhere in the recorded area. The gradient of the P-fields is not so steep as is usually seen in seizure waves. After local application of penicillin, the positive maximum propagates but in a much more irregular manner than do seizure waves and not to

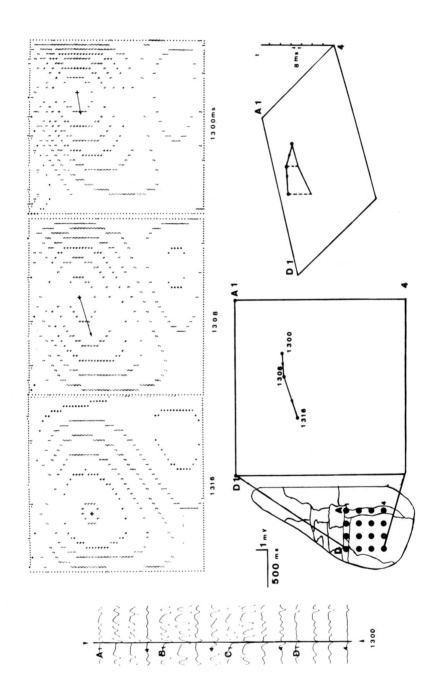

the same extent, whereas the maximum of the negative field of the spike seems to remain stationary (Fig. 2A–D). Spike activity takes place not only prior to seizures, but may also be interspersed in fully developed seizure activity (Fig. 2E). Nevertheless, the fundamental properties of the P-fields of ECoG spikes remain unchanged. The ECoG of Fig. 2E was recorded with 1-mm interelectrode distance over the area striata. It shows a regular seizure pattern which is interrupted by a single PNC spike. Two following P-fields (1 and 2 in Fig. 2E) are shown on the right. It is seen that the path of the first field has no relation at all to the path of the second positivity, whereas the seizure activity mostly takes place rostrally and medially outside the square.

This behaviour allows a clear distinction between spike activity and seizure patterns from the topographical point of view, because as will be seen later on, seizure activity is characterized by a clearly determined spatial sequence of the positive or negative P-fields of the half-waves out of which it is composed. It should be remembered, however, that, even in seizure patterns, there are sudden changes in the spatiotemporal behaviour of surface P-fields. These sudden changes reflect lack of stationarity and are believed to be due to some cortical or subcortical influences, which disturb the regular behaviour of surface P-fields.

The Beginning of a Penicillin-Induced Seizure

PNC-induced seizures usually start with a PNC spike followed by sinusoidal waves of lower voltage and of high frequency (Fig. 3). Then the frequency slowly decreases. The spatiotemporal analysis of the P-fields shows that these are first restricted to a relatively small region of the cortex. Although the visual analysis of the ECoG indicates a continuous decrease

---

FIG. 1. Description of the procedure. **Left:** Sixteen ECoG signals (calibration: 500 msec/ 1mV), recorded from 16 Ag-AgCl electrodes from the area striata of rabbit's cortex against a common reference electrode on the nasal bone. These electrodes are labelled A to D and 1 to 4, and correspond to the ECoG signals. The electrodes are arranged in a square, the interelectrode distance between adjacent electrodes being 2 mm (only 1 mm in Figs. 2, 3, 6, 10, and 11). The exact position of the electrodes on the cortex is shown by the black dots on the inset in the middle of the figure, which represents a dorsal view of the rabbit's brain, according to Rose (17). **Upper:** From those 16 ECoG traces, equi-potential maps are calculated at 8-msec intervals, each of them representing the potential distribution over the cortical region covered by the electrodes at a certain instant. These maps are to be read from right to left. The first shows that, at time 1,300 **(vertical bar in the ECoG),** a large positivity is present with its maximum somewhere in the region of electrode B2. This positive potential field is not stable, but propagates over the cortex. **Lower:** The square represents the cortical region covered by the 16 electrodes. The coordinates of the maxima of the positive potential fields, seen in the equipotential maps of the upper part of the figure, are marked on the square and connected by lines, these lines being speed vectors. **Right lower:** The square seen from left behind. Time is indicated on the z axis. The dots indicate the position of the maximum of the potential field every 8 msec.

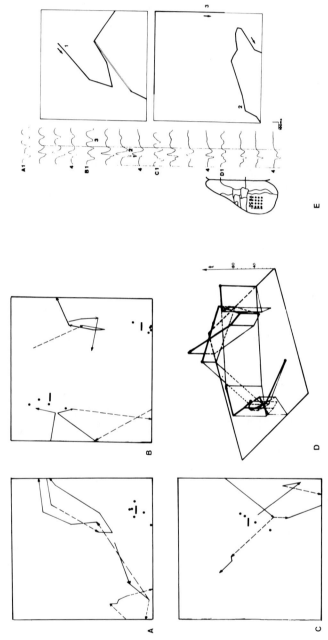

FIG. 2. Five individual penicillin spikes from one experiment were analyzed (**A** to **E**). The corresponding ECoG pattern is shown only for **E** (calibration: 1mV, 100 msec). Each square represents the cortical area covered by the 16 electrodes (9 mm²). The equipotential maps were calculated at 8-msec intervals and the location of maximum positivity of the fields were marked. These locations were connected by lines so that speed-vector graphs result. In **E**, the corresponding events in the ECoG and in the vector graphs are indicated by the numbers 1 to 3. The vectors were drawn as dashed lines when the computer did not give an unambiguous location of the maximum. In **D**, the same was presented, but with time on z axis. Note the complicated configuration the positive P-field maxima describe with time. In contrast to this, the negative P-field maxima (dots with "—" sign) remain almost stationary. **A–D:** Interseizure spikes. **E:** A spike, superimposed on a seizure activity fading away, their maxima being outside the square.

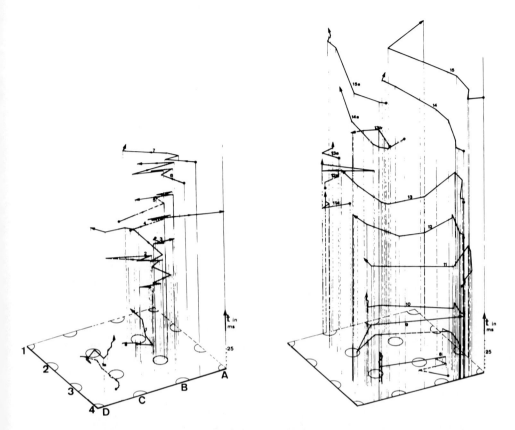

FIG. 3. Three-dimensional representation of the beginning of penicillin-induced seizure activity, recorded as in Fig. 1. Time on the z axis (to be read from left to right). The numbers correspond to the waves of the accompanying ECoG (not in the figure). From wave numbers 3 to 7, the positive P-field maxima are concentrated on a small place; from 7 to 14 the maxima propagate in about the same way, with increasing range. At 14, the spatiotemporal behaviour abruptly changes.

of the frequency, the analysis of the P-fields shows that their spatial pattern of propagation makes some abrupt changes, as was also previously observed (9).

Such nonstationarities of the spatiotemporal behaviour, i.e., moments in which the P-fields behave in an unforeseeable manner, are illustrated by the beginning of the seizure in Fig. 3. First, there are a few irregular components (waves numbered by 1, 1a, and 2) the propagation of which does not show any tendency. Then, beginning with wave number 3, the amplitude maxima tend to remain concentrated in a relatively small part of the recording square; however, during the further development of the activity (about between wave numbers 7 and 13), the amplitude maxima seem to concentrate in two regions where they show a tendency to remain quasistationary (corresponding to the electrodes A,B4, and C3). These two regions, however, become more and more separated from each other. Beginning with wave number 14, a quite new spatiotemporal behaviour begins insofar as the two regions described above do not anymore initiate each other but act independently, which illustrates a spatiotemporal non-stationarity.

Tonic Pattern

The most regular activity the cortex is able to produce is the tonic seizure. The spatiotemporal analysis of this pattern has demonstrated that the surface P-fields appear to describe almost circular pathways (10). An example of this activity is shown in Fig. 4. It must be emphasized that in regular patterns the negative maximum exactly follows the path of the maximum of the positive P-field. Moreover, one has the impression that this property is even characteristic for regular seizure activities. In the case of Fig. 4, the electrode grid covers 36 mm² of the striatal area, i.e., the interelectrode distance is 2 mm. The figure shows the superimposition of the paths of the positive maxima of all the ECoG waves. The distance between two points reflects the propagation within 8 msec. At first sight, all P-fields seem to describe an almost circular path around a point somewhere in the middle of the square grid. No single positive maximum propagates across the square.

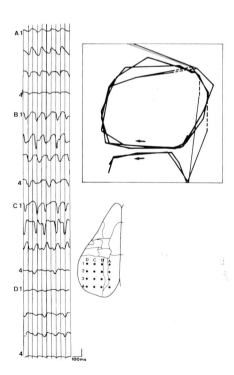

FIG. 4. Speed-vector graphs of the positive P-field maxima of a tonic seizure. The electrode grid covers 36 mm². As in all regular activities, the propagation of the negative P-field maxima (not drawn) exactly follows the paths of the positive ones. Note the almost circular propagation of the P-field maxima for all three waves. Two of them show an additional circling of another maximum in the lower part of the recording square.

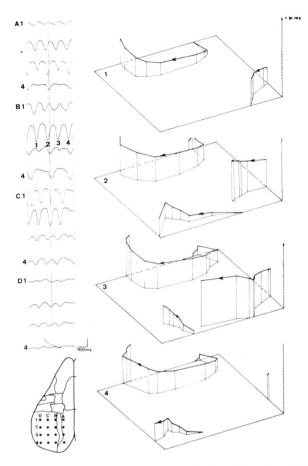

FIG. 5. Tonic seizure as in Fig. 4, but 30 sec later, in three-dimensional view (as in Fig. 1, 2D and Fig. 3). Again a circular propagation of the P-field maxima is found, but now the circles have shifted rostrally. Each P-field is accompanied by a P-field propagating counterclockwise in the lower part of the area striata, but, in contrast to Fig. 4, the medial and the lateral parts of the caudal region seem to act independently of each other.

Some of them are accompanied by other P-fields in the lower part of the cortical square that also move circularly but counterclockwise.

A closer inspection reveals that the distances between two successive maxima are not equally distributed along their paths over the cortex. Obviously, there do exist cortical regions in which a P-field tends to remain more or less stationary. These special regions coincide with those, where the amplitude maxima of the P-fields repeatedly attain the highest voltage (not shown in the figure because of data reduction and simplification, but see below).

Figure 5 shows an example of the change of tonic activity with time. It is from the same animal and the same seizure as the preceding figure and shows another tonic pattern but 30 sec later. The four squares represent the cortical area and the spatiotemporal behaviour of each of the four positive half-waves. Time is registered on the z axis. It turns out that the main activity has now shifted rostrally with respect to the situation in Fig. 4. The highest amplitudes of the ECoG are found at the same electrodes as before but now the P-fields behave differently. Most likely, there still exists a circular clockwise propagation. The center of the circle, however, has shifted rostrally. Each positive P-field that moves in this direction is followed by another, smaller one, that crosses the caudal part of the striatal area anticlockwise. On closer examination a phase shift is found between the rostral and the caudal parts of this special cortical activity. It is best seen in the ECoG between electrodes C2 and C3. This time shift was already present in Fig. 4 but only for the two positive transients 2 and 4.

There is, in the cortical activity, still another difference between these two examples of tonic seizures: in Fig. 4, the P-fields behave in the same way in the caudal part of the area striata, but this regularity has vanished 30 sec later (Fig. 5). In fact, one gets the impression that the medial and the lateral parts of this region now act largely independently from each other. In other words, a strong linkage of different cortical regions has been replaced by a weaker one.

It is interesting to follow this disintegration of tonic activity over time. An example of this is shown in Fig. 6. The ECoG shows three different stages of a tonic seizure at 3-sec intervals, recorded with an interelectrode distance of 1 mm. It is part of the end of an experiment after the administration of a low dose of diazepam (0.5 mg/kg) that is known to regularize the cortical activity at low dosages (11). The frequency decreases with time from 6.3 to 5.2 Hz and the ECoG pattern slightly changes its shape (see channel 9). The behaviour of the P-fields also changes: the first three P-fields still describe nearly circular paths, whereas the other P-fields tend to curve around a spot in the left upper part of the electrode grid, and even this place does not remain stable but is slowly displaced rostrally. It is evident that this information cannot be acquired by visual inspection of several ECoG curves, even if one carefully observes the phase relationships with higher paper speed. The significance of this finding will be discussed later in the light of the results of other authors.

Looking at the speed-vector graphs, we got the impression that there might be an interdependence between the amount of the propagation of the P-field maxima and their amplitudes. Therefore, correlation functions were calculated between amplitude of the P-field maximum and speed vector for three different parts of a tonic seizure (Fig. 7). Autocorrelation of both the speed vector and the amplitude of the P-field maxima shows a rhythmic oscillation of both parameters with time. The periodicity of the amplitudes of the P-field maxima is best seen in part III of the seizure: this is probably due to the fact that, in this sample, the ECoG frequency is most stable.

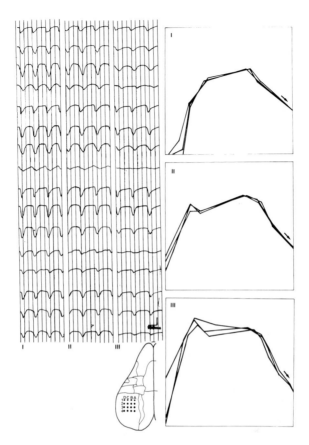

FIG. 6. Speed-vector graphs of the tonic activity in another experiment after 0.5 mg/kg diazepam administration. Interelectrode distance, 1 mm; the electrode covers now 9 mm². Three stages, 3 sec apart, are shown. The main frequency decreases from 6.3 to 5.2 Hz. Almost circular propagation of the P-field maxima in stage I of the sample is illustrated. In stages II and III, a distinct cortical region becomes predominant (corresponding to electrode position C2) around which the P-field maxima seem to curve during their propagation. Besides, this particular place seems also to shift rostrally.

The speed vectors, on the other hand, do not show such a good correlation with the ECoG frequency. In the cross correlation, a significant correlation between speed vector and amplitude of the P-field maxima is found for all three parts of the seizure. Moreover, for parts I and II, a time delay of 16 msec between amplitude of the P-field maximum and speed vector is found, the speed vector being the leading one. This means that the amplitude maximum appears at the leading edge of the speed vector. This finding suggests that the speed of propagation of the P-field maxima may be determined by the amplitude this maximum is attaining. In contrast to the first two parts, the third part is ambiguous: according to the cross correlation, there may be

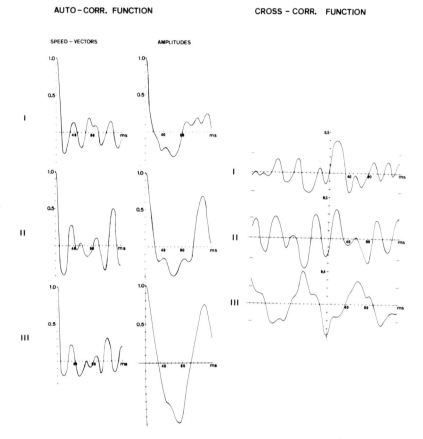

FIG. 7. Correlation functions between the amplitude of the P-field maximum and its speed vector from the three different stages (I to III) of the tonic seizure shown in Fig. 8. **A:** Autocorrelation function. As was to be expected, a clear rhythmic oscillation of the amplitude of the P-field maximum is visible, especially in stage III. The speed vectors do not show such a clear oscillation with the rhythm of the ECoG frequency. **B:** Cross-correlation function between amplitude of the P-field maxima and the speed vector of the same three stages of tonic activity as in **A.** The correlation between the two parameters is significant (significance levels indicated by bars). For stages I and II, a cross-correlation coefficient of 0.37 is found between these parameters with a time delay of 16 msec, thus indicating that the speed of the propagation of the P-field maxima is determined by the amplitude the P-field maximum is attaining. Stage III is ambiguous (see text).

either a negative correlation between amplitude maximum and speed vector or the amplitude is leading by about 50 msec.

For graphical representation, the histograms of both the speed vectors and the amplitudes of the P-field maxima were drawn. Figure 8 shows the ECoG, the circular shifting of the P-fields, and the histograms of the two parameters during three different stages of a tonic pattern. The histograms show the distribution of the maximal amplitude of the P-fields and the

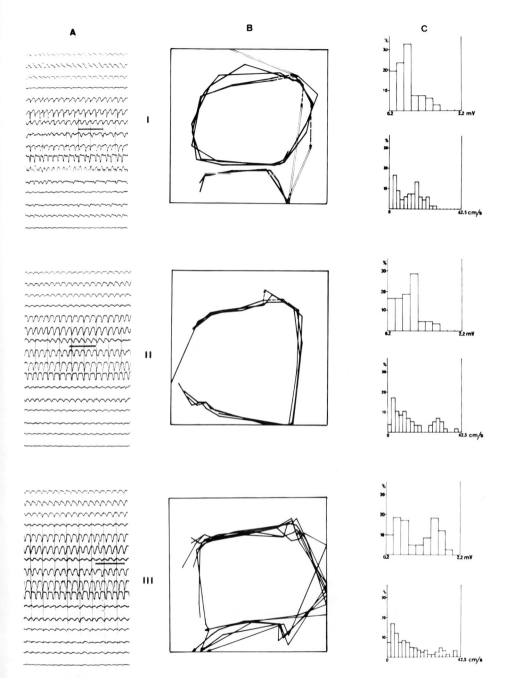

FIG. 8. Speed-vector graphs of the same tonic seizure stages as in Fig. 7. ECoGs on the left side. Electrode position as in Fig. 4. Calibration: 500 msec, 1 mV. Note the decrease in frequency from 9.5 to 8.5 Hz. The speed-vector graphs of the positive P-field maxima of four to five subsequent waves are shown in the middle of the figure. The circles change their shapes during the three stages of the tonic seizure, which were recorded 3 sec apart. On the right, the histograms of both the amplitude of the P-field maximum and the speed vector are shown. Note that there are two modes of speed vector in stage I and two modes of the amplitude in stage III.

speed vectors; it is remarkable that the distributions vary widely in the different stages of this self-sustained activity.

There is another interesting feature: one may see that the modes of the distributions of the amplitudes of the P-field maxima and the modes of the distribution of the speed vectors follow different laws. In stage I there is one mode in the amplitude histogram and there are two modes in the speed vector histogram; in stage II the two modes of the speed vector histogram are more separated than in stage I; and in stage III, different distribution curves exist for both parameters – two modes for the amplitude and only one for the speed vector. It was thus tempting to pick up two ranges of the parameters and to compare them. In this way four possible combinations of amplitude maximum and speed vector were obtained:

A: low-amplitude P-field maxima, low speed vector
B: high-amplitude P-field maxima, high speed vector
C: high-amplitude P-field maxima, low speed vector
D: low-amplitude P-field maxima, high speed vector

The next step was to prove the spatial distribution of these four different groups. As demonstrated in Fig. 9, only such points show a distinct spatial and temporal distribution, where the speed vectors are low, independent of the amplitude of the field maximum. This means that there are preferred regions on the cortex where the P-fields remain quasistationary. The black points in Fig. 9 designate the high-amplitude maxima in their spatial distribution, while the small circles indicate the low ones.

In Table 1, the relative frequency of occurrence of the four groups is shown. Group A occurs most frequently in the first stage, whereas group C is found to be most frequent in the third stage of the seizure. The other two ranges show, in all three stages of the seizure, the same frequency of occurrence.

A closer examination of the spatial distribution of the clusters of Fig. 9 shows that they change their position in the square with respect to time. This is clearly seen in the cluster in the right lower part of the square, which disappears between stage II and stage III. One thus gets the impression that these clusters are related to special cortical regions that do not seem to be stable but alter their position with time. This assumption is corroborated by the observation that, within the first stage, there are only clusters of group C around electrode C2, while the region of the electrodes A,B2 contains only clusters of group A. There is a cluster of group C in the lower part of the electrode arrangement that disappears during the development of the seizure. At the end of the observation period, however, there are mostly group C clusters around electrodes C2 and A,B2, the former being somewhat displaced medially.

The same figure (right side of Fig. 9) shows (for all measured data) the change of the speed vector with time and its spatial representation. It turned out that these places are also clustered and that these clusters

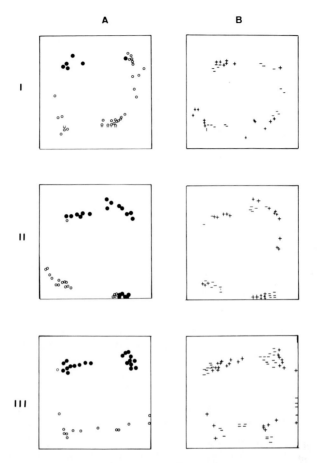

FIG. 9. Same tonic seizure as in Figs. 7 and 8. Demonstration of the spatial distribution of sites in the A. striata where P-fields with either a high-amplitude maximum or a low-amplitude maximum propagate over short distances only. **A:** The three stages again represent the electrode grid in the three different stages of the seizure. The black dots designate the P-field maxima with high amplitudes; the circles indicate maxima with low ones. Note the increasing clustering of the black dots during the development of the seizure, indicating that the amplitudes of the P-field maxima increase over distinct regions with the ongoing seizure. In these regions, the fields tend to remain stationary. **B:** Spatial distribution of all measured speed vectors of the three stages. An increase of these vectors is indicated by a "+" sign and vice versa. The speed vectors, too, are not distributed at random, but are clustered on the same regions as in Fig. 9A. Regions where the speed vector decreases are followed by such where an increase takes place. Note for both parts of the figure that such a particular region (near the right lower corner of the square) disappears between stages II and III, and that the two other clusters change both their shapes and their relative positions in the square.

coincide with the clusters of groups A and C. It is remarkable that places where the speed vector diminishes are always followed by such areas where an increase takes place. These findings seem to indicate that, during their travel, propagating P-fields seem to slow down in velocity, simul-

TABLE 1. *Relative frequency of occurrence of the four possible combinations of amplitude maximum and speed vector in the three stages of seizure*

	Stage		
Group	I	II	III
A	53.7%	29.3%	22.0%
B	22.4%	19.0%	23.2%
C	9.0%	36.2%	40.2%
D	14.9%	15.5%	14.6%

taneously increase in amplitude, then decrease in amplitude and again travel over a longer distance, but with increasing speed.

It is interesting to note that the frequency of the tonic seizure from stage I to stage III slowed down from 9.5 to 8.5 Hz. This seems to indicate that, at the beginning of a seizure, almost exclusively low-voltage P-fields are present, which travel only short distances, but, at the end of the tonic seizure, when its frequency has decreased, these P-fields propagate over short distances, attain high amplitudes, and, then suddenly, propagate over long ones. And third, if, at the beginning of the tonic seizure, three clusters were present where the activity seemed to be concentrated, this does not hold true anymore for the end of the seizure, although these clusters are more distinct than they were at the beginning of the seizure (see Fig. 9). The possible functional meaning of these findings will be discussed later on in this chapter.

One further remarkable observation concerning the extent of the cortical surface taken by the propagating P-fields has to be added: there are some indications that this extent largely depends on the amplitude of the P-fields. As Fig. 10 demonstrates, the tonic pattern in this stage has occasionally been interrupted by positive transients that are very similar, in their amplitude distribution, to the main transients but have lower amplitudes (wave numbers 2 and 5). These waves not only follow the main transients at shorter intervals but also have been caused by potential fields whose radius of circling is smaller than that of the main transients. This is sketched in the inset at the lower right of Fig. 10. This is a further and impressive sample for the fact that, in self-sustained activities, the ECoG frequency is determined by the length of the path the propagating potential field is covering.

Clonic Pattern

A special seizure pattern consisting of groups of waves interrupted by isoelectric intervals of up to 1 sec is called clonic. Although its waves sometimes look sinusoidal, they clearly differ in their spatiotemporal behaviour

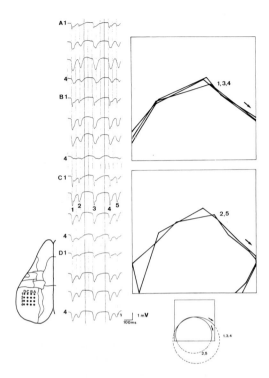

FIG. 10. Example of the mutual interdependence of amplitude, velocity of propagation, and the spatial distribution of propagating P-fields. Positive transients of the end of a seizure. Two of the main transients (wave numbers 1 and 4) are immediately followed by other positive transients with lower amplitude (wave numbers 2 and 5), the paths of both groups being circular. However, the lower transients follow smaller circles than the higher ones.

from the sinusoidal tonic seizure. Optical similarity does not mean that the underlying P-fields behave equally, as Fig. 11 shows. No obviously preferred way of propagation exists for this pattern, but three different sources seem to emerge in this sample almost simultaneously, as can be shown by the analysis of the single-surface P-fields.

Irregular Seizure Pattern

Seizure patterns that look irregular on the ECoG may be irregular in two different aspects, when looked at from the topographical point of view: irregular in space and irregular in time. These two dimensions of irregularity are in most cases combined. The P-field analysis of such patterns allows a clear distinction between these two possibilities: if the irregularity in shape concerns only the time dimension, the fields are mostly well represented by the position of their maxima, and speed vector graphs may be drawn as in the cases of clonic patterns. But if the irregularity additionally concerns the

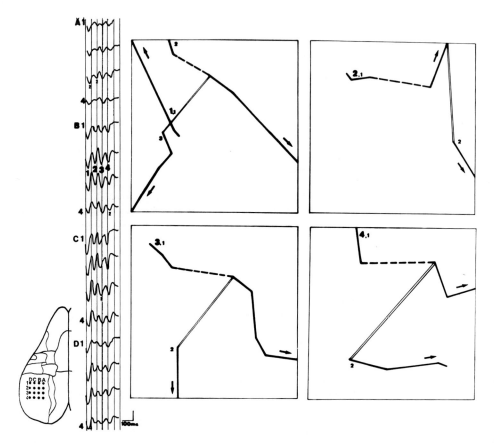

FIG. 11. Speed-vector graphs of clonic seizure patterns. PNC-induced seizure. Although the clonic pattern much resembles a regular tonic activity, a topographical analysis by means of speed-vector graphs reveals completely different behaviour of the positive P-field maxima. No regular propagation can be seen, but the simultaneous emergence of several P-fields can. In this case, as in the case of irregular seizure patterns, negative and positive P-field maxima behave independently from one another.

dimension of space, the equipotential lines are often complicated curves and the position of the maxima of the P-fields (that are given by the computer) cannot be considered any longer as representative for the whole field. Speed-vector graphs of such fields, therefore, will yield an apparently random behaviour of their propagation. A more detailed analysis of this pattern, therefore, was not attempted in this chapter.

DISCUSSION

These studies, the purpose of which was to obtain a better knowledge of the phenomena underlying the ECoG, namely the interweaving of potential fields, both confirm previous results and yield some new suggestions for a few rules controlling synchronization. From this point of view, it is worth discussing the essential differences between the spatiotemporal behaviour of interseizure phenomena such as "spikes," the beginning of self-sustained activities, and the different kinds of seizure patterns. In the time domain, the spikes differ mainly in two aspects from the waves of self-sustained activity: the duration of their individual constituents is by far shorter than the duration of the waves in self-sustained activities (except interspersed spikes) and their voltage is much greater: PNC spikes may attain amplitudes up to several millivolts, whereas the seizure waves are seldom more than 2 mV. In the space domain, spikes are often caused by P-fields or larger extent than seizure waves (10). As far as the propagation of their points of maxima is concerned, there is a consistent difference between negative and positive P-field maxima: a propagation of the maxima is seen only for the positive half-waves whereas the negative half-waves appear stationary. The reason for this is still obscure. One may assume, it is true, that the fast positive part of the epicortical spike is connected to neuronal discharges in deep cortical layers (1–3), and it may be assumed that the following slow negativity could accompany inhibition. But the nature of this inhibition is uncertain: it is in most cases even unlikely that the cells that are involved in the formation of the positive phase are the same that produce this negativity, because, as Fig. 2 demonstrates, the moving of the positive maxima of the P-fields often occurs outside the negative field. Since the spatial distribution of the positive and the negative maxima of the P-fields does not coincide, no direct dependence between these two events may be assumed.

One of the most remarkable features of the P-fields of spikes is the arbitrary shifting of their maxima. Even if a greater number of P-fields is measured, there is no possibility to foresee the path the following potential field will take. Another difference with respect to self-sustained seizure waves is the short range of the shifting of the maxima. Other than in seizure waves, these maxima tend to remain fairly constant before shifting to another point. Although this shifting may raise the impression of a true propagation of the maxima (an impression that is even stronger in seizure waves), two other possibilities have to be considered. One is that the margin of error of the calculation of the coordinates of the P-field maxima is so large that no decision can be made about the possible physiological nature of this displacement. But there is one main reason against this, namely the observation that the negative maxima of the P-fields often remain stationary within a fraction of 1 mm^2 over fairly long periods. The other possibility is that the generator zone underlying a P-field remains stationary for a couple of milliseconds and then is replaced by another generator zone apart from this; this alternating activation of different generator zones can raise the impression of a propagation particularly if the number of these activated generator zones is high and their distance is small. We understand "generator zone" to mean "that volume of cortical tissue that gives rise to one distinct grapho-element in the ECoG." The term is merely descriptive (11)].

In summary, the spikes, in their spatiotemporal aspect, seem to be composed of the activation of generator zones, the position and the shifting of which is not foreseeable.

The beginning of self-sustained activities has been mainly studied in PNC-induced seizures in the striate area, because they are a good model of the focal seizures with generalization in humans. The spikes do not vanish immediately at the beginning of the seizure but fade within the first few seconds. They may reappear before the end of the seizure, but never occur during the full seizure activity. From this, one may conclude that, for the emergence of a spike and of self-sustained activities, different neuronal circuits seem to be involved.

It is tempting to bring this finding into context with the degree of synchronization. Although general agreement about the meaning of this concept has not yet been achieved, these results shed new light on this phenomenon; that, in seizures, a high degree of spatiotemporal organization is maintained for relatively long periods of time. In 1972, we postulated taking the similarity of shape rather then synchrony as a criterion (13). This raises the question of how this similarity of potentials in different recording points may be produced. The beginning of a seizure is a good example from which to discuss this mechanism. As may be seen in Fig. 3, the seizure starts after a transient (wave numbers 1 and 1a), the P-fields of which behave unpredictably. Then, two centers of alternating activity develop (wave numbers 7 to 13) with increasing distance. At wave number 14, a sudden change of the spatiotemporal organization occurs, the new organization being maintained for another few waves. Two phenomena are to be considered in this context: (a) the question of propagation of P-fields and (b) the possible significance of this sudden spatiotemporal new organization ("switching") that may best be studied in tonic seizure patterns.

To (a): If, in this context, the words "movements of P-fields," "propagation," or "shifting" are used, we always understand an apparent displacement of the points of maximum of the P-fields within a range of centimeters per second, the nature of it does not need to be discussed at present. These words are only used to describe the phenomenon.

However, another phenomenon is usually observed: there are preferred regions where the speed vectors decrease to a minimum. A dislocation of these regions in the course of several waves is also observed, but at much lower speed (a few mm/min, see Figs. 6, 8, and 9). Therefore, the "propagation" of the P-fields has to be clearly distinguished from the "dislocation" of those regions where the propagation is minimum.

To (b): The switching phenomenon, a sudden change of the ECoG pattern, is obviously related to the problem of synchronization itself, since it can be found simultaneously in depth recordings during different stages of the seizure (see this volume). Thus, it seems that it does not concern only the most superficial layers but involves the entire cortex profile. Depth recordings seem to indicate that sudden changes of the ECoG pattern are due to sudden changes of the linkage of different generator zones. Since this must be projected toward the surface one can assume that the switching phenomenon, seen at the surface, represents a new linkage of different generator zones.

The tonic seizure pattern, a special case of cortical synchronization, also reflects some principles underlying cortical synchronization. A topographical analysis of P-fields of tonic seizure patterns shows that these P-fields travel more or less circularly over the cortex (Figs. 4 and 8). It is evident that the speed of the displacement of the P-field maxima is not uniform but that there are regions where they seem to slow down and others where they seem to speed up (Fig. 9). The spatial distribution of the maximum amplitudes of the P-fields is not random, but clustered (see Fig. 9, stage III). This can even be concluded from the ECoG pattern in Fig. 8. The change of the amplitude maxima of the P-fields and the change of the speed vectors are fluctuating phenomena and are correlated to each other, as was shown by the correlation function (Fig. 7). This correlation however, changes with time (compare Fig. 7/1 and 7/3). It may be assumed from the correlation function that either P-fields with low amplitude travel short distances or vice versa. On the other hand, toward the end of the tonic seizure, high-amplitude P-fields travel short distances and vice versa. Furthermore, Fig. 9 shows that two out of groups A to D are clustered at distinct cortical regions, namely, groups A and C (see also Fig. 8 and Table 1). Moreover, it can be concluded that the relatively high correlation between amplitude and speed vector at a time shift of 16 msec is determined mostly by group A (compare Fig. 7/1 and Fig. 9/1).

From all these observations it is reasonable to conclude that a tonic pattern is likely to be produced by the successive activation of different neuronal populations or generator zones, pulsing in the same rhythm, but shifted in time. To assume a successive activation is logical because the P-fields never reverse in their propagation. Thus, a highly ordered sequence of the activation of different generator zones must take place. This successive activation is, in our case, of such a kind that an almost circular propagation of the P-fields appears. It is possible that other kinds of propagation also exist, at least in the striate area. It may be, however, that the striate area as the largest region of a homogeneous cortical structure is particularly prone to produce this kind of propagation. In this context it should also be mentioned that the longest tonic patterns are found in this region.

It is a common experience that the cortex is not able to maintain tonic patterns for very long periods of time. Thus, it seems likely that the high regularity of the activation of different generator zones may easily be dis-rupted. In this context, some speculations about the possible nature of such disturbing influences might be in order.

The idea that cortical synchronization is due to the sequential or mutual initiation of different electrical sources was first proposed by Fessard (6) who arrived by theoretical considerations at the conclusion that the model of pacemakers beating in the same rhythm would best fit the known results. But this model requires some assumptions: the rhythm of a single pace-maker must not be disturbed by other influences and the phase lag between it and the following one has to be constant, i.e., provided that the speed of the information transport is the same, the spatial distance between these two pacemakers must also be the same. None of these assumptions is veri-fied for the tonic activity of the intact cortex, because it is under the steady influence of subcortical regions. Therefore, it is likely that these influences may easily disorganize the high regularity of the successive activation of different generator zones, either by changing the rhythm of a single generator zone or by creating a new one by additional synaptic bombardment of a certain cortical region already under the strong influence of the epilepto-genic region in the neighborhood. This may be one of the main reasons why P-fields suddenly change their direction of propagation. This seems also to be the reason why the undercut cortex is better able to produce long-lasting tonic patterns than the intact cortex (16).[1]

That even an unexpected extraneous intracortical influence is able to disturb the highly balanced relationship between different cortical popula-tions may be assumed from Fig. 2.

But there is still another reason why tonic activity cannot be maintained for longer periods of time, namely the unstable nature of the generator zones (or "pacemakers" according to Fessard) themselves. It is evident from Figs. 8 and 9 that the clusters of groups A and C are not stable. They also change with time. In the last seconds of the tonic seizure, the combination between high amplitude and low speed vector becomes more prominent (Fig. 9/3). This can only mean that, in this special region, a closer syn-chronization of underlying elementary events of still unknown nature takes place. It seems, therefore, that at the beginning of a tonic seizure there are several generator zones present that give rise to a successive activation of their neighbors, whereas at the end of a tonic seizure there are only a few (Fig. 9/3), the other being devoured by the increasing synchronization of the former.

There is reason to believe that still another mechanism is involved in the breakdown of a tonic seizure. A close inspection of the paths of the P-fields

---

[1] Hirsch, J. (1975): Contribution à l'Étude de l'Activité Spontanée et Paroxystique d'un Gyrus Cortical Isolé. Thesis, Université Paris VI.

and the clustering phenomenon in subsequent time intervals during a tonic seizure reveals that these clusters change their position with time (Figs. 4, 6, 8, and 9). In Fig. 9, this dislocation is clearly seen in the clusters in the region of electrode B3, which vanishes between stage II and stage III of this seizure. It is evident that such dislocations, if they exceed a certain distance, are able to impair the stability of the cooperation of the different generator zones. The result is a decay of the pattern.

Furthermore, it is evident that the frequency of the pattern is determined by the speed of the circling. This is still corroborated by the observation that the decrease of frequency in such patterns is accompanied by an enlargement of the diameter of the circle (Fig. 8).

As for the very nature of this dislocation, we can only speculate. A slow shifting of the place of origin of the waves during epileptic activity was reported by Scherrer and Calvet (18) and later thoroughly analyzed by Hirsch.[1] This author recorded epileptic activity of the undercut cortex of cats by several transcortical leads. The electrodes were arranged in a row and the time intervals between the different leads were calculated. It was shown by phase analysis that the place of origin of the waves slowly shifted over the cortex at a velocity of several millimeters per minute. This phenomenon may be compared with our observation of the slow displacement of the clusters ("dislocation"). DC potential measurements made by Hirsch revealed that this displacement was accompanied by a DC shift and there was also a concomitant increase of single unit activity. Since it is known that epileptic seizures are accompanied by an increase of extracellular potassium concentration and that such an increase may facilitate epileptic discharges (7), and since the excitability of neurons is known to increase with increasing extracellular potassium concentration, it may be that this phenomenon of "dislocation" is related to the local spreading of extracellular potassium.

Multidimensional analysis of the ECoG has shown that there are sequences where a striking similarity of the paths of both positive and negative P-fields is found. Such patterns are characterized by a high regularity. In a previous paper (10) we have suggested that such regularities may be due to a path of facilitation caused by the pathway of one P-field, thus increasing the probability that the next P-field follows the same route. This behaviour of the P-fields can be explained by the assumption that a highly coordinated and successive activation of different generator zones takes place (see above). In terms of cellular activity, however, it has been reported that no clear relationship exists between cellular behaviour and ECoG waves in the tonic stage of a seizure (18). This may be due to the fact that even the activity of a group of neurons need not be representative for the total population involved in the surface ECoG. Therefore, it could be that pluridimensional single unit analysis would reveal a closer relationship between the discharges of a neuronal population and the surrounding ECoG, as has been described by Verzeano for thalamic and cortical neuronal populations during epileptiform activity (20).

It is known from previous experiments that cortical incisions are able to interrupt the regular pathways of P-fields during seizures only if they reach down to the sixth cortical layer (12). Since more superficial incisions do not seem to alter significantly the cortical interconnectivity, i.e., to alter it in such a way that surface P-fields cannot cross these incisions, it is reasonable to look for structures necessary for the propagation of P-fields during seizures in deep cortical layers. Thus, it seems that groups of large pyramidal cells with their dendrites are the histological substrate for large P-fields, that an emerging P-field reflects their simultaneous de- or hyperpolarisation, and that the propagation of those fields is due to the activation of a second group of pyramidal cells by the activity of the first group. In this way, activity spreads out through the cortical network. For our model, no subcortical influence is necessary for the propagation of P-fields. Moreover, additional influences from subcortical centers seem to be able to disturb the high regularity in the propagation during tonic seizure activity. However, further experiments with reversible suppression of subcortical centers are necessary to prove this assumption.

These results concern the largest cortical region of almost equal laminar structure, namely the A. striata. This region was chosen because recordings from nonhomogeneous cortical regions have turned out to raise problems that cannot be solved by this method of representing the spatiotemporal behaviour of the P-fields by speed-vector graphs. It may be presumed that architectonic nonhomogeneity and anisotropism are the main reasons. This probably also holds true for other modern approaches to the understanding of the EEG, such as field-potential analysis or current-density analysis. Therefore, a sufficient knowledge of the histological organization of the recording region is indispensable.

ACKNOWLEDGMENT

This research was supported by the Fonds zur Förderung der wissenschaftlichen Forschung (Nr. 2186 and M 3/1726) and by the European Training Program in Brain and Behaviour Research (ETPBBR). The calculations were performed in the Rechenzentrum der Medizinischen Fakultät der Universität Wien. The authors wish to thank Dr. B. Schlesinger for his careful reading and comments on this chapter.

REFERENCES

1. Calvet, J., Calvet, M. C., and Scherrer, J. (1964): Etude striatigraphique corticale de l'activité EEG spontanée. *Electroenceph. Clin. Neurophysiol.*, 17:109–125.

2. Creutzfeldt, O. (1966): Neuronal mechanism underlying the EEG. In: *Basic Mechanisms of the Epilepsies*, edited by H. Jasper, A. Ward, and A. Pope, pp. 397–410. Little, Brown, Boston.
3. Creutzfeldt, O. (1974): Neuronal generation of the electroencephalogram. In: *International Handbook of Electroencephalography and Clinical Neurophysiology, Vol. 2*, Editor-in-chief, A. Rémond. Elsevier, Amsterdam.
4. Elul, R. (1968): Brain waves: Intracellular recordings and the origin of the EEG. In: *Data Acquisition and Processing in Biology and Medicine, Vol. V*, edited by K. Enslein, pp. 93–115. Pergamon Press, Oxford.
5. Elul, R. (1972): The genesis of the EEG. *Int. Rev. Neurobiol*, 15:227–272.
6. Fessard, A. (1958): Les mécanismes de synchronisation interneuronique par leur intervention dans la crise épileptique. In: *Bases Physiologique et Aspects Clinique de l'Epilepsie*. Masson et Cie, Paris.
7. Hoston, J. R., Sypert, G., and Ward, A. A. (1973): Extracellular potassium concentration change during propagated seizures in neocortex. *Exp. Neurol.*, 38:20–26.
8. Jami, L., Fourment, A., Calvet, J., and Thieffry, M. (1968): Etude sur modèle des methodes de détection EEG. *Electroenceph. Clin. Neurophysiol.*, 24:130–145.
9. Petsche, H., Nagypal, T., Prohaska, O., Rappelsberger, P., and Vollmer, R. (1975): Approaches to the spatio-temporal analysis of seizure patterns. In: *CEAN-Computerized EEG Analysis*, edited by G. Dolce and H. Künkel. Gustav Fischer, Stuttgart.
10. Petsche, H., Prohaska, O., Rappelsberger, P., Vollmer, R., and Kaiser, A. (1974): Cortical seizure patterns in multidimensional view: The information content of equipotential maps. *Epilepsia*, 15:439–463.
11. Petsche, H., Prohaska, O., Rappelsberger, P., and Vollmer, R. (1975): The possible role of dendrites in EEG—synchronization. In: *Advances in Neurology, Vol. 12, Physiology and Pathology of Dendrites*, edited by G. W. Kreutzberg. Raven Press, New York.
12. Petsche, H., and Rappelsberger, P. (1970): Influence of cortical incision on synchronization pattern and travelling waves. *Electroenceph. Clin. Neurophysiol.*, 28:592–600.
13. Petsche, H., Rappelsberger, P., and Frey, Z. (1972): Intracortical aspects of the synchronization of self-sustained bioelectrical activities. In: *Synchronization of EEG Activity in Epilepsies*, edited by H. Petsche and M. A. B. Brazier, pp. 263–284. Springer, Berlin.
14. Petsche, H., Rappelsberger, P., and Trappl, R. (1972): Properties of cortical seizure potential fields. *Electroenceph. Clin. Neurophysiol.*, 29:567–578.
15. Petsche, H., and Shaw, J. (1972): EEG topography. In: *International Handbook of Electroencephalography and Clinical Neurophysiology, Vol. 2*, edited by A. Rémond. Elsevier, Amsterdam.
16. Petsche, H., and Sterc, J. (1972): The significance of the cortex for travelling phenomena of brain waves. *Electroenceph. Clin. Neurophysiol.*, 25:11–22.
17. Rose, M. (1931): Cytoarchitektonischer Atlas der Groβhirnrinde des Kaninchens. *J. Psychol. Neurol. (Leipzig)*, 43:353–440.
18. Scherrer, J., and Calvet, J. (1972): Normal and epileptic synchronization at the cortical level in the animal. In: *Synchronization of EEG Activity in Epilepsies*, edited by H. Petsche and M. A. B. Brazier, pp. 112–132. Springer, Berlin.
19. Trappl, R. (1970): Die näherungsweise graphische Darstellung von Isopotentiallinien aus EEG-Mehrkanalregistrierungen mittels EDV-Anlage. *Experientia*, 26:329–331.
20. Verzeano, M. (1972): Pacemakers, synchronization and epilepsies. In: *Synchronization of EEG Activity in Epilepsies*, edited by H. Petsche and M. A. B. Brazier, pp. 154–188. Springer-Verlag, Wien.

Architectonics of the Cerebral Cortex,
edited by M. A. B. Brazier and H. Petsche.
Raven Press, New York © 1978.

Mathematical Quantification of EEG Records from Architectonically Different Areas

P. Rappelsberger

Neurophysiological Institute of the University of Vienna, and Brain Research Institute of the Austrian Academy of Sciences, Vienna, Austria

For many years we have been dealing with the spatiotemporal properties of the electrocorticogram using different methods (5–11,13,14). Our experiments have been performed on the lissencephalic rabbit. The results of the experiments are sets of bioelectrical signals that are to be interpreted with respect to a special working hypothesis to be discussed below. In clinical electroencephalography the interpretation of the EEG signals is usually made by the mere visual inspection of the recordings. This is a very coarse method, most influenced by subjective factors that yield only a small part of the information content. For diagnostic purposes this may be sufficient, but the more complex the scope of the investigation the more exact and objective the methods of extracting information from the signals have to be. Therefore, mathematical methods have been used and have been found to be successful for this purpose. However, there is an essential difference between quantification or measurement in for example physics and quantification of the information contained in bioelectrical signals. Because these are very variable, only statement of a certain probability can be given. This means that methods of mathematical statistics are more useful than pure mathematical methods.

The aims of investigating bioelectrical signals from the surface of the cortex is to examine their relationship to known or hypothetical morphological structures. Therefore, the mathematical methods are used to build up links between known structural data and bioelectrical findings on the one hand, and, on the other hand, to lay down appropriate bioelectrical models from which inferences to anatomical structures can be made. In detail, the recordings from the cortical surface are made to study the electrical properties of the different cortical areas and to investigate the effect of the boundaries between such areas on these properties. Two examples are shown and the results obtained by a simple mathematical method are presented. These findings are compared with the results of the more complicated spectral analysis.

Very closely connected to the cortical structure seems to be the problem of synchronization of the bioelectrical signals. The term "synchronization" is frequently used in electroencephalography, not only in its literal sense that two or more events appear exactly at the same time, but also that the activities from different regions have a similarity in shape (synmorphism). In electroencephalography, the criterion of synmorphism seems to be more relevant. As a consequence, signals of the same shape recorded at different sites of the cortex are usually called synchronous but without taking into account possible time relations between them. The close connection between electrical activity and underlying cortical structure is shown by the observation that boundaries between different cortical areas influence the synchronization mechanism of the electrical activities. Therefore, we assume that within an area of synchronous activity there is also a morphological homogeneity, i.e., a cortical area of uniform structure.

Synchronized activities do not appear very frequently in the spontaneous EEG especially if the electrode distance is relatively large with respect to the brain size, as in our case. Epileptic seizures, however, result in strong synchronization. Therefore, we have been using the model of the epileptic seizure as a generator of appropriate signals for our study. The seizures were elicited by local application of penicillin or contralateral electrical stimulation.

METHODS

As mentioned above, the lissencephalic rabbit has been used as the experimental animal because the surface of the cortex is open to any manipulation, since no sulcus interrupts the continuity. The electrodes used for surface recordings are silver wires with a diameter of 0.3 mm. The wires are arranged in a row of seven electrodes embedded in artificial resin. The electrodes are at 1-mm distances. To obtain better recording properties the contact areas of the electrodes were chlorided before. After preparation of the skull and opening of the dura, the electrodes are placed directly on the cortex. The electrode holder is fastened on the bone by means of screws. The method of preparation is described in detail by Vollmer et al. (14). For orientation for the application of the electrodes the atlas of Rose (12) was used. The recordings were made with respect to a common-reference Ag-AgCl electrode on the nose bone. By experience, this is a site with negligible electrical activity, so that the recorded signals may be considered to be identical with the electrical activity of those areas of the cortex where the electrodes were placed. The signals were amplified by means of a Schwarzer EEG machine, recorded on EEG paper, and stored on an Ampex analog tape (FR 1300) for further processing. Computations have been performed by means of an IBM 370/145 computer.

To find the boundaries between different cortical areas, a special but relatively simple mathematical method was developed. To verify the results obtained by this method they are compared with the results obtained by means of spectral analysis. The method is described in ref. 11. It is based on a comparison of the shape of two signals recorded from different cortical sites. For this purpose the signs of the first derivatives of those two signals are multiplied. If the two signs are equal, that means both of them +1 or −1, the result is +1. In the other case, the result is −1. An averaging over a chosen time interval, in our case 10 sec, yields a number between +1 and −1 that we call the S value. It may be interpreted as follows: "+1" means that the two signals are identical in shape within the chosen time interval and therefore they are synchronous, not only in the electroencephalographic sense but also in the strict sense of the literal meaning. The value "−1" means that the two signals are completely phase-reversed. If the two signals are sine waves, phase reversal corresponds to a phase shift of 180°. A value between +1 and −1 can be caused by a time delay between two signals of the same shape or by the two signals having different shapes. Therefore, "0" can indicate either asynchrony in the sense of electroencephalography, or, if the two signals have the same shape, a time delay corresponding to 90°. From experience one can say that the second case is very unlikely if surface electrodes of the kind as described are used.

The method described enables the degree of synchronism as defined above to be quantified. For the quantification of structural differences this so-called S method can be completed by a statistical test based on confidence limits. As can be shown, the calculated S values are distributed binomially $B(p = (S + 1)/2, N)$ (2). N is the number of the discrete values +1 and −1 over the epoch averaged. Using this fact, corresponding confidence limits can be calculated. The confidence limits show whether or not significant differences between two S values exist. Thus, structural differences may be inferred from the S values.

Power spectra and coherence spectra were computed in the frequency range 0 to 32 Hz. Smoothing was performed in the time domain using a Papoulis window (4) with a truncation point M = 1 sec (3) yielding a frequency spacing of 0.5 Hz. For comparison, the same 10 = sec samples were analyzed as with the S method. According to the above parameters, spectral estimates with 34 degrees of freedom were obtained. Statistical tests for coherences were performed using confidence intervals as suggested by Benignus (1).

RESULTS AND DISCUSSION

In the first example, Figs. 1–3, a 160-sec sample of an EEG (interseizure activity consisting of penicillin spikes followed by a seizure at second 70) was analysed. The electrode arrangement is parallel to the midline as demonstrated in Fig. 1, where the results of the application of the S method are presented in a three-dimensional graph. In the X direction the electrode sites are indicated. The electrodes are numbered and their approximate position is shown in the lower right part of the figure where the left half of

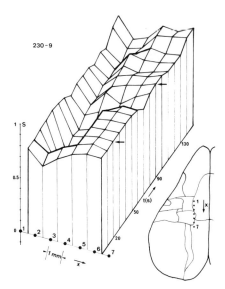

FIG. 1. Three-dimensional graph of S values. The dots in the X direction represent the electrodes. The approximate sites of the electrodes on the rabbit's cortex are indicated in the lower right part. The S values were calculated between adjacent electrode pairs for 16 successive samples of 10 sec each. Two types of S profiles can be distinguished: first, profiles with steep decreases from S_{1-2} to S_{2-3} on the one hand and from S_{4-5} to S_{3-4} on the other hand due to EEGs consisting of penicillin spikes, and second, during a seizure lasting from about second 70 to second 130, V-shaped profiles with the minimum at S_{2-3}. Samples of the two types of S profiles are shown in Fig. 2 (arrows).

the rabbit's brain with the different cortical areas as given by Rose (12) are drawn. The S values were calculated between adjacent electrode pairs for 16 successive samples of 10 sec each. The S scale is in the Y direction.

If one considers the S values (Fig. 1) it is remarkable that between second 20 and 60 and between second 130 and 160 there is a steep decrease from S_{1-2} to S_{2-3} on the one hand and from S_{4-5} to S_{3-4} on the other hand, so that a U-shaped valley results. This decrease is significant ($2\alpha = 0.01$) as can be seen in the upper part of Fig. 2. A sample of the corresponding EEG (second 20, arrow in Fig. 1) is also presented. Almost no differences can be observed between, for example, EEG traces 3 and 4 by the naked eye if one neglects the amplitude differences which do not influence the results of the S method. But because of the extreme sensitivity of the method, such differences can be discovered. From the results one can conclude that there may be structural inhomogeneities between electrodes 2 and 3 on the one hand and between 3 and 4 on the other hand. This means that the area under electrode 3 is to some degree independent of the surrounding areas. The electrodes 4, 5, 6, and 7 seem to be situated on an approximately homogeneous area. At second 70, a seizure starts which lasts about 60 sec. During this seizure the observed U-shaped valley becomes V-shaped, with only the S values between 2 and 3 differing significantly from the adjacent S values. This may be interpreted by assuming that the cortex under electrode 3 now has become synchronized by the seizure activity that dominates at the electrodes 4 to 6.

In the lower part of Fig. 2, a sample of the seizure can be seen together with the corresponding S values and their confidence limits. The confidence limits of S_{2-3} and S_{1-2} on the one hand and S_{2-3} and S_{3-4} on the other hand

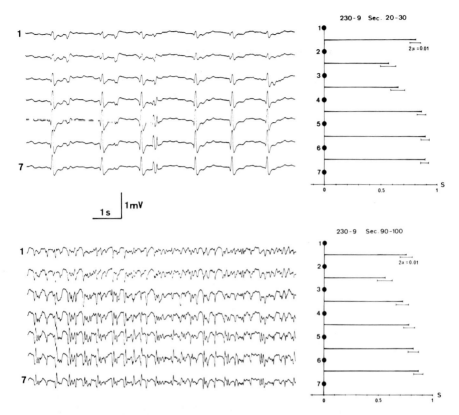

FIG. 2. EEG samples and S profiles (see Fig. 1, arrows). The upper part shows an EEG sample consisting of penicillin spikes. Almost no differences in the shapes of the signals can be observed if one compares the traces 3, 4, and 5. But due to the extreme sensitivity of the S method, such differences can be discovered. Significant differences between S_{1-2} and S_{2-3} and between S_{4-5} and S_{3-4} can be stated by means of the confidence intervals. In the lower part of the figure, an EEG sample of the seizure is presented. During the seizure the significant decrease observed between S_{4-5} and S_{3-4} (upper S profile) shifts and is now evident between S_{3-4} and S_{2-3}.

do not overlap each other so that a significant difference with probability 0.99 can be stated between them. There is nevertheless great similarity between the activities at the electrodes 2 and 3 but the superimposed high-frequency components with spatially limited generator zones (from electrode 3 to 7) are responsible for these differences.

The division into different cortical areas as given by Rose (12) is very coarse and raises the erroneous impression of sharp architectonic boundaries. In reality, the cortical structure does not change abruptly from one region to another but the transition is gradual. However, there are a few boundaries which are very clear as, for example, between the area praecentralis and the area Rsgβ or between Rsgβ and area striata. Taking into

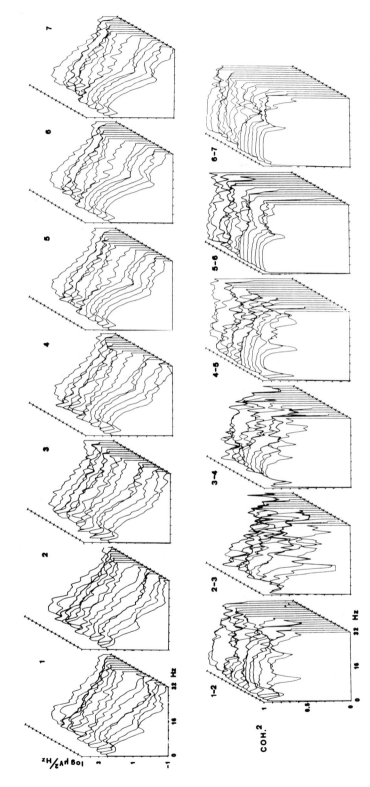

FIG. 3. Plots of autospectra and squared coherence spectra of the same 10-sec EEG samples are analysed by means of the S method (see Fig. 1). The most striking feature is the relatively low coherence spectra between 2 and 3, which differ significantly ($2\alpha = 0.05$) from 1–2 on the one hand and 4–5 on the other hand almost within the entire frequency range. The coherence values 3–4 lie about in between the coherence values 2–3 and 4–5. In the autospectra, the beginning of the seizure clearly can be perceived by the increase of power at higher frequencies.

account as a first approach the cortical organization stated by Rose (12) as shown in Fig. 1, it can be assumed with some probability that the discontinuity found in this example agrees with the boundary between area praecentralis agranularis and Rsgβ.

In the following, these results obtained by the S method are to be compared with the results obtained by means of spectral analysis. In Fig. 3, spectra and coherences are presented. For comparison, the same 10-sec samples were analysed as in Fig. 1. In the upper row of Fig. 3 the autospectra for the successive samples are plotted, whereas in the lower row the squared coherence spectra between the adjacent electrodes are shown. In contrast to the S method, which only yields one value characterizing the degree of synchronization, i.e., the degree of relationship between two signals, the result of coherence analysis is a set of frequency-dependent values, the coherence spectrum. Therefore, a simple three-dimensional presentation as in Fig. 1 would be only possible for one distinct frequency. If one considers the coherence spectra 4–5, 5–6, and 6–7, their shapes are fairly uniform with high coherence over the entire spectrum. However, the spiking period of the first 60 sec clearly differs from the seizure period, which is accompanied by a distinct increase of higher frequency components as is clearly seen in the autospectra. Similar trends show the coherences between 1 and 2. The coherences between 3 and 4 are somewhat lower than those between 4 and 5, but the differences are not significant. Only in the range between 0.5 and about 4 Hz the coherences between 3 and 4 are significantly ($2\alpha = 0.05$) lower except the first 20 sec. All coherences between 2 and 3 are much lower with a significance extending over the entire frequency range. As with the S method, significant differences can be determined by means of the confidence intervals (1). Because of the complicated procedure only confidence limits for $2\alpha = 0.05$ were applied. In summary, it can be stated that both methods essentially yield the same results about the detection of local differences of electrical brain activities from which the structural differences can be inferred.

The second example is from another experiment. In this case the electrode row was placed perpendicular to the midline. The seizure analysed in this example was elicited by contralateral electrical stimulation (2 msec pulse width, 100 Hz, 10 mA, 10-sec duration) via two screws in the skull. The results obtained by the S method are presented in Fig. 4. The electrode arrangement is indicated in the lower right part of the figure. In the graph of the S values, three parts can be distinguished: in the first 50 sec (from second 30 to 80 of the time scale) there is a distinct significant ($2\alpha = 0.01$) step in the S values from about 0.65 over the area striata to about 0.9 over the area Rsgβ. From about second 80 on, the S values 2–3 considerably decrease but from about second 130 no significant differences can be observed anymore. EEG samples of each of these three parts are demonstrated in Fig. 5. The relatively low S values between the activities of the lateral

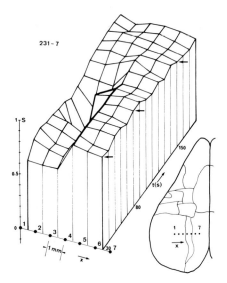

231-7

FIG. 4. Three-dimensional graph of S values as in Fig. 1. In this experiment the electrodes were placed perpendicular to the midline as indicated in the lower right part. During the first 50 sec there is a significant ($2\alpha = 0.01$) decrease between S_{4-5} and S_{3-4}. For the next 40 sec (seconds 80–120 of the time scale) an additional decrease of S_{2-3} occurs and, finally, during the last 60 sec no significant differences can be observed anymore. Samples of S profiles are shown in Fig. 5 (arrows).

electrodes during the first 50 sec can be explained by the very high frequent and localized activities which are superimposed on the basic rhythm (see electrode 3 in the upper part of Fig. 5). The EEG traces 4 to 7 look much more uniform, indicating a higher degree of synchronism in the electroencephalographic sense, as is also shown by the S values. The steep decrease of S_{2-3} at about second 80 to 110 is due to the considerable time delay of the tonic patterns in electrode 2 and 3. Such tonic patterns occasionally occur, lasting some seconds. An EEG sample is shown in the middle part of Fig. 5. The time delay is not visible at this recording speed. With ongoing seizure this time delay becomes smaller and smaller and vanishes from about second 130 on. That means an increase of the degree of synchronism. Also, the spatially limited generators under the lateral electrodes have synchronized so that the significant differences in the degree of synchronism found during the beginning of the seizure disappear (lower part of Fig. 5). It is true that there is a distinct decrease of the EEG amplitudes between traces 3 and 4, but as mentioned above the S method is not sensitive to amplitude differences.

As in Fig. 3, the corresponding results by means of spectral analysis are presented in Fig. 6. The coherence spectra 1–2, 2–3, and 3–4 clearly show a negligible nonsignificant coherence at higher frequencies. That means that the small superimposed high-frequency activities are independent from one another. The increase of the degree of synchronism toward the end of the seizure is indicated by the increase of coherence at higher frequencies. In contrast to the lateral activities the coherences of the medial activities are high over the entire frequency spectrum throughout the whole seizure, thus indicating a highly synchronized state.

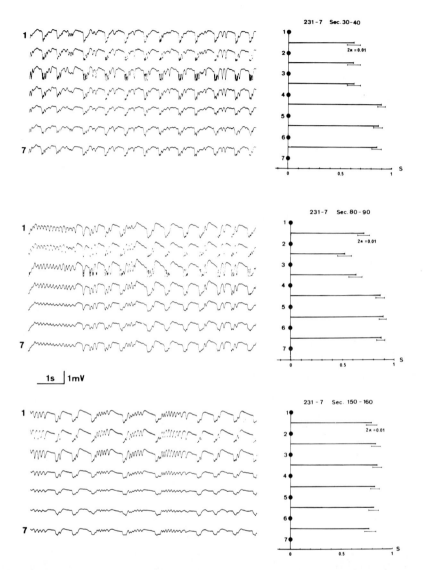

FIG. 5. EEG samples and S profiles (see Fig. 4, arrows). The uppermost S profile shows significant lower S values between the lateral electrodes 1, 2, 3, and 4 due to high frequent and localized activities as clearly can be seen in trace 3 of the EEG sample. In the second profile a time delay between the tonic activities in electrodes 2 and 3 are responsible for the additional decrease of S_{2-3}. The time delay is not visible at this recording speed. In the lowest profile no significant differences can be observed anymore. Amplitude differences in the EEG as between trace 3 and trace 4 do not influence the S values, which are only sensitive to differences in shape.

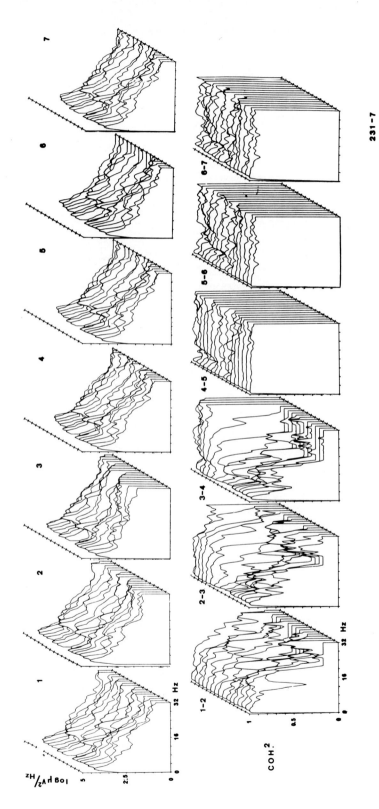

FIG. 6. Plots of autospectra and coherence spectra of the same 10-sec EEG samples as analysed by means of the S method (see Fig. 4). During the first 100 sec at higher frequencies the coherences 1–2, 2–3, and 3–4 are mostly below the 5% significance level. This is reflected in the S graph (Fig. 4) by the lower S values within this cortical area. Toward the end of the seizure, the coherences at higher frequencies increase so that significant differences not only between frequency bands but also between the different coherence spectra vanish. Note the peaks in the power spectra at about 10 Hz indicating periods of tonic activities.

231–7

If one compares the results by means of the two methods with the cyto-architectonics of Rose (12) one can assume with great probability that the discrepancy found between electrodes 3 and 4 is due to the structural differences between area striata and area Rsgβ.

At this point some remarks about the recording of bioelectrical signals from the cortical surface have to be made. As a first approach the activity recorded from a single-surface electrode can be considered as the sum of the potentials within a cone below the electrode. If the cones of two adjacent electrodes overlap one another, in both records a share of the activities of the overlapping zone appears. The larger the aperture of the cones the larger the overlapping zone and the larger is the common portion of the two signals. That means with increasing aperture of the cones the degree of synchronism increases too and in the limit with an aperture of 180° complete synchronism is obtained. This theoretical case can be compared to two electrodes being situated within a uniformly discharging region, that is what we call "generator zone." However, the case of S = 1 could not be observed in the examples discussed above. Also the coherences are not exactly "1" over the entire frequency range as they should be in the completely syn-chronized case, that is, inclusion of the entire neuronal networks below two electrodes into the synchronization mechanism.

Because of the agreement of the results by means of the S method and the results of the well-established spectral analysis it is justifiable to apply the S method to the investigation of the relationship between cortical morphol-ogy and electrical activity. The advantage of the S method is that it is simpler and yields only a single value for a chosen time interval, which can serve as a quantitative measure for the degree of synchronism between the two sig-nals investigated. To quantify any differences between two S-values, con-fidence intervals can be calculated. From those differences, structural differences responsible for the recorded signals may also be inferred.

ACKNOWLEDGMENT

This research was supported by the Fonds zur Förderung der wissen-schaftlichen Forschung (M3/1726). The calculations were performed in the Rechenzentrum der Medizinischen Fakultät der Universität Wien. I would like to thank Dr. Vollmer for performing the experiments.

REFERENCES

1. Benignus, V. A. (1969): Estimation of the coherence spectrum and its confidence interval using the Fast Fourier Transform. *IEEE Trans Audio Electroacous.* AU-17, No 2:145–150.
2. J. R. Geigy A. G. (ed.): Pharmazeutische Abteilung, Basel. *Documenta Geigy. Wissen-schaftliche Tabellen.*
3. Jenkins, G. M., and Watts, D. G. (1969): *Spectral Analysis and its Applications.* Holden-Day, San Francisco.

4. Papoulis, A. (1973): Minimum-bias windows for high resolution spectral estimates. *IEEE Trans. Inform. Theory*, IT-19, No 1:9–12.
5. Petsche, H., and Rappelsberger, P. (1970): Influence of cortical incisions on synchronization pattern and travelling waves. *Electroenceph. Clin. Neurophysiol.* 28:592–600.
6. Petsche, H., Rappelsberger, P., and Trappl, R. (1970): Properties of cortical seizure potential fields. *Electroenceph. Clin. Neurophysiol.*, 29:567–578.
7. Petsche, H., and Rappelsberger, P. (1973): The problem of synchronization in the spread of epileptic discharges leading to seizure in man. In: *Epilepsy, Its Phenomena in Man*, edited by M. A. B. Brazier, pp. 121–151. Academic Press, New York.
8. Petsche, H., Prohaska, O., Rappelsberger, P., Vollmer, R., and Kaiser, A. (1974): Cortical seizure patterns in multi-dimensional view: The information content of equipotential maps. *Epilepsia*, 15, 439–463.
9. Petsche, H., Nägypal, T., Prohaska, O., Rappelsberger, P., and Vollmer, R. (1975): Approaches to the spatio-temporal analysis of seizure patterns. In: *CEAN-Computerized EEG Analysis*, edited by G. Dolce and H. Künkel. Gustav Fischer Verlag, Stuttgart.
10. Rappelsberger, P., and Petsche, H. (1975): Spectral analysis by means of autoregression. In: *CEAN-Computerized EEG Analysis*, edited by G. Dolce and H. Künkel. Gustav Fischer Verlag, Stuttgart.
11. Rappelsberger, P., Prohaska, O., Petsche, H., and Vollmer, R. (1976): Application of a special time domain technique for epi- and intracortically recorded epileptic seizures. In: *Quantitative Analysis of the EEG*, edited by M. Matejcek and G. K. Schenk, Verlag AEG-Telefunken, Konstanz, BRD.
12. Rose, M. (1931): Cytoarchitektonischer Atlas der Großhirnrinde des Kaninchens. *J. Psychol. Neurol. (Leipzig)*, 43:353–440.
13. Vollmer, R., Prohaska, O., Petsche, H., Rappelsberger, P., and Kaiser, A. (1974): Kreisende kortikale Potentialfelder beim epileptischen Anfall. *Experientia*, 30:156–157.
14. Vollmer, R., Petsche, H., Pockberger, H., Prohaska, O., and Rappelsberger, P. (1977): Spatiotemporal analysis of cortical seizure activities in a homogeneous cytoarchitectonical region (*this volume*).

Architectonics of the Cerebral Cortex,
edited by M. A. B. Brazier and H. Petsche.
Raven Press, New York © 1978.

The Cortical Alpha Rhythm in Dog: The Depth and Surface Profile of Phase

F. H. Lopes da Silva and W. Storm van Leeuwen

*Brain Research Department, Institute of Medical Physics TNO,
Utrecht, The Netherlands*

The question as to what the intracortical sources of alpha activity are has not yet been settled, notwithstanding the fact that this type of electrophysiological activity is of paramount importance in electroencephalography. A clear answer to this question is of importance for understanding the basic neurophysiological mechanisms responsible for the generation of alpha activity. The lack of precise information on this problem probably stems from the fact that the neurophysiological basis of alpha rhythms, as commonly defined in electroencephalography, has been studied in animals with intracranial electrodes in only a few instances (13,17,20,21). The uncertainty regarding the neural basis of alpha rhythms has even led to claims that alpha rhythms may have an extracerebral origin (15).

A generally followed approach to search for intracortical sources of neuroelectrical activity is to determine the distribution of the corresponding potential within the cortex, i.e., the cortical depth profile. The basic assumption is that the neuronal population generating the activity in question should form a dipole field oriented perpendicularly to the cortical surface. The interpretation is that the site of inversion of polarity of the field potential should indicate the location of the underlying postsynaptic activity on the soma-dendritic membrane (4,11). In spite of the fact that this model certainly represents a much too simplified hypothesis, we thought that it would be important to determine the cortical depth profile of spontaneous alpha activity as a necessary first step in the establishment of the intracortical sources of this type of EEG activity. Thus, the main purpose of the present investigation was to determine whether alpha waves showed potential reversal within the visual cortex. The experiments were carried out in dogs because they have an alpha rhythm which is similar to that of man in localisation, frequency band, and reactivity to eye closure (17). It must be recognized that alpha waves vary appreciably as a function of time; they can only be characterized by statistical methods of signal analysis. Thus, we made use of general methods of spectral analysis in this study. In this way, the cortical profile of the alpha waves was determined by studying the phase relations between alpha activity recorded simultaneously at the surface and in the depth of the cortex.

MATERIALS AND METHODS

Recordings

The EEG measurements were made in unrestrained dogs (German boxers) using chronically indwelling electrodes. It should be emphasized that the recordings had to be obtained from unanesthetized dogs in order to avoid the influence of anesthetics, which alter the characteristics of the spontaneous rhythms as shown previously (17). The stereotaxic atlases of Lim et al. (14) and of Adrianov and Meringe (1) were used for guidance in placing the electrodes. Two types of electrodes were implanted under anesthesia and aseptic conditions.

The intracortical electrodes consisted of bundles of insulated stainless steel wires (100 μm diameter) with a bare tip of 100–200 μm and an interelectrode distance of 300–400 μm, or of single wires of 200 μm diameter. Electrodes were placed in three dogs. The dura was incised and the electrode bundles were lowered into the cortex using a microdrive in such a way that the last electrode of the bundle (counting from the tip) was just at the level of the pia-mater. The other type of electrodes were placed on the pial surface; these consisted of arrays of stainless steel wires with uninsulated surfaces of 0.04–0.15 mm^2, imbedded in a polyethylene sheet less than 0.5 mm thick. The sheet was placed under the dura over the posterior marginal gyrus. All electrodes were placed under visual inspection (sometimes aided by a dissecting microscope) after removal of a flap of occipital bone. After placement of the electrodes, the removed occipital bone was substituted by an inert plastic material, which was fixed to the surrounding bone by using acrylic cement. Postmortem histological verification revealed that an optimal placement of the intracortical electrodes was obtained in the case shown in Fig. 1, where the electrodes were placed along a line about perpendicular to the cortex, spanning the whole cortical width from the surface down to the white matter. In other cases, the placement of the electrodes was involuntarily restricted to only a part of the cortical layers. Recordings were carried out by means of a multichannel radio-telemetering system over a period of a few months following the operation. The EEGs were recorded against a common reference electrode (a screw in the frontal bone) or between adjacent electrodes, for control. Alpha rhythms were obtained as the dog closed its eyes in a quiet, dimly illuminated room as previously reported (17,18). The EEGs were recorded by means of an Elema-Schönander apparatus using a time constant of 0.3 sec and a high-frequency cutoff of 40 or 70 Hz. The EEGs were written on paper and recorded on

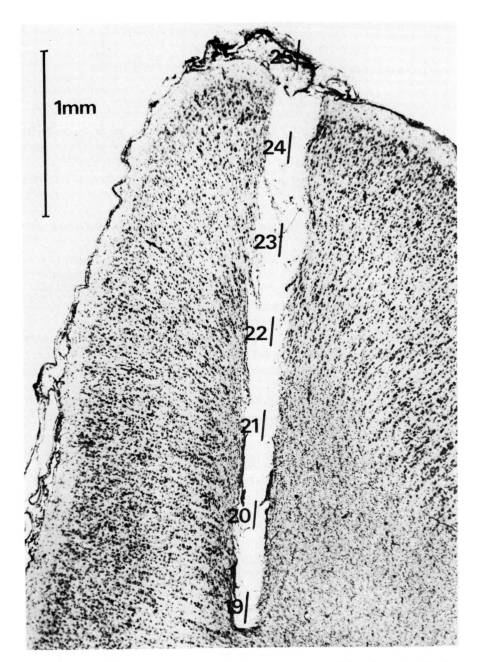

FIG. 1. Photomicrograph of a section of the marginal gyrus (dog Oki) at about the following stereotaxic coordinates: F = −2; L = 3.5. The electrode bundle is schematically indicated; the distance between electrodes is given according to the scale. The electrode numbers refer to the same electrodes represented in the other figures.

magnetic analogue tape. A time code signal was recorded both on paper and on tape.

Analysis

Suitable epochs of EEG in which alpha activity was present were selected by visual inspection and digitized by an eight-channel analogue-to-digital converter. These epochs were made up of 256 sample points; they had a duration of 3.2 sec (sampling rate 80 samples/sec). Before being digitized, the EEG signals were bandpass-filtered between 0.5 Hz and 40 Hz (18 dB/octave). The digitized signals were stored on digital tape and analysed off-line by a PDP-9 computer using Fourier analysis. This mathematical method serves essentially the same purpose as analogue filter analysis. Here one uses the mathematical operation of multiplication with sine and cosine waves in order to simulate very narrow digital filters. In this way, a distribution of the power as function of frequency or power spectrum, can be obtained. Using similar principles one may calculate the relationships between two signals in the frequency domain. This is done by calculating the cross-power spectrum between two signals. The cross-power gives similar information to the cross-correlation function in the time domain. It has a magnitude and a phase angle. The magnitude is usually normalized so that it is independent of the amplitudes of the two signals; this normalized magnitude is called the coherence function. Coherence and phase thus give information on the relationships between two signals. It should be noted that here we used the estimate of squared coherence function defined as

$$\gamma^2(f) = \frac{|\hat{C}_{xy}(f)|^2}{\hat{A}_{xx}(f)\,\hat{A}_{yy}(f)}$$

where $\hat{C}_{xy}(f)$ is the estimate of the cross-power spectrum between the signals $x(t)$ and $y(t)$ which have as estimates of the power spectra $\hat{A}_{xx}(f)$ and $\hat{A}_{yy}(f)$; in our case $x(t)$ and $y(t)$ are the electrocorticograms from any two derivations. A large value of coherence (near to unity) indicates that the two signals tend to vary in harmony; a coherence of zero or near to zero indicates that they vary independently of each other and thus are probably not related; an intermediate value of coherence within a certain frequency band indicates that, in that band, the two signals share a common component, which accounts for a part of the energy in the band. In short, the value of coherence is a measure of the relation within a certain frequency band, between the energy of the components shared by two signals, and that of the unrelated components. The phase angle is only reliable when coherence is significantly different from zero. It indicates the time relations between the two signals. Two EEG signals having opposite polarity (one is a mirror image of the other) would present a phase shift of 180°. One signal, within a frequency band centered at the frequency f, which would lead another by a certain time delay (Δt) would have a corresponding phase shift (in degrees) $\Delta \psi = \Delta t \, 360°/T$, where T is the period at frequency f ($T = 1/f$ in seconds). Power spectra, coherence, and phase functions were computed according to a FFT (Fast Fourier Transform) program by ensemble averaging of 4 to 30 epochs, in order to increase statistical reliability. The 95% confidence intervals of phase were computed according to the procedure of Jenkins and Watts (12).

The analysis of nonlinear properties of the EEG signals was performed by means of a program for computation of bispectra, bicoherence, and biphase (method developed at this Institute by J. M. Valeton). The quantity used here is the bicoherence $\hat{\text{bic}}_{xx}(f_1, f_2)$ of the signal $x(t)$, defined as follows:

$$\hat{\text{bic}}_{xx}(f_1, f_2) = \frac{\hat{B}_{xxx}(f_1, f_2)}{\sqrt{\hat{A}_{xx}(f_1)\, \hat{A}_{xx}(f_2)\, \hat{A}_{xx}(f_1 + f_2)}}$$

where $\hat{B}_{xxx}(f_1, f_2)$ is the estimate of the bispectrum of the signal $x(t)$; it is obtained by estimating the triple product: $A_{xx}(f_1)\, A_{xx}(f_2)\, A_{xx}{}^x (f_1 + f_2)$, where $A^x (f_1 + f_2)$ is the complex conjugate of $A_{xx}(f_1 + f_2)$.

The bicoherence $\hat{\text{bic}}_{xx}(f_1, f_2)$ is an estimate of the relations between harmonic frequency components and of their phase locking, which has been used previously in EEG analysis (5).

Visually Evoked Potentials (VEPs)

In order to compare the intracortical distribution of alpha waves with evoked potentials, the latter were studied using sine-wave-modulated light (SML). Stimulation was by diffuse illumination of a white screen at 0.5 m from the dog's eyes, which were kept open. Averages of these evoked potentials were computed in a Mnemotron CAT-400 C computer (see ref. 16 for details).

RESULTS

Morphology of Intracortical Alpha Waves

A typical record is shown in Fig. 2. Three main points emerge from this figure: (a) An alpha rhythm of 12 to 13 cycles/sec was found in all leads but with considerable differences in waveform; (b) the morphology of the alpha rhythm recorded from the intracortical electrodes showed an arcuate waveform in which one may distinguish a sharp wave element occupying about one-third of the period, i.e., with a duration of about 30 msec. The sharp waves at the superficial electrodes (particularly at E24 in Fig. 2) were, although not always, negative-going, whereas those at the deep lying electrodes (for example E22) were in the opposite direction. Thus, the waveform of the intracortical alpha rhythm was far from sinusoidal. (c) The extra-

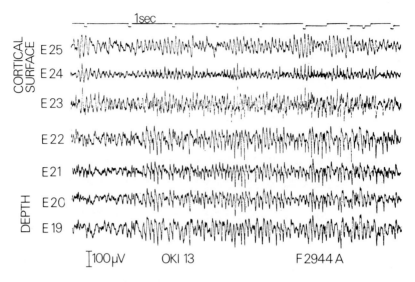

FIG. 2. Dog's alpha rhythms recorded simultaneously from seven cortical electrodes; E25 is just outside the cortical surface; E19 is placed at the greatest depth. The electrodes (100 to 200 μm uninsulated) are placed at a distance of 300 to 400 μm from each other along a line almost perpendicular to the surface of the posterior gyrus marginalis. Note that the alpha rhythm waveform is rather smooth at E25, but is peaky and arcuate in the deeper-lying electrodes. The polarity of these "peaks" is negative-going at E24, but positive-going at E22 and deeper electrodes. At E23 a transitory type of waveform is apparent (negativity upward).

cortical electrode (E25) placed at the level of the pia and the next most superficial electrode (E24) presented an alpha rhythm with a smoother waveform than that recorded from the deeper-lying electrodes. Spectral analysis of the records with alpha activity is shown in Fig. 3. In this case it can be seen that particularly at the deeper-lying electrodes (white matter), there was considerable variability of the frequency spectrum from epoch to epoch and from electrode to electrode. At some of the intracortical electrodes there were some epochs where two components with different peak frequencies were encountered as shown more clearly in the ensemble averages of Fig. 4. At these electrodes, there were apparently two types of rhythms with peaks at 8.1 cycles/sec and 12.5 cycles/sec; at the more superficial electrodes only the latter was present. In some epochs a clear spectral component at the second harmonic of the alpha peak was found as shown in Fig. 5. By using bispectral analysis it was shown that indeed the alpha rhythm in such cases is a complex signal with a second harmonic component phase locked to the component at the fundamental frequency.

Phase Relationships Between Surface and Deeper Layers

By simple visual inspection, it was difficult to establish clearly the phase relationships among the different electrodes. It was necessary to approach

SPECTRA OF ALPHA RHYTHMS SIMULTANEOUSLY RECORDED IN DIFFERENT CORTICAL ELECTRODES

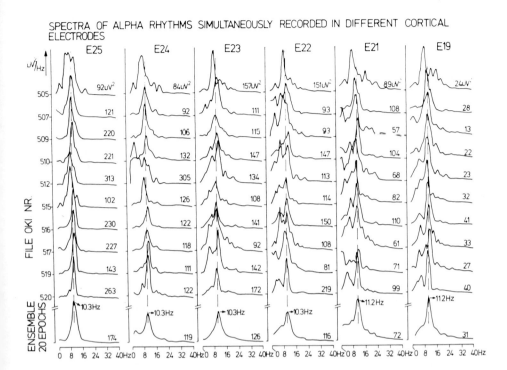

FIG. 3. Frequency spectra of 10 epochs of alpha rhythms recorded simultaneously from the same seven electrodes of Fig. 1. An epoch was 3.2 sec long; each spectral value was computed using a frequency window three points wide so that the frequency resolution is approximately 0.94 Hz. The maximal value (μV^2) is indicated at the right-band side of each spectrum. The lowest row shows ensemble spectra computed from 20 epochs, which included the 10 shown in the figure. Note that in the depth (E23 to E19) the spectra are more complex and variable than on the surface (E25 to E24). The spectral values are the lowest in the deeper-lying electrodes. Note that the peak frequency, even in the surface, is not constant. Of course, the variance of the spectra computed for each epoch is large (the number of degrees of freedom, dF, associated with each smoothed estimator is only 6, but in the case of the ensemble it increases considerably (no dF = 60).

this problem statistically by computing the phase of the cross-power spectrum between pairs of derivations as shown in Fig. 6. In this example, there are differences between the two electrode sites with regard to the spectral composition of the alpha rhythms. The coherence is only moderate, although significantly different from zero, implying that besides some common spectral components there are also unrelated components in the two electrodes even within the alpha frequency band.

The most striking result, however, is that the phase between the two electrodes fluctuates around 180°. This holds not only for the alpha frequency range but also for other frequency bands. In order to study the depth profile of the alpha activity more accurately, the phase between the most superficial electrode (E25) and all others was computed. The result is shown in Fig. 7. It is evident that there is a gradual and small phase shift between

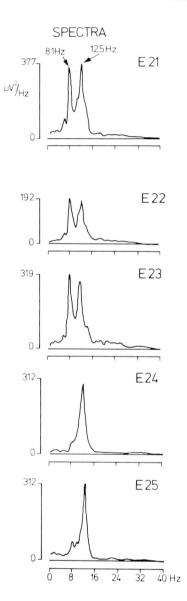

FIG. 4. Frequency spectra computed by ensemble averaging five epochs of alpha rhythms showing the double-peaked spectra at the deep-lying electrodes (E23 to E21), whereas at the surface electrodes only one peak is present. Frequency smoothing as in Fig. 3.

E25 and the two other superficial electrodes (E24 and E23), but that between E23 and E22 there is a sudden phase shift that reaches values not significantly different from 180°. In this case the phase reversal takes place at about 1,100 μm below the cortical surface; this level corresponds to layer V. In other animals, we also obtained phase differences between different intracortical electrodes: for example, in one dog, a phase difference of 97° ± 6° within the alpha frequency range was encountered between two electrodes placed within the visual cortex and separated by 400 μm. In this

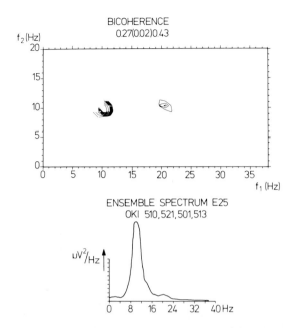

FIG. 5. Frequency spectrum computed by ensemble averaging of four epochs of alpha rhythms at a cortical surface electrode showing a peak at 10.3 Hz and a smaller one at 20 to 21 Hz. The corresponding bicoherence (defined in text) shows a maximum at the intersection of 10.3 Hz and 10.3 Hz, which indicates phase locking between the component at 10.3 Hz and the second harmonic; a smaller maximum at the intersection between 10.3 Hz and 20.6 Hz indicates that there is also phase locking with the third harmonic. The values of bicoherence are plotted above 0.27 in steps of 0.02. In the conditions of this analysis, a value of bicoherence is significantly different from zero above 0.12 ($p < 0.01$, for a signal with a flat spectrum).

case, however, the electrode bundle was almost tangential to the cortex; one of the electrodes was found in the deeper cortical layers and the other in the subjacent white matter. In other cases, phase differences of about 30° were obtained between electrodes placed within the superficial cortical layers. In these records, however, it was not possible to find a complete phase reversal, i.e., 180°.

Depth Profile of VEPs

It appeared to us that it was of general interest to compare the intracortical phase depth profile of the spontaneous alpha rhythm with that of VEPs recorded from the same electrodes. The VEPs were investigated at different stimulation frequencies of SML. As expected, the largest VEP amplitudes were encountered as a stimulating frequency of 30 Hz in accordance with the phenomenon of beta frequency selectivity characteristic of the lateral gyrus of the dog (16) when stimulated with SML with the eyes

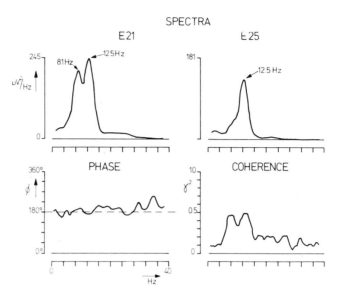

FIG. 6. Average spectra of five epochs recorded from two electrodes: E25 (cortical surface) and E21 (intracortical) with an interelectrode distance of about 1,400 μm. There is a clear difference in spectra, but the squared coherence attains peak values of 0.5 within the alpha frequency range. Note that the phase fluctuates about 180° over a wide frequency band. In this case, extra smoothing was introduced by using a wider frequency window (10 sample points).

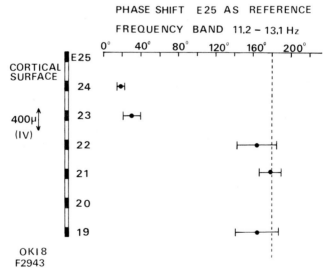

FIG. 7. Phase shift between the electrode at the cortical surface, E25, and the other deeper-lying electrodes computed from several epochs of alpha rhythms. The mean value and its standard deviation are indicated. Note the gradual increase in phase shift as a function of depth down to electrode E23 and the sudden jump to a mean phase of about 180° at the level of E22. The value of 180° is indicated by the broken line.

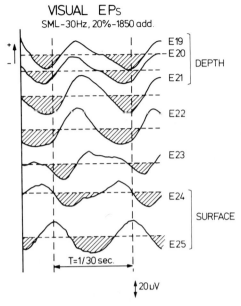

VISUAL EPs
SML-30Hz, 20%-1850 add.

FIG. 8. Average evoked potentials to a 30-Hz SML (20% modulation depth) recorded from electrodes as in Fig. 1. Note the gradual phase shift from the deeper-lying electrodes to the more superficial ones.

open. It should be noted that the spontaneous activity of the dog's electrocorticogram recorded from the visual cortex when he is alert and with the eyes open is dominated by frequencies in the range of 20 to 40 Hz (beta activity). A characteristic result is shown in Fig. 8: the VEPs also show a phase reversal as in the case of the alpha rhythm. The opposition of phase between the surface and the depth of the cortex is clear; however, one is not a simple mirror image of the other, probably owing to the coexistence of several sources at different depths.

Phase Relations of Alpha Rhythms in a Tangential Direction over the Cortical Surface

In a number of cases, the phases (and coherences) between alpha rhythms recorded from arrays of subdural electrodes lying directly on the cortical surface (marginal gyrus) were computed as summarized in Fig. 9. The aim was to determine whether consistent patterns of phase could be demonstrated, namely whether any evidence for a sweep of alpha rhythm over the cortex (3,10) could be found. Indeed, stable phase relations were encountered between adjacent electrodes within the alpha band. However, the sign of the phase differences measured along a row of cortical electrodes was not always the same. Thus, Fig. 9 shows that the alpha activity (dog R) recorded at E18 was apparently leading that recorded at the neighbour electrodes both in anterior (E17) and posterior (E19) directions; similar results were obtained in other animals.

Phase shifts (Δf) were transformed into the time domain (Δt). From the

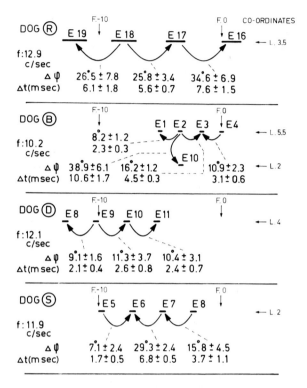

FIG. 9. Schematic representation of the phase relations for alpha rhythms (frequency indicated by f) recorded from rows of electrodes placed on the cortical surface of the marginal gyrus of four dogs. The electrodes are indicated approximately in scale within the stereotaxic coordinates: F0 and F-10, which correspond to the frontal planes passing through the ear bars and 10 mm behind the latter, respectively; the lateral plane is indicated on the right-hand side. The arrows indicate the sign of the phase shift; for example, in dog R, E18 (electrode) is leading both E19 and E17. The phase shift ($\Delta\Psi$, in degrees) has been transformed into the time domain (Δt, in m/sec).

"time delays" (*t*) "velocities of propagation" were computed. In the cases of Fig. 9 the "velocities of propagation" varied within the following limits: dog R, 0.3 to 0.4 m/sec; dog B, 0.3 to 0.7 m/sec; dog D, 0.8 to 1.0 m/sec; dog S, 0.3 to 1.2 m/sec.

It should be stressed that these "velocities" are only *apparent* since phase shifts of this type do not necessarily result from propagation of neural activity in only one direction (see below).

DISCUSSION

The fact that opposition of phase exists between alpha rhythms recorded at different depths within the visual cortex is proof of the cortical origin of this EEG rhythmic activity. A complete depth profile of alpha rhythms with a 180° phase shift had not been, to the best of our knowledge, previously reported. It should be noted that the reversal level, in this case at about 1,100 μm below the cortical surface (Fig. 7), may not give precise information concerning the exact location of the corresponding neuronal generators. This is due to the fact that different sources that can give rise to field potentials with different spatiotemporal characteristics may coexist. Indeed, a clear understanding of depth profiles of field potentials in terms of precisely defined neuronal activity depends on different factors: (a) the geometric characteristics of the neuron populations; (b) the underlying membrane processes, such as postsynaptic potentials, length, and time constants of soma-dendritic membranes; and (c) the electrical properties of the conductive extracellular medium. A detailed knowledge of such factors in relation to the generation of alpha waves has not yet been obtained. However, it may be advanced that the depth profile of the alpha rhythm shows a general similarity to that of some spindle waves found in cats (2).[1] Extrapolating also from findings of correlations between intracellular and surface cortical recordings obtained in other conditions (4,9), it can be hypothesized that the negative-going waves found at the cortical surface may correspond to summated postsynaptic potentials of cortical neurons. According to this view, the superficial cortical layers would appear as sinks; the sources would be in deeper layers at the level of the bodies and basal dendrites of neurons of layers IV and V.

The phase gradients encountered between electrodes placed on the cortical surface do not support, for the dog at least, the idea of an alpha rhythm sweeping all over the cortex, as has been suggested for the alpha rhythm recorded at the scalp in humans (3,10). On the contrary, it appears that in dog over the marginal gyrus there are different *epicenters* of alpha activity from which this activity spreads in several directions just like water springing from small fountains.

The *apparent* velocities of propagation that have been calculated, however, do not necessarily indicate that alpha activity spreads from discrete epicenters as a *travelling* wave with that velocity. For example, phase shifts could also be related to differences in the orientation of the neurons contributing to the alpha activity with regard to the recording electrodes. It should, however, be noted that the recordings analysed here have been obtained from electrodes placed on a rather even cortical surface, the posterior part of the marginal gyrus. This justifies thinking of these phase differences in terms of propagation. The relatively slow velocities encountered would correspond to propagation along slow paths, most likely dendrites or thin axon collaterals; the possibility of dendrodendritic interactions may also

---

[1] Calvet, M. C. (1967): Etude Quantitative et Organisation des Décharges Unitaires du Cortex Cérébral en Fonction des Niveaux de Vigilance et du Comportement. Thesis, Faculté de Médecine de Paris, 88 pp.

be taken into account. In this way the phase gradients could be interpreted as due to delays in the activation of different cortical domains, similarly to what has been demonstrated to occur in the prepyriform cortex (8). Such phase gradients would also be compatible with Elul's interpretation that thalamic neuronal populations in some way scan the cortex (7). However, one should be careful in interpreting phase shifts because they are not unambiguous.

The VEPs obtained using SML at 30 Hz showed a similar phase reversal between the surface and the deeper layers. This demonstrates that the depth profiles of the alpha rhythm are akin to those of steady-state VEPs characteristic of cortical beta selectivity. Furthermore, signal analysis of the alpha activity has shown that the process of generation of the alpha rhythm is characterized by clear nonlinear properties. Measurements of alpha rhythms from the skull of dog (17) show that such nonlinear components may be much attenuated; however, even in scalp derivations in man Dumermuth et al. (6) have shown, in some special cases, alpha activity with peaks at harmonically related frequencies as shown by the bispectrum. Attenuation of these higher harmonics at the skull can be expected due to spatial averaging caused by the tissues and cerebrospinal fluid interposed between the cortical source and the recording electrodes. Moreover, it is likely that in recordings obtained with larger electrodes, at greater distance from the sources, other factors, such as phase differences between different cortical sites, may play a role in the attenuation of higher frequencies such as shown by Pfurtscheller and Cooper (19).

SUMMARY

The question of the intracortical sources of the alpha activity of the EEG has been investigated in dogs, using (a) intracortical electrodes placed along a direction perpendicular to the cortical surface and (b) subdural electrodes placed on the cortical surface.

Alpha rhythms have been quantified using spectral analysis, namely the phase relationships between alpha activities recorded between several electrodes has been computed. It was demonstrated that opposition of phase exists between alpha rhythms recorded at different depths within the visual cortex.

The phase reversal (180°) was found at about 1,100 μm below the cortical surface.

It was found that the phase gradients between electrodes placed on the cortical surface do not support the idea of an alpha rhythm sweeping all over the cortex. It appears, rather, that different "epicenters" of alpha activity exist on the cortex from which activity spreads in several directions.

The neurophysiological basis of such alpha activity is discussed.

REFERENCES

1. Adrianov, O. L., and Meringe, T. A. (1959): *Atlas of the Dog's Brain* (in Russian), 237 pp. Medgiz, Moscow.
2. Calvet, J., Calvet, M. C., and Scherrer, J. (1964): Etude stratigraphique de l'activité EEG spontanée. *Electroenceph. Clin. Neurophysiol.*, 17:109–125.
3. Cooper, R., and Mundy-Castle, A. C. (1960): Spatial and temporal characteristics of the alpha rhythm: A toposcopic analysis. *Electroenceph. Clin. Neurophysiol.*, 12:153–165.
4. Creutzfeldt, O., and Houchin, J. (1974): Neuronal basis of EEG-waves. In: *Handbook of Electroencephalography and Clinical Neurophysiology*, Editor-in-Chief, A. Rémond, Vol. 2, Part C, *The Electrical Activity from the Neuron to the EEG and EMG, The Neuronal Generation of the EEG*, edited by O. Creutzfeldt, pp. 5–55. Elsevier, Amsterdam.
5. Dumermuth, G., Huber, P. J., Kleiner, B., and Gasser, T. (1971): Analysis of the interrelations between frequency bands of the EEG by means of the bispectrum. *Electroenceph. Clin. Neurophysiol.*, 31:137–148.
6. Dumermuth, G., Gasser, T., and Lange, B. (1975): Aspects of EEG analysis in the frequency domain. In: *CEAN Computerized EEG analysis*, edited by G. Dolce and H. Künkel, pp. 432–460. Gustav Fischer Verlag, Stuttgart.
7. Elul, R. (1972): The genesis of the EEG. *Int. Rev. Neurobiol.*, 15:227–272.
8. Freeman, W. (1975): *Mass Action in the Nervous System*, 489 pp. Academic Press, New York.
9. Frost, I. D. (1968): EEG-intracellular potential relationships in isolated cerebral cortex. *Electroenceph. Clin. Neurophysiol.*, 24:434–443.
10. Grey Walter, W. (1962): Oscillatory activity in the nervous system. In: *Neural Physiopathology*, edited by R. G. Grenell, pp. 222–257. Hoeber Medical Books, Harper & Row, New York.
11. Hubbard, S. I., Llinás, R., and Quastel, D. (1969): *Electrophysiological Analysis of Synaptic Transmission*. Edwards Arnolds, London.
12. Jenkins, G. M., and Watts, D. G. (1968): *Spectral Analysis and its Applications*, 525 pp. Holden-Day, San Francisco.
13. Lanoir, J. (1972): *Etude Electrocorticographique de la Veille et du Sommeil Chez le Chat*, 520 pp. Université de Marseille.
14. Lim, R. K. S., Lin, C. N., and Moffitt, R. A. (1960): *A Stereotaxic Atlas of the Dog's Brain*, 93 pp. Thomas, Springfield, Ill.
15. Lippold, O. C. J. (1973): *The Origin of the Alpha Rhythm*, 267 pp. Churchill Livingstone, London.
16. Lopes da Silva, F. H., Van Rotterdam, A., Storm van Leeuwen, W., and Tielen, A. M. (1970): Dynamic characteristics of visual evoked potentials in the dog. II. Beta frequency selectivity in evoked potentials and background activity. *Electroenceph. Clin. Neurophysiol.*, 29:260–268.
17. Lopes da Silva, F. H., Van Lierop, T. H. M. T., Schrijer, C. F. M., and Storm van Leeuwen, W. (1973): Organization of thalamic and cortical alpha rhythm: Spectra and coherences. *Electroenceph. Clin. Neurophysiol.*, 35:627–639.
18. Lopes da Silva, F. H., Van Lierop, T. H. M. T., Schrijer, C. F. M., and Storm van Leeuwen, W. (1973): Essential differences between alpha rhythms and barbiturate spindles: Spectra and thalamo-cortical coherences. *Electroenceph. Clin. Neurophysiol.*, 35:641–645.
19. Pfurtscheller, G., and Cooper, R. (1975): Frequency dependence of the transmission of the EEG from cortex to scalp. *Electroenceph. Clin. Neurophysiol.*, 38:93–96.
20. Rougeul, A., Corvisier, J., and Letalle, A. (1974): Rhythmes electrocorticaux caractéristiques de l'installation du sommeil naturel chez le chat. Leurs rapports avec le comportement moteur. *Electroenceph. Clin. Neurophysiol.*, 37:41–57.
21. Storm van Leeuwen, W., Kamp, A., Kok, M. L., de Quartel, F. W., Lopes da Silva, F. H., and Tielen, A. M. (1967): Relations entre les activités électriques cérébrales du chien, son comportement et sa direction d'attention. *Actual. Neurophysiol.* (Paris), 7:167–186.

Architectonics of the Cerebral Cortex,
edited by M. A. B. Brazier and H. Petsche.
Raven Press, New York © 1978.

Static and Dynamic Components of Object Representations in the Central Nervous System

Gerhard Werner

University of Pittsburgh, School of Medicine, Pittsburgh, Pennsylvania 15261

Few themes have proven to be as pervasive and fundamental in the neurobehavioral sciences as the polarity between specificity and diffuseness of the neural mechanisms that assure the representation of environmental events and organismic states in the nervous system. Experimental paradigms and idiosyncratic conceptualization of different investigators have traditionally tended to emphasize the role of one or the other type of neural mechanism. In contrast, von Economo's contributions are a remarkable exception: not only did his work on encephalitis lethargica set the stage for identifying a neural control system of generalized influence on the brain's transactional capability with the external environment, but he also developed the concept of progressive cerebration on the basis of extensive cytoarchitectonic work that demonstrated discreteness and specificity, at least in terms of cell morphology. The perceptiveness for significant observations and the circumstances facilitating this elucidation of a principle of duality in the organization of the nervous system have been charmingly rendered by von Economo's devoted biographer, his wife. But there remains some awe and wonder by virtue of the fact that von Economo's work took place in the same physical setting in which some 20 years prior and without anyone's knowledge (with the possible exception of Fries in Berlin) Sigmund Freud had drafted a manuscript entitled, *Project for a Scientific Psychology,* which remained hidden until some time after his death. In this theoretical treatise, Freud developed a conceptual model of a nervous system in which both discrete (projection) and diffuse (core nuclear) neural systems were assigned their respective roles in ways that are in astonishing harmony with von Economo's findings and with contemporaneous thought, except for some difference in terminology. One cannot help but muse about the intellectual climate in which such fundamental insights could come to fruition.

Advances in experimental methodology and conceptual refinements permit us now to reexamine the discreteness–diffuseness spectrum in regard to extracting and processing of information available in environmental events. In the regulation of behavior (which includes in man verbal reports of subjective experiences), external stimuli can be categorized along a multitude of dimensions, of which place, intensity, shape, direction of change, and context are some. Depending on which of these aspects of the stimulus is the particular topic of inquiry in the study of neurophysiology of sensory systems or of behavior, the conceptual tools of traditional psychophysics or those of cognitive psychology become applicable: the former in regard to proximal stimuli as quantifiable events in isolation, the latter in reference to the organism's apparent capability of constructing representations of scenes or objects by drawing on past experiences of temporal or spatial regularities in the external world.

The subsequent examples are intended to illustrate some of the principles by which information contained in external events comes to be represented as neural activity. These principles will primarily be exemplified by findings with the somesthetic, notably tactile, sensibility with but a limited attempt to marshall corollary evidence from other sense modalities; the reason for this restriction being that systematic investigations in several laboratories during the past decade or so have aimed at deliberate comparisons of the diversity of mechanisms for the encoding of tactile stimuli relative to psychophysical stimulus attributes and acquired significance of such stimuli in discrimination learning.

One of the best established operating principles for identification and analysis of different forms of stimuli by the nervous system involves the availability of receptors, pathways, and central projection areas that signal selectively specific types of stimuli, at least within a limited range of stimulus intensities. This concept of "labeled lines" implies that the particular pathway over which a neural discharge train arrives signifies to the central nervous system certain attributes of the stimulus; moreover, it connotes that the anatomical organization constitutes structural information inherent in the central nervous system which permits the "decoding" of certain stimulus attributes (see ref. 10). This well-established principle obtains with varying degrees of specificity in the visual, somesthetic, and auditory systems in regard to stimulus modality and place of the stimulus on the respective peripheral receptor sheet.

As far as the representation in primary cortical receiving areas is concerned, parcellation into an anatomical mosaic of regions, each with emphasis on the registration of a different aspect of the stimulus (i.e., depth, contour, color, and movement) is most prominent in primate visual cortex (20); but existing data with the somesthetic system furnish additional insight into the sorting processes along afferent pathways that are significantly involved in setting the stage for the pattern of cortical representation (18).

At the level of the afferent pathways that project to the somatic sensory area I (S-I) in the postcentral gyrus, there occurs an anatomical separation of "labeled lines," which are distinguished not only by the receptors they subserve, but also by their cortical destination. For instance, afferents from guard hairs (type T) by far prevail over those supplying hair follicles of down hairs (type D) at the cervical level of the cat's dorsal column relative to their proportional distribution in the spectrum of cutaneous myelinated afferents in peripheral nerve (2). On the other hand, afferents from type D receptors populate the spinal cervical system. For the primate, Whitsel et al. (17) established that slowly adapting afferents from types I and II cutaneous receptors and also from the joints, fascia, and periost from the hind limb enter, at first, the dorsal columns at their respective segmental levels, ascend in the dorsal columns for a few segments, and then proceed to their rostral destination outside the dorsal columns. The same process of progressive elimination of slowly adapting afferents from the dorsal columns is also initiated, although not brought to completion, at forelimb levels.

These processes at the spinal level foreshadow the cortical modality distribution: S-I consists of a central and predominantly cutaneous core zone (area 1 and area 3), which is dominated by input from the cervical fasciculus gracilis, and a posterior and anterior border zone (area 1–2 and area 3-A), receiving cutaneous as well as deep input from pathways ascending outside the dorsal columns. These conclusions are based on the ability of spinal lesions to dissociate the S-I map of the hind limb into minimally overlapping projection fields associated with different spinal projection pathways and signify that each spinal path contributes uniquely to the body representation in S-I (3). Hence, different types of mechanoreceptive afferents come to project differentially to the different cytoarchitectural fields which comprise S-I.

This and other related evidence speaks to the segregation of afferents in spinal ascending tracts and cortical projection areas according to receptor properties, i.e., the signals they carry and receive (see ref. 16). In addition, body topography is also operative as an organizing principle in bringing about a rearrangement of afferents along their ascending spinal course: shortly after entry into the dorsal columns, the ascending collaterals of the fibers in each dorsal root arrange to a fiber laminar with a dorsolateral to ventromedial orientation in the columns. Within each segmental laminar thus formed, fibers are characteristically ordered: this is demonstrated by the fact that a recording microelectrode which advances perpendicular to the long axis of the laminar encounters a sequence of fibers whose receptive fields describe a continuous path on the body (the "dermatomal trajectory," see ref. 14). Furthermore, each time the tip of the electrode crosses the boundary between consecutive segmental fiber laminae in the lumbar dorsal column, there occurs an abrupt jump in the receptive field location which backtracks part of the peripheral path mapped in the preceding lamina, reflecting overlap in the peripheral segmental innervation. As dorsal column fibers ascend from lumbar to cervical levels, a significant change occurs, apart from the separation of submodalities referred to earlier. The fibers of consecutive dermatomes rearrange to the extent that an electrode advancing through the cervical fasciculus gracilis encounters a sequence of fibers whose receptive fields form a smooth and continuous path on the body periphery (17). This process brings afferents from the same body regions into neighborhood and proximity relations that approach those of the neurons in S-I.

A schematic overview over the details of the body representation in S-I brings several general aspects into focus: One essential ingredient of the cortical map is the fact that each dorsal root projects to an anteroposterior band of cell columns extending across all the cytoarchitectural areas comprising S-I (Fig. 1). Within each dermatomal band, the receptive field sequence of the dermatomal trajectories of upper spinal levels is preserved. In their totality, the consecutive dermatomal bands compose sequences of neurons in the mediolateral traverse of the cortical map, whose receptive fields align in the body periphery to characteristic pathways, as shown schematically in Fig. 2.

For the purpose of conceptualizing the mapping of body periphery to S-I in the framework of topology, Werner and Whitsel (15) proposed to visualize the body as an aggregate of receptive fields which combine to ordered sets in the form of the dermatomal trajectories. Similarly, the cortical map can be considered as an aggregate of neurons which also combine to ordered sets, each set receiving afferents from one dermatomal trajectory. The relationship between body periphery and cortical map is then one of topological equivalence, for each set of elements in the periphery corresponds to one set of elements in the cortex and vice versa. As a consequence, the neighborhood of two receptive fields in the periphery is also preserved in the projection when these receptive fields are adjacent members of one trajectory; but two adjacent receptive peripheral fields which do not belong to the same trajectory need not be neighbors on the cortical map. The same mapping principle encompasses also in all details the trigeminal projection area as S-I (4).

FIG. 1. Schematic unfolded view of the body representation in the postcentral gyrus of *Macaca mulatta*. Labels positioned external to the map **(medial, lateral, anterior, and posterior)** indicate the orientation of the map of the cortex. Brackets to the left of the figure identify the serially overlapping anteroposterior regions to which the dorsal roots project. Labels contained within the map designate the body parts represented by the cell columns occupying that cortical location. The overlap of the face and radial hand areas in the central portion of the map (areas 1 and 3) is intended to reflect the disjoint character of the RFs observed at this location. **preax.,** preaxial; **post.,** postaxial; **ant.,** anterior; **DA,** dorsoaxial line; **VA,** ventroaxial line; **AM,** anterior midline; **PoM,** posterior midline. The numerals **(2, 1, 3, and 3a)** along the cut lateral edge of the map indicate the cytroarchitectural fields which comprise S1. Lines subdividing the foot and hand areas overlie those cell columns that represent the very tips of digits. If the map were refolded to the configuration of the postcentral gyrus, its anterior edge would be like at the fundus of the central sulcus (areas **3a and 3** comprise the anterior wall of the gyrus); and its posterior edge would occupy the fundus of the intraparietal sulcus laterally and the postcentral sulcus medially. (From ref. 19a.)

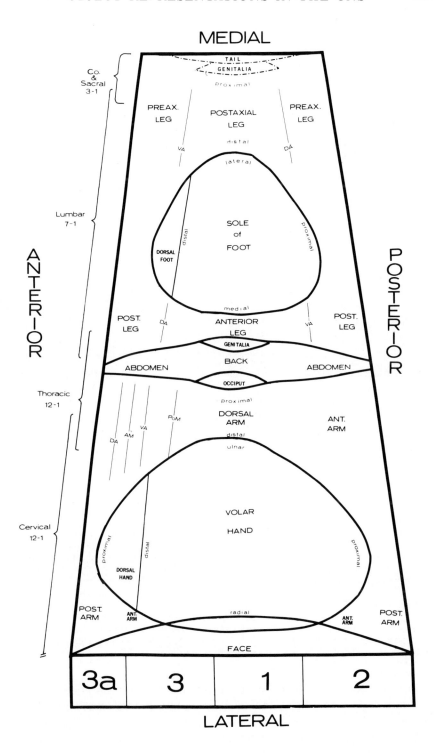

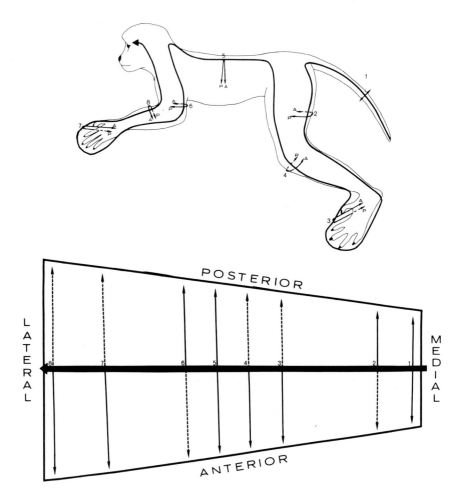

FIG. 2. The lower portion of the figure is a composite map designed to illustrate the local neighborhood relations of the S1 map in finer detail than Fig. 1. Labels located external to the map indicate its orientation on the cortex. The heavy uninterrupted arrow crossing the map corresponds to a continuous mediolateral array of cell columns which (a) extends across the entirety of S1, and (b) maps the sequence of body regions encountered along the heavy arrow drawn on the figurine displayed at the top. The narrow arrows drawn orthogonal to the heavy arrow in the lower portion of the figure correspond to linear arrays of neurons aligned in the anteroposterior dimension of S1. The interrupted portion of these narrow arrows corresponds to those parts of the body surface hidden from the view illustrated at the top and indicate the cortical cell columns representing those same regions. Labels at the extremes of the peripheral paths drawn orthogonal to the heavy arrow indicate the body regions encountered as one moves either anterior or posterior in the S1 map. **A,** anterior in S1; **P,** posterior in S1. (From ref. 19a.)

The principal point of this necessarily cursory overview is the juxtaposition of evidence for the concomitant operation of two seemingly opposing organizational principles in the somesthetic projection system: one, consisting of progressive parcellation and segregation according to peripheral receptor properties at all levels up to and including S-I; the other, represented by the concept of the dermatomal trajectory, which insures that certain sets of receptive fields maintain their neighborhood relations in the mapping from body periphery to S-I.

While the principles of place and modality representations are at least in certain, typical instances realized in the form of "labeled lines" and topographically organized projection patterns, there remains the fundamental question of the interpretation of the signals carried over these channels in the form of neural spike discharge trains. However, unlike the communication engineer, the neurophysiologist is not in the position to examine the transmission of messages over these channels on the basis of established principles in information theory, namely: prior knowledge of the statistical structure of both signals and noise. Instead, one of the questions neurophysiological studies seek to answer is, "What is the signal, what is the noise?" One approach to addressing this question consists of the selection of certain aspects of the neural responses which can be measured and which permit one to determine quantitative relations between them and physical stimulus parameters. Accordingly, a primary concern in the quantitation of neural responses is the selection of scales and of a metric which will result in a monotonic functional relation between the neural response and the corresponding stimuli which evoke them. One might then expect that there are some scales among these fulfilling this criterion which tally with psychophysical scales. This would tend to validate the relevance of the particular neural response scale in the sense that it reflects the manner in which the nervous system "encodes" certain stimulus parameters.

Under appropriate experimental conditions, it is possible to show that the frequency of discharges of slowly adapting myelinated afferents innovating the glabrous skin of the monkey's hand and also of neurons in the postcentral gyrus meets this criterion at least in the first approximation. In this case, the relation between stimulus and response (the former measured in terms of mechanical skin displacement, the latter in the form of a steady-state frequency of neural discharges) is described with a high degree of statistical validity by a power function of the general form $R = K \cdot S^n$ (13). This general relationship falls into the same class of stimulus response relationships that also pertain generally in psychophysical judgments to stimulus intensity in man (12).

A more stringent criterion can be applied by measuring in informational terms the accuracy of stimulus identification in a manner analogous to that introduced into psychophysics by Garner (5). This approach eliminates the need for defining a metric scale for the stimulus and response domain, and merely requires a method of stimulus and response classification. In the experiments that lead to the data illustrated in Fig. 3, responses were categorized in terms of frequency of discharges elicited during the steady-state periods of skin indentation. Stimulus uncertainty, plotted on the abscissa of Fig. 3, is a function of the number of categories into which the entire range

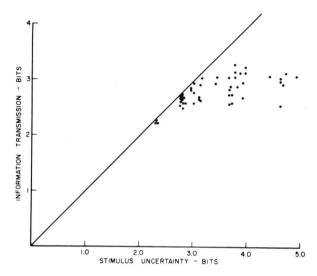

FIG. 3. Information transmission calculated from a series of stimulus-response data obtained for each of 17 mechanoreceptive fibers ending in the palm of the hand (macaque). The stimuli were applied at a rate of 6 or 12 per minute: observation times were 500 msec or longer but not exceeding 1 sec. (From ref. 16a.)

of the stimulus continuum is divided, and the relative frequency of which stimuli of each category are applied at the level of peripheral cutaneous afferents. This method of analysis results in the computation of information transmitted from the stimulus to the response domain, amounting to 2.5 to 3 bits per stimulus. The surprising correspondence between this result and information transmission in regard to stimulus intensity in psychophysical tests in man appears to validate the assumption of a frequency code for stimulus intensity. This comparison also suggests two further implications: one, that the human central nervous system is capable of preserving all the information it receives over first-order fibers; and second, that, in principle, information about the intensity of the stimulus could be conveyed by a single or at least very few peripheral nerve fibers.

The next step in the analysis of information handling by the nervous system can be taken by increasing the complexity of the stimulus over and above the relatively artificial limitation to time in variant punctate stimuli. One way of accomplishing this is to introduce a periodic time-varying parameter in the form of vibratory stimuli. A sinusoidally vibrating stimulus applied to the body surface evokes in human subjects at frequencies from 5 to 40 Hz the sensation of an easily localized cutaneous flutter. Higher frequencies elicit a deep, poorly localized, but very characteristic hum of vibration. Human subjects in psychophysical, and rhesus monkeys in behavioral, experiments perform alike in terms of detection threshold, sensitivity range, and frequency discrimination of sinusoidal stimuli (7,9). One of the important results of neurophysiological studies in Mountcastle's laboratories (8) was the identification of two different sets of receptors and afferents, one subserving the range of subjective flutter sensation and signaling mechanical deformation which could be attributed to Meissner corpuscles in dermal ridges of the glabrous skin; the other mediating the high-frequency vibratory hum attributable to Pacinian corpuscles. The two sets of afferent fibers differ radically in their tuning points (i.e., the minimal amplitude of mechanical skin deformation at which the neural discharges occur in the dominant frequency of the vibratory stimulus). Nonetheless, in the psychophysical tests in monkey and man, the threshold function for the detection of vibratory stimuli is continuous over the entire frequency range, in spite of the two separate neural channels with distinctly different response parameters. The intriguing aspect of this mode of stimulus representation is that the nervous system separates stimuli that belong to the same physical continuum (i.e., periodically recurring deformation of body surface) into two separate transmission channels, distinguished by the frequency characteristics of their respective mechanoreceptive organs.

In the projection to S-I, the two classes of afferents remain essentially distinct and activate different cortical neurons. One class of quickly adapting cortical neurons follows readily the sinusoidal mechanical stimulus with a periodic recurrence of impulses at intervals close to the cycle lengths of the vibratory stimulus, as is the case for the first-order afferents from the glabrous skin. Thus, information on stimulus frequency remains preserved in the temporal discharge pattern of these cortical neurons. This suggests that the capability of discriminating frequencies of vibratory stimuli in behavioral and psychophysical tests may be attributable to a central neural mechanism that can detect differences between the period length in impulse trains of this class of neurons. The situation is entirely different with another class of cortical neurons, which receives its afferent input from the Pacinian corpuscles. Vibratory stimuli at the high-frequency range, which entrain periodic discharges in the afferents originating from pacinian corpuscles, are reflected merely by the increase of discharge rates in these cortical neurons. But there is no relation between the magnitude of the increase in firing rate and the stimulus frequency, nor is there any periodicity in the discharges, which would reflect the stimulus frequency (8). Yet, the human observer and the monkey in behavior tests are both capable of discriminating between different frequencies of vibratory stimuli, irrespective of whether the stimuli engage, according to their frequency, the quickly adapting system of afferents from the glabrous skin or the pacinian elements.

The general implication is that the certain stimulus attributes which by virtue of the choice of the selected physical measure (e.g., frequency, as in the case under consideration) can be represented on a continuous and monotonic scale, need not be processed by the nervous system in an equally continuous and homogeneous fashion. Instead, different ranges of a particular attribute may be represented by the nervous system through different transmission channels, each using a different code.

The examples cited so far illustrate instances in which discharge rate in spike trains or temporal patterning of consecutive discharges satisfies at least some of the criteria that would enable these quantitative parameters of spike trains to serve the role of neural codes in labeled lines. However, there is now also a number of instances well documented that attest to different principles. These principles relate to the reduction of redundancy in stimulus information.

The underlying notion is that an adaptation of the organism to certain types of redundancies that are always present in the environment would have occurred during evolution. The guiding principle in these considerations is Shannon's concept of "optimal codes," which match the statistical structure of regularities in the available repertoire of messages. To begin with, two mechanisms were identified as being available to the nervous system for the purpose of reducing redundancy of information in stimulus. These were, in the temporal domain, mechanisms specifically sensitive to onset and cessation of a stimulus; and in the spatial domain, lateral inhibition. The potential significance of such redundancy-reducing codes consists of economy in signal transmission, because these codes exploit lawful regularities in the stimulus source. For instance, the duration of the stationary stimulus is uniquely defined by the moments of its beginning to end, and thus, there is no need for generating neuronal impulses in the interval between these points in time.

The concept of the "stimulus feature" can be considered a generalization of this principle. This concept becomes applicable whenever a neuronal discharge signals with relatively high selectivity the occurrence of an input state that contains in its specifications the concomitant occurrence of certain regularities in the stimulus space, in addition to being specific for a certain place of the receptor sheet and stimulus modality. For instance, because matter is cohesive, objects can be fully characterized in terms of their boundaries; hence, boundaries (that is, edges, corners, and angles) become the "features" in terms of which the spatial layout of a stimulus object can be unambiguously represented.

Carried to its logical consequence, this principle implies that the central nervous system takes the information available in the proximal stimulus on receptor sheets out of its original context and imposes a classification into disjunctive entities. The general principle appears to be that the number of neurons available to signal stimulus information increases with progression along the afferent pathway, but that any given neuron is less frequently activated as the constraints of its stimulus feature become more severe (1).

The neurophysiological reality of the feature detection is by now amply substantiated. The relative selectivity with which certain neurons in S-I respond to cutaneous stimuli moving in a particular direction across the receptive field of the skin is an example of this type of coding (19). Such neurons can be "triggered" to discharge at a high rate when a fine hair or brush is moved across the receptive field at constant velocity in certain directions, but not in others. There is some gradation of the density of discharges with variation of the direction of stimulus motion, but there exists for these neurons a clearly defined direction of stimulus movement which elicits a maximal discharge (Fig. 4). Thus, such neurons can be classified according to their "best" stimuli. A response less than maximal indicates only departure from the optimal stimulus, but not the direction of departure. The occurrence of the maximal discharge in a neuron of this kind can be thought of as the "code" for a conjunction of stimulus properties; namely, stimulus movement in a particular direction on a particular place of the skin. To the extent to which a neuron exhibits this property, it is capable of representing a relatively large amount of information in regard to stimulus used, since a vigorous response, when it occurs, not only reflects the presence of the mechanical event, but also the spatiotemporal progression of a mechanical ascent traversing the neuron's receptive field. Hence, a response in a direction-specific neuron reduces the uncertainty in regard to nature of the stimulus much more than does a response in a first-order afferent fiber or, for that matter, in a cortical neuron lacking this discriminative capability. Reduction of uncertainty, and correspondingly, the gain of information, is the more marked than narrower in the range of stimulus orientations with directional preference.

Of all cortical neurons in S-I, those situated in lamina IV are closest to the specific thalamocortical input. Neurons in this lamina lack any appreciable transformation of the stimulus-evoked activity, other than convergence of afferents to larger receptive fields. Hence, except for a reduction in the dynamic range of discharge rates, responses of lamina IV neurons — with rare exceptions — replicate the activity in first-order afferents. Likewise, there occurs by and large much less information processing by lamina IV neurons of visual cortex (notably lamina IVB) compared to the specificity of response properties in more superficial and deeper cortical laminae (6). In contrast to the relative paucity or, at least, lesser degree of stimulus feature specification by neurons in lamina IV, there is a prevalence of feature extracting neurons and, at least in the visual cortex, also increasing refinement of such features, both in more superficial and deeper cortical laminae. The implication is that the elaboration of feature specificity of cortical neurons results from intracortical synaptic interactions.

The occurrence of feature-analyzing neurons in cortical projection areas has led to much speculation on their role in perception, notably in connection with some classes of pattern-recognizing machines that also make use of feature-analyzing elements. However, despite substantial successes in certain circumscribed areas of application, analysis and identification of patterns and shapes by machines fall far short of the perceptual capabilities

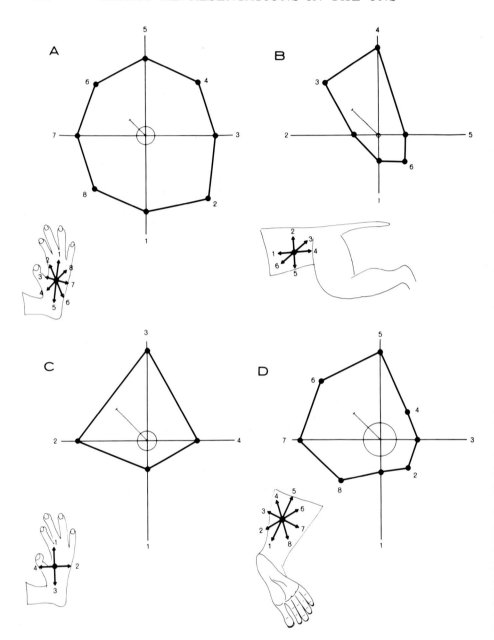

FIG. 4. Contribution of a selected region of the receptive field to the cortical neuronal response as a function of the direction of stimuli motion. To generate each of the polar plots of this figure, the moving stimuli were applied at a variety of intersecting orientations within the receptive field, as is indicated in the accompanying schematic drawing. The response profiles obtained from each stimulus orientation were arranged to permit identification of those "bins" corresponding to the point of chord intersection in the receptive field. The mean discharge rate per stimulus (expressed in impulses per second)

of organisms. A discussion on this issue must take cognizance of the fact that perception of organisms is for the most part action-oriented: both in the sense of motor acts enabling the acquisition of snapshots of scenes following each other serially in time, and also with regard to purposeful actions to be carried out with the objects of perception. Hence, the analogy is more with the program control of a robot than it is with the computer program that labels and categorizes patterns. But even disregarding for the moment the motor component in perceptual activity, there is need for postulating additional operational principles and neural mechanisms in the attempt to account for the perceptual achievements of organisms. Neisser's concept of "figural synthesis," Simon's "noticing," and Pribram's emphasis on the organism's competence in dealing with alternatives by the mechanisms of "selective attention" are some of these explanatory postulates. To this, current neurophysiological investigations in our laboratory add evidence that the neural representation of the peripheral stimulus may vary greatly depending on the behavioral context in which the stimulus is received, as may the ongoing neural activity preceding the arrival of a next stimulus in a programmed sequence. We shall now turn our attention to this.

One experimental paradigm used for the exploration of these relationships was modeled after the test situation for contingent negative variation (Fig. 5). In this task, a brief tone appears and 2.5 sec later a red light comes on and stays on for 500 msec, during which time the monkey must hit a bar. For this action he receives a reward. After a 10-sec pause, the same cycle is repeated. A cutaneous stimulus is then applied to the palm of the hand that is not involved in the execution of the movement for rewards. The entire behavior cycle is repeated many times in succession in order to obtain averaged values for the neural responses. Figure 6 is a display of average neural responses obtained from one neuron in S-I studied under these conditions. The important point to note is that the response to identical cutaneous stimuli differs, depending on the timing of the cutaneous stimulation in the behavioral cycle which is controlled by the tone-light sequence. It must be emphasized that the cutaneous stimulus has in these experiments no

---

in these bins reflects the contribution of that portion of the receptive field to the neuronal response as the direction of brush advance is varied. Each direction of stimulus motion (identified by the direction of the arrowheads on the schematic drawings) is assigned a number corresponding to one of the heavy points on the circumference of the polar plots. The distance of these points from the origin of the coordinate system measures the neuronal response (in impulses per second) generated by traversing the receptive-field center in the direction identified by the appropriate number. Each stimulus was replicated 25 times. The circle around the origin of the coordinate system represents the level of spontaneous activity. The length of the interrupted radial line in each plot represents a calibration value of 50 impulses/sec/stimulus. **A**: A symmetrical S-I neuron, for the magnitude of neuronal response is independent of stimulus direction. **B, C, and D**: Asymmetric S-I neurons which displayed direction selectivity at certain chord orientations. The stimulus velocities employed were 63 mm/sec (neuron **A**); 56 mm/sec (neuron **B**); 39 mm/sec (neuron **C**); and 236 mm/sec (neuron **D**). (From ref. 19.)

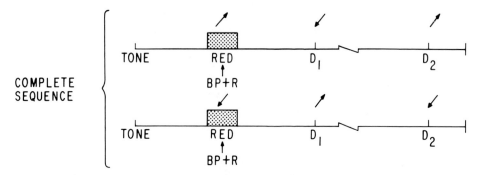

FIG. 5. CNV paradigm with neutral test stimuli. Schematic display of the complete test cycle, beginning with a brief tone and followed 2.5 sec later by a red light of 500-msec duration, during which time a reward is available if the subject presses a bar **(BP + R).** During this period, a cutaneous stimulus moves in one direction, indicated by arrow, across a cutaneous receptive field on the palm of the hand opposite to the hand working for the reward. This period is followed by a 10-sec pause, during which at the points D_1 and D_2 cutaneous stimuli are applied with alternating directions of stimulus motion (as indicated by the directions of the arrows). In the second line, the same sequence is repeated, except that the directions of cutaneous stimulus motion are now reversed at corresponding points in the behavioral cycle. As a result, there are now two sample periods of neural activity for each epoch in the behavioral cycle available, each with opposing directions of stimulus motion. This entire sequence is repeated 50 to 100 times. Code signals are stored by the computer for each cutaneous stimulus, permitting retrieval of neural data according to timing and direction of the cutaneous stimuli.

behavior-controlling function. Instead, these stimuli merely serve as behaviorally neutral test probes, which are, as it were, injected into the neural network to test its responsiveness to the stimuli. The general point to which these experiments speak is as follows: an identical stimulus is signaled by a given cortical neuron in S-I by a different magnitude of the evoked activity, depending on which point in time in the behavioral cycle this stimulus is applied. Most significantly, the point in the behavioral cycle at which a stimulus is registered with maximal response differs for different neurons which, in every other respect, appear to have identical response characteristics: for some neurons, the response may be maximal in the expectancy period that intervenes between the tone and the light signal, in others con-

FIG. 6. Display of averaged neural responses to cutaneous stimuli moving in opposite directions **(DIR 1 and DIR 2,** top and bottom row, respectively) across a cutaneous receptive field on the palm of the hand of a macaque while performing in the behavioral paradigm of Fig. 1. The test stimuli are applied during the phase RED **(Bp + R)** and at the point labeled D_1 in Fig. 1 (i.e., 5 sec after the red light goes off). The neural activities are displayed as mean number of impulses per stimulus in each consecutive bin of 50-msec duration throughout the traverse of the receptive field by the moving cutaneous stimulus. The vertical bars in each bin represent standard errors of the mean number of spikes per stimulus (expressed as impulses per second). Note the difference in response to direction 1, as contrasted to the equality of responses in direction 2, at the respective reference points of red-light-on and D_1 in the behavioral cycle.

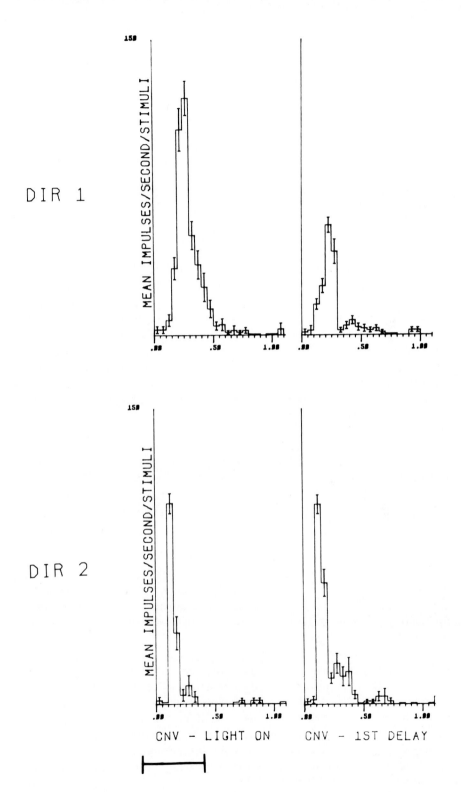

comitantly with or immediately following the bar-press response, and in others in the 10-sec pause that intervenes between consecutive behavioral cycles.

In a second experimental paradigm, the cutaneous stimuli themselves are used as behavioral controlling cues (Fig. 7). The basic plan of the experiment consists of the following: the red light comes on, cutaneous stimulus is applied, whereby the direction of stimulus motion across the receptive fields is now crucial. One of the two directions indicates to the monkey on the basis of previous training that a reward is available and he can press the bar with the nonstimulated hand to obtain it. The other direction of stimulus motion is not rewarded, and he has learned that the red light in the on position is an instruction that indicates that, given the latter direction of cutaneous stimulation, no reward is available. Having the light off is another instruction telling him that no matter what the direction of the stimulus motion is, rewards are not available. Thus, there is one out of four conditions that is interesting to the monkey in the sense of telling him of the availability of the reward whereas three other conditions indicate to him the unavailability of reward. This experiment is performed in three different variants. In variant I, the number of consecutive repetitions of the same direction of stimulus motion is equal, constant, and 10. Hence, the expectancy structure of the task permits a high degree of anticipation: if the stimulus moves in one direction, the likelihood of the same direction to occur with the next stimulus is very high. In a second variant, the numbers of repetitions of equal stimulus motion vary in a random manner between three and eight. Thus, there is an intermediate degree of expectancy. Finally, there is a third variant in which the direction of motion of the next stimulus is either identical with, or opposite to the preceding stimulus. Thus, there is a 50% probability that the next stimulus will be opposite to the preceding one.

In contrast to the previously described paradigm, the stimulus responses are entirely identical, irrespective of the particular behavioral situation that prevails at any one moment: for instance, availability or nonavailability of reward. However, there are considerable differences with respect to the neural activity that occurs in the periods between application of cutaneous stimuli. Figure 8 is intended to schematically illustrate the sampling periods for the interstimulus activity. In a review of the data obtained in our laboratory for 90 neurons studied in this manner, it becomes apparent that there exists one class of neurons, exemplified by Fig. 9, which displays a substantial difference between the neural activity samples obtained between application of cutaneous stimuli, depending on whether or not the animal is involved in the behavioral task. It appears for this category of neurons that involvement of the animal in the behavioral tests is accompanied by setting the spontaneous activity to a reduced level throughout the entire behavioral period, irrespective of what the specific stimuli and the instructions (i.e., light signals) are. Another category of neurons is more discriminative: Fig. 10 shows discharge interval histograms for the intertrial periods under

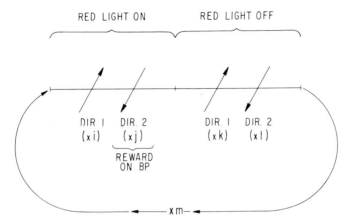

FIG. 7. Schematic representation of the conditional discrimination task for direction of cutaneous stimulus motion. The red light instructs the subject that stimulus motion in direction 2 signals availability of a reward by bar press **(BP)**, but unavailability of reward for stimuli moving in the opposite direction. Absence of the red light signals unavailability of reward irrespective of direction of stimulus motion. The entire cycle is repeated several hundred times **(xm)**; the values of **i, j, k, and l,** indicating numbers of repetitions of cutaneous stimulus motions of equal directions, differ in accordance with the expectancy structure of the task (see text).

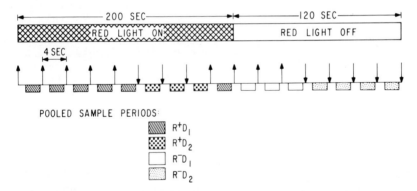

FIG. 8. Schematic diagram of intertrial activity sampling in the discrimination task of Fig. 4. The periods of red light on (200 sec) and red light off (120 sec) are indicated at the top. These sequences are repeated 50 or more times. Throughout the entire test period, brush strokes are applied at 4-sec intervals to the receptive field of the neuron under study. The arrows on the bottom line of the figure signify the direction in which the brush moves across the receptive field. The specific instance depicted in the figure refers to random order of the direction of motion of consecutive stimuli (see text). The intertrial activity of the neuron is sampled beginning 1 sec after the termination of the last brush movement to just prior to the beginning of the next cutaneous stimulus. For the analysis of the neural data, the neuronal discharges of identical instructions (**R+**, red light on; **R−** = red light off) and direction of stimulus motions (**D$_1$**, direction 1; **D$_2$**, opposite direction) are averaged. Thus, four sets of data are obtained, corresponding to the four pooled sample periods listed in the figure.

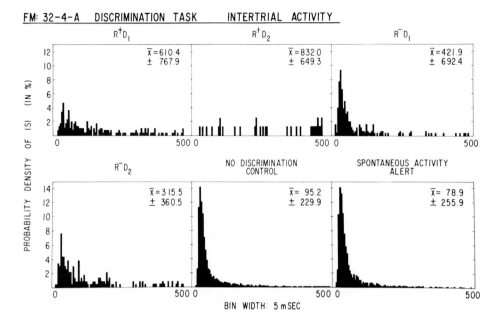

FIG. 9. Interspike interval histogram of a neuron obtained for the four intertrial activity periods of the discrimination task illustrated in Figs. 4 and 5, and also for two additional sample periods. "No discrimination control" refers to samples of neural activity collected in the manner shown in Fig. 4 (i.e., extending from 1 sec after end of last cutaneous stimulus to just prior to next stimulus), except that the discrimination performance was not required. The panel labeled "spontaneous activity, alert" refers to neural activity in the absence of any intentional stimulation of the cutaneous receptive field while the animal was in a state of alert wakefulness. The numbers in each panel express the mean interspike discharge interval ($\bar{x}$) and the standard deviation of the interspike interval distribution. The ordinate marks the probability density for each 5-msec bin of the histograms in percent.

different conditions labeled in the figure $R + D_1$, etc. In the evaluation of the discharge interval histograms, use was made of the well-established fact that gamma functions represent interspike interval distributions adequately and permit their description in terms of appropriate numerical parameters. By comparing the parameters of the best-fitting gamma curves for the different intertrial periods illustrated in Fig. 10, it becomes apparent that sampling period $R + D_2$ is distinctly set aside from all other sampling periods. Accordingly, the neural activity following the $R + D_2$ condition (i.e., red light on and cutaneous stimulus motion in direction two) is distinctly different from the activity occurring subsequent to all other stimulus conditions. Data on intertrial activity of this nature, which are independent of the particular variant in the expectancy structure of the behavioral task suggests that neurons of this latter class are capable of reflecting in their posttrial activity their last instruction (light signal) and the direction of movement of the last cutaneous stimulus. Different neurons appear to have

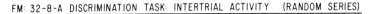

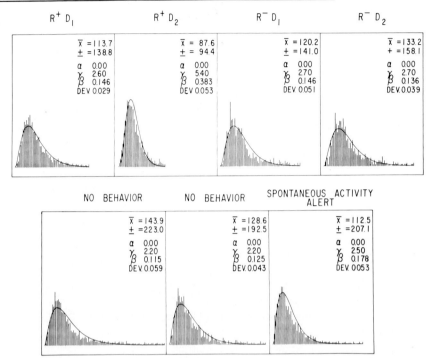

FIG. 10. Interspike interval histograms and fitted gamma distributions (solid contours of histograms) of a neuron's activity studied in the discrimination paradigm illustrated in Fig. 7. The expectancy structure of the task was that of random numbers of repetition of cutaneous stimuli with equal direction of motion. In the top row, the activities in the four sample periods listed in Fig. 5 are displayed. In the bottom row, the two histograms labeled "no behavior" were obtained from control periods with cutaneous stimulation, but no provision for discrimination behavior. The last panel in the bottom row (spontaneous activity) refers to ongoing neural activity in the absence of any cutaneous stimulation. The numbers in all panels list mean interspike discharge interval, standard deviation of the mean, and parameters of the fitted gamma distributions. Note the distinct difference of the activity sampled under $R + D_2$ from all other conditions. Bin width of the histograms: 5 msec; ordinate probability density in percent.

acquired in the training period for the task the capacity to "specialize" in some sense for one or another of these stimulus-instruction combinations. As a result of this selective retention of information on the behavior condition prevailing at the last stimulus application, such neurons will signal the next stimulus against different backgrounds of intertrial activity. Accordingly, some neurons in the pool of neurons representing the tactile sensibility of the hand area in S-I will enhance the contrast for stimuli occurring after $R + D_2$ situation, others after $R + D_1$ situation, etc. In other words, a new stimulus-instruction conjunction is evaluated against some residual information as to the last stimulus-instruction combination which was held over in the form of "buffer memory," to use an analogy from computer technology. This line of thought further supports the contention that at least some aspect of "selective attention" may be related, in neural-mechanistic terms, to generating contrasts and loss of redundancy in signaling physically identical stimuli that have acquired behavioral significance in the course of past learning.

In pursuing the leading theme of the duality between discreteness and diffuseness in the nervous system, we have been led to speak at great lengths of various forms of specificity: due to the selectivity of peripheral receptors for narrow ranges of physical parameters of stimuli; due to labeled lines; due to topological mappings; and due to intracortical transformations for generating neuronal specificity for temporal or spatial stimulus context (i.e., features). Diffuseness of neural controls entered the picture in a subtle and indirect way: namely, in the form that certain behavioral conditions are accompanied by either a phasic or a tonic change of neuronal activity patterns. But direction and extent of such changes are individualistic and different for different neurons, not otherwise distinguishable on the basis of their specific and discrete properties. Seen in that light, diffuseness refers to the extent of the neuron pool affected at any one time, rather than to the manner in which each individual neuron's activity in that pool is affected.

The two behavioral paradigms studied, namely the situation created by variation in the expectancy in the CNV sequence and the conditional discrimination of cutaneous stimuli, entail different consequences: in the first case, the stimulus response *per se* is subject to phasic changes; in the second case, the neural activity between stimuli is affected in a tonic manner. This duality of nonspecific changes in the activity of neuron pools compares with the classic finding of Sharpless and Jasper (11) on diffusely organized tonic and phasic neural systems, one attributable to the lower portion of the ascending reticular system, the other involving the unspecific thalamic system.

According to this conception, diffuse neural control mechanisms are capable of bringing about a diversification of neural responses between neurons sharing commonplace and modality labels. This diversification appears related to the acquisition of expectations and anticipations through learning of environmental regularities, i.e., behavior-controlling contingencies. The result is a reduction of the redundancy of stimulus representation which is inherent in the labeled line principle. There is a parallel between this effect of diffuse neuronal systems on the one hand and feature extracting mechanisms on the other: the latter is concerned with adaptation to environmental regularities in phylogeny and, to some extent at least, early ontogeny when the synaptic connections of feature-extracting neurons are formed to last throughout the subject's life span; the former is attributable to learning of environmental regularities prevailing under certain conditions and at certain times in the individual's life history. The common denominator of both feature mechanism and the function of the nonspecific neural systems lies in their ability to augment the information-processing potential of the place and modality-specific projection systems by reducing the redundancy of stimulus encoding and by allowing temporal and spatial contexts of stimuli to be reflected in the neural activity these stimuli evoke in the specific projection systems.

REFERENCES

1. Barlow, H. B. (1969): Trigger features, adaptation and economy of impulses. In: *Information Processing in the Nervous System,* edited by K. N. Leibovic. Springer, Berlin.
2. Brown, A. G. (1968): Cutaneous afferent fiber collaterals in the dorsal columns of the cat. *Exp. Brain Res.,* 5:293–305.
3. Dreyer, D. A., Schneider, R. J., Metz, C. B., and Whitsel, B. L., (1974): Differential contributions of spinal pathways to body representation in postcentral gyrus of *Macaca mulatta. J. Neurophysiol.,* 37:119–145.
4. Dreyer, D. A., Loe, P. R., Metz, C. B., and Whitsel, B. L. (1975): Representation of head and face in postcentral gyrus of macaque. *J. Neurophysiol.,* 38:714–733.
5. Garner, W. R. (1962): *Uncertainty and Structure as Psychological Concepts.* Wiley, New York.
6. Hubel, D. H., and Wiesel, T. N. (1968): Receptive fields and functional architecture of monkey striate cortex. *J. Physiol. (Lond.),* 195:215–243.
7. LaMotte, R. H., and Mountcastle, V. B. (1975): Capacities of humans and monkeys to discriminate between vibratory stimuli of different frequency and amplitude; a correlation between neural events and psychophysical measurement. *J. Neurophysiol.,* 38: 539–559.
8. Mountcastle, V. B., Talbot, W. H., Sakata, H., and Hivarinen, J. (1969): Cortical neuronal mechanisms in flutter vibration studied in unanesthetized monkeys; neuronal periodicity and frequency discrimination. *J. Neurophysiol.,* 37:452–484.
9. Mountcastle, V. B., LaMotte, R. H., and Carli, G. (1972): Detection thresholds for stimuli in humans and monkeys; comparison with threshold events in mechanoreceptive afferent nerve fibers innervating the monkey hand. *J. Neurophysiol.,* 35:122–136.
10. Perkel, D. H., and Bullock, T. H. (ed.) (1968): Neural coding. *Neurosci. Res. Program Bull.,* 6:227–348.
11. Sharpless, S., and Jasper, H. (1956): Habituation of the arousal reaction. *Brain,* 79: 655–680.
12. Stevens, S. S. (1957): On the psychophysical law. *Psychol. Rev.,* 64:153–181.
13. Werner, G., and Mountcastle, V. B. (1965): Neural activity in mechanoreceptive afferents: Stimulus response relation, Weber functions and information transmission. *J. Neurophysiol.,* 28:359–397.
14. Werner, G., and Whitsel, B. L. (1967): The topology of dermatomal projection in the medial lemniscal system. *J. Physiol. (Lond.),* 192:123–144.
15. Werner, G., and Whitsel, B. L. (1968): Topology of the body representation in somatosensory area I of primates. *J. Neurophysiol.,* 31:856–869.
16. Werner, G., and Whitsel, B. L. (1973): Functional organization of somatosensory cortex. In: *Handbook of Sensory Physiology, Vol. II,* edited by A. Iggo, pp. 622–700. Springer, Berlin.
16a. Werner, G., and Mountcastle, V. B. (1968): Quantitative relations between mechanical stimuli to the skin and neural responses evoked by them. In: *The skin senses,* edited by D. R. Kenshalo, pp. 112–137. Charles C Thomas, Springfield, Ill.
17. Whitsel, B. L., Petrucelli, L. M., and Sapiro, G. (1969): Modality representation in the lumbar and cervical fasciculus gracilis of squirrel monkeys. *Brain Res.,* 15:67–78.
18. Whitsel, B. L., Petrucelli, L. M., Ha, H., and Dreyer, D. A. (1972): The resorting of spinal afferents as antecedents to the body representation in the postcentral gyrus. *Brain Behav. Evol.,* 5:303–341.

19. Whitsel, B. L., Roppolo, J. R., and Werner, G. (1972): Cortical information processing of stimulus motion on primate skin. *J. Neurophysiol.,* 35:691–717.
19a. Whitsel, B. L., Dreyer, D. A., and Roppolo, J. R. (1971): Determinants of body representation in postcentral gyrus of macaques. *J. Neurophysiol.,* 34:1018–1034.
20. Zeki, S. M. (1974): The mosaic organization of the visual cortex in monkey. In: *Essays on the Nervous System,* edited by R. Bellairs and E. G. Gray, pp. 327–343. Clarendon Press, Oxford.

Architectonics of the Cerebral Cortex,
edited by M. A. B. Brazier and H. Petsche.
Raven Press, New York © 1978.

The Neocortical Link: Thoughts on the Generality of Structure and Function of the Neocortex

O. D. Creutzfeldt

Abteilung für Neurobiologie, Max Planck-Institut für Biophysikalische Chemie, D-3400 Göttingen, Federal Republic of Germany

HISTORICAL CONTEXT AND THESIS

The weight and thus the volume of the brain are, within a given order and also between orders, proportional to the body weight. The same holds for the volume of the cerebral cortex. But since this is a sheet of tissue, with a nearly constant thickness of about 2 to 3 mm, its surface also increases with the same proportionality. Since the smooth inner surface of the skull only grows in proportion to the weight raised to the power of two-thirds, this large sheet needs to be folded in the larger animals.

As a consequence of this evolutionary rule, the cerebral cortex of man is conspicuously large and anatomically complicated because of its foldings. It is, therefore, usually considered the most human part and at the same time the most noble evolutionary achievement of the brain. Because of the cerebral cortex's large size, localized lesions of circumscribed, functionally homogeneous volumes (and thus areas) caused by disease or injury are more frequently observed than in other parts of the brain where functionally different volumes are packed close together. Since such lesions, placed appropriately, may interfere with specific human performances of the brain such as language, cognition, ethics, and aesthetics, it is not surprising that the areas of the cortex whose destruction leads to such symptoms are considered the actual "seat" of these functions.

This idea, first expressed highly speculatively in the romantic period of research in cortical function by neurologists like Gall and Spurzheim and others at the beginning of the 19th century (phrenology), gained further support in the middle of the last century with the clinical observation of speech loss (aphasia) after a lesion of the frontal cortex (Broca) and of "psychische Blindheit" after experimental ablation of the occipital pole (Munk). The discovery during this period of morphological differences of various districts (or areas) of the cortex during the last century (Baillarger, Vicq-d'Azir, Meynert, Betz) started a systematic search for correlations between these apparently specific morphological differences and functional properties of the different areas. The art of this classification of cortical areas based on morphological criteria reached its height in the work of neuroanatomically oriented physicians such as Campbell (6), the Vogts (74,75), Brodmann (5), and von Economo (22) during the first quarter of this century.

The fruit of this research is, in its basic findings, a very useful method of distinguishing various parts of the cerebral cortex. Its shortcoming is the neglect of the functional aspects of cortical neuronal organization, since the methods used were appropriate for making visible distinguishing features of the various areas (e.g., Nissl stain of cell bodies, myelin stains for myelinization patterns) but were deficient in demonstrating the processes and contacts of individual neurons. They thus gave only a highly abstracted picture of cortical anatomy, overemphasizing differences and underestimating similarities. This abstract picture could in no way be correlated functionally to the actual symptoms seen after destruction of such areas but by coincidence or by statistical correlations as in more recent attempts by neuropsychologists. Nevertheless, the hope was maintained that the cytoarchitectural dissection of the cortex might yield a key to its function.

This view may be exemplified by a few allusions to the work of Constantin von Economo (1876–1932), to whose memory these thoughts are dedicated. In 1927, Economo published a series of lectures, *Zellaufbau der Großhirnrinde des Menschen* (22), based on his extensive studies with Koskinas, which had appeared 2 years earlier. This small booklet had, because of its sensible reductionism, a large influence on neurology and neuroanatomy, and at the same time reflects ideas and knowledge of the time in this area. Economo wrote in this book: "Meynert, the Viennese psychiatrist, is, by pointing out in the 1860's the partially very significant differences in the cellular structure of the cerebral cortex, the real founder of modern cytoarchitectonics. He assumed, long before the discoveries of Fritsch and Hitzig, that because of the different structure of the cortical surface, the latter can virtually be broken up into single organs, to each of which may be assigned a different function according to its structure; and he[Meynert] foresaw that the exact determination of the areation of the cortical surface will lead us to a new, anatomically well founded, *organology of the brain,* which he brought in contrast with the then fashionable organology of Gall" (22, p. 1, translated).

Economo then describes the differences of the five types of neocortex (Fig. 1: homotypical frontal, parietal, and polar; heterotypical granular and agranular) and divides the cortex into fields accordingly. Although realizing that the heterotypical agranular and the koniocortices are the typical efferent and afferent cortical structures, respectively, the analysis remains fully descriptive, and Economo surmised—along with his contemporaries—that the cytological differences of the neurons in the various cortical areas are the morphological basis for their different functions.

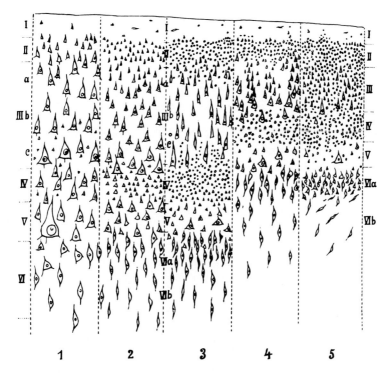

FIG. 1. The different cytoarchitectonic Bautypen of the cerebral neocortex as defined by von Economo (1925, 1927). In the homotypical isocortex **(2, 3, 4)** the six layers can well be recognized in the Nissl picture. It shows three major types: the frontal **(2)**, the parietal **(3)**, and the polar type as found in the frontal and occipital pole **(4)**. On both sides of these types of the homotypical isocortex extremes are found, in which the six-layered structure is difficult to recognize in the Nissl picture. These heterotypical isocortical areas may either show extremely few small cells (agranular cortex as found in the area praecentralis, **1**) or an extreme abundance of small cells (the granular or koniocortex as found in area striata or other sensory cortices, **5**). Whereas the two heterotypical cortical structures are characteristic for the efferent (motor, **1**) and the afferent (sensory, **5**) cortical areas, respectively, the six-layered isocortex serves the commemorative and associative functions of the cortex.

It follows from this that the ideal cortical map should be a layered map which also takes into account the local variations in the structure of the various laminae, so that "one would see in front of oneself in such an ideal map, consisting of various leaflets superimposed on each other the variations of each layer at each point of the cortex" (22, p. 14). Since this was not possible, Economo had to restrict himself for practical reasons to the areal cerebral map. Intercortical fibre patterns, although known to him through Weigert's cortical "Markscheidenbild" (myelinization picture), were interesting to him only insofar as this Markscheidenbild might allow another system for interareal distinction. The Vogts had, some years earlier, combined both methods for their more elaborate cytoarchitectonic map of the cortex. Economo's myeloarchitectonic atlas of the brain was not finished and the manuscript got lost, unfortunately.

In the succeeding 100 pages, Economo describes the local variations of the cortex, not spending more than maximally one page, *in toto,* on the afferent input (of the koniocortex only, of course) and on some efferent connections of the temporal cortex; and maybe five lines each on the functional significance of the different lobes (frontal, temporal, parietal, occipital, central) as derived from neuropathology. In fact, the various "cortical organs" were to him (and many colleagues of his time) virtually the seat of the soul. He wrote: "As we know, the koniocortex is the sensory cortex, i.e., that part into which flow, after being relayed in the diencephalon, the impulses [*sic!*] from the sense organs and the spinal cord, in order to be received and further *apperceived.*" This is clearly meant in the philosophical tradition of Descartes, Leibniz, and Kant, probably in the form of the then widely read psychology of Wundt, who defined apperception as the "single process, by which any psychical content (psychischer Inhalt) is brought to a clear understanding (Auffassung)" (and into consciousness), in contrast to perception, which is not accompanied by attention and consciousness (81).

In this context, the general concept of cortical functions, current at that time, must be recalled. It was, in principle, Flechsig's concept (24); he divided the cortex into areas of afferent, efferent, and intercortical connections, i.e., sensory, motor, and association areas. This terminology reveals the philosophy behind the concept, i.e., a hierarchy of mental processes from perception, to apperception, association, judgment, and executive command, best expressed again by the "apperception psychology" of Wundt (81). and the aphasia scheme of Wernicke (79). Simultaneously in the following years, the functionally white association areas were filled with more and more psychologically or philosophically defined functions as derived from observations after circumscribed cortical lesions and during electrical stimulation on the operating table.

Basic to this concept is the assumption that the actual morphology of a cortical area is specific to its function, or in other words that — at some future time — the complete anatomical description of a "cortical organ," say, the speech area, will be equivalent to its actual function and, in this case, will explain speech. This view, of course, has often been challenged since. But in spite of the long and often vehement discussion between localization and holism advocates (for further reference see Creutzfeldt, refs. 12,13), modern thinking about the cortex still reflects to some extent these concepts either directly or indirectly, or by emphasizing findings which were unexpected in this context. For example, in the context of specific functions given to each lamina of the cortex, the failure to see significant laminar differences of cell responses in the somatosensory cortex (55,58) was such an unexpected finding. The argument is still not settled whether there is sequential invasion of neurons up or down the cortical laminae or not. The "apperception" and "association" model lies clearly in the hierarchical concept of the primary visual cortex (36,37) and of subsequent visual areas, or – for that matter – in many psychological concepts of perception. And the explicit model of cortical columns as basic functional units each being specialized for a certain function can be seen as a consequent extension of Meynert's and Economo's "organologie" to the microscopic level.

I shall try to defend the thesis that *the morphological differences of the different cortical areas are not essential and that the functional distinctions of the various cortical areas are their various connections with afferent projection systems and with efferent target structures* but not due to fundamental differences of their functional structures. I shall restrict myself to the neocortex because of its common developmental history and shall not consider the various allocortical areas, which are indeed, due to the organization of their afferent and efferent connections as well as due to their ontogenetic development morphologically and functionally, as different from the neocortex as the cerebellar cortex, although those different cortical structures also share some important general principles (14).

IDENTICAL ANATOMICAL AND FUNCTIONAL PRINCIPLES OF THE DIFFERENT NEOCORTICAL AREAS

This thesis will meet immediately with the objection that the cytoarchitectonic differences between cortical areas argue against it. In a recent review, Sanides (63) has shown that cytoarchitectonic borders indeed match satisfactorily the "functional" borders between different brain areas. It is obvious that the koniocortex (of primates), for example, is the typical morphological aspect of sensory areas and that the agranular cortex is typical for the motor cortex, etc. There is also no doubt that the sensory cortices receive their afferent input from sensory organs via specific thalamic relay nuclei, and the motor cortex sends its axons down, *interalias,* to the anterior horn nuclei via the pyramidal tract. Thus, the sensory cortices "have to do" with the respective senses, the motor cortex with motor execution, and one tends to argue that these cortical structures are specifically designed for their respective tasks. On the other hand, the homotypical frontal and parietal cortices, which are involved in complex cerebral performances may be specifically designed to analyse, as association areas, various outputs from other primary cortical areas. But in spite of their different morphological and functional appearances, all these areas have basic anatomical and functional properties in common. Some of these will be sketched in the following paragraphs.

The Afferent Input into Cortical Areas with Special Emphasis of the Thalamocortical Loop

What might have first appeared specific for the sensory areas, i.e., that they receive *thalamic input* over the radiation fibres, does not distinguish them from any other cortical area: basically all neocortical fields receive a thalamic input (Fig. 2). This may come from a "specific" relay nucleus, which transmits signals from the sense organs, or an intrinsic nucleus, which receives its input from other cerebral structures such as the tectum, the cerebellum, or the limbic system. In addition to the global demonstration of this general principle with classic degeneration methods (52,77,78), the evidence is now increasing and fills up the yet "white" association areas like the peristriate area in primates and parietotemporal association areas, which are shown to receive a topographically ordered thalamic afferent input from the various lateral posterior and the pulvinar nuclei; the other classic "association fields," the frontoorbital areas receive ordered thalamic afferents from the different medial and lateral ventral thalamic nuclei (31,46). Whether the athalamic lower temporal areas may in the future also get assigned their appropriate thalamic projection nucleus or whether they will remain, in this respect, distinct from the rest of the neocortex and, there-

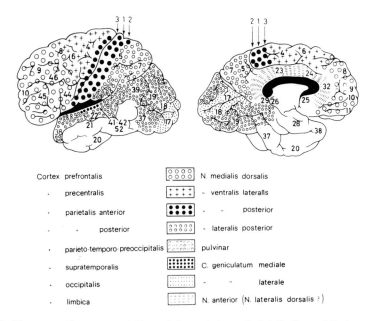

FIG. 2. Diagrammatic representation of the origin and distribution of thalamocortical connections in the neocortex of man. The symbols signify the projection areas of the various thalamic nuclei as indicated below on the right-hand side, which coincide with the different cortical fields **(left).** The numbers on the cortical maps correspond to the fields according to Brodmann. (From ref. 52.)

fore, not classified as neocortex, has to be awaited. Even the most outspoken "efferent" cortex (area 4), receives a specific thalamic input.

Anatomically and functionally, the thalamocortical input appears to be similarly or even identically organized in all neocortical areas. The main termination sheet of the thalamocortical projection fibres is the middle cortical layers (III and IV). The primary action of these fibres is excitation of the cells, with which they establish monosynaptic contacts (see refs. 9,10). These monosynaptically excited cells are not the only cells in which the somata are located in these laminae. Pyramidal cells from the fifth and sixth layers in the motor cortex are shown with neurophysiological methods to receive monosynaptic thalamocortical excitation (19,20), and in area 17, this has been suggested from anatomical (29,49,69,76) and from electrophysiological findings (44). However, in the apical dendritic shafts of the fifth and sixth layers, pyramidal cells do not appear to receive direct thalamocortical afferents (57).

There is no reason to assume a difference in those areas, which have not been investigated yet. However, there might exist some phylogenetic differences inasfar as the proportion of neurons above the main termination zone of thalamocortical fibres receiving a direct thalamic input may be smaller in the primate neocortex than in cortices of lower animals (my observations).

An essential anatomofunctional property of the thalamocortical input is its *topographical orderliness.* The thalamocortical fibres grow essentially vertically into the cortex and are thus parallel to each other. They branch within the cortex, and the branches may take an oblique course to their place of termination. In the visual cortex it has been demonstrated that the width of this branching is independent of visual field eccentricity (1,2,40–42). This spread determines the preciseness and the overlap of the cortical representation of the functional topography of the respective afferent system, i.e., the diencephalic projection nucleus and thus in the sensory projection areas the preciseness of somatotopy. It may be that there are some quantitative variations in the various projection fields, especially between species, but the principle of branching and thus impreciseness and mutual overlap is general.

It is usually assumed that many thalamocortical fibres converge on individual cortical cells. But neurophysiological evidence rather indicates that a sizable proportion (maybe up to 50%) of cortical cells receives their main excitatory specific thalamic input from only few, if not single, thalamocortical fibres (18,32) (Fig. 3). The size and form of excitatory receptive fields of cortical neurons are not significantly different from that of their afferent thalamic neurons, and we need not invoke complicated anatomical models such as the "dendritic" domain in order to explain the form of excitatory cortical receptive fields. Even in the visual cortex, the size of excitatory fields of simple and many complex cells do not differ significantly from those

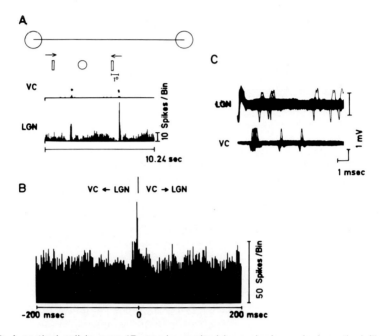

FIG. 3. A cortical cell in area 17 may be excited by a single geniculocortical fibre, as demonstrated by simultaneous recording from a cell in the lateral geniculate body and one in the visual cortex, which is excited by this LGB cell. **A:** Location of the receptive fields of both cells **(small circle)** relative to the blind spots **(large circles).** Line stimulus moves across receptive field back and forth. The poststimulus histograms of the two cells show responses appearing simultaneously and only over a narrow area. The small response of the cortical cell is indicated by a dot. **B:** Cross correlogram between the spontaneous activities of both cells, showing a positive correlation between the discharges of the LGB cell and the visual cortex cell at a latency of about 1.2 msec latency. **C:** If the oscilloscope beam is triggered by each spontaneous discharge of the LGB cell, discharge of the VC cell **(bottom record)** follows frequently at a fixed latency. (From Tsumoto et al., *in preparation.*)

of retinal ganglion cells of the x and y types, and in the somatosensory cortex the types of afferent fibre responses can still be recognized in the responses of a large proportion of cortical cells (64). However, some efferent cells in the lower layers (V and VI) of the visual cortex may have larger receptive fields, which suggests excitatory convergence from a wider input area (67,73,80).

The Functional Maps of Cortical Areas Reflect the Topographical Organization of Their Afferent Thalamic Nuclei

This leads, in the primary and also in so-called secondary sensory areas, to a somatotopic representation of the body surface. This somatotopy is, in the sensory projection areas, completely determined by the peripheral sense organs in such a way that the amount of cortical tissue available for a peripheral sensory neuron is constant within the receptive sensory projection area (1,9,40–42,60). From the fact that the density of receptor neurons varies considerably in the different parts of the receptor surfaces (e.g., fovea and peripheral visual field) result the characteristic distortions of sensory surfaces in their cortical representation such as homunculi, various magnification factors in the visual field, etc.

On the microscopic level, the projection maps are fuzzy due to the intracortical branching and the overlap of receptive fields of the afferent fibres, but also partly due to the impreciseness of representation of sensory space already in the thalamic relay nucleus (61). Therefore, if one looks closer into the afferent input of individual cortical cells, which are lined up in a vertical row throughout the cortex, one discovers that each cell appears to have its individual excitatory input line from the thalamus (Fig. 4A). This may be an individual fibre or a combination of a few fibres. The excitatory receptive fields of these individual cells within a vertical penetration are all situated roughly in the same receptor area (visual field, tone frequency, or body surface, respectively) and they may be overlapping, but each neuron is excited only by one or a few peripheral receptor nerve cells from within this homogeneous group. A vertical array of cells thus looks on a relatively wide area of the receptor surface, but with the individual receptor cells from within this field that each cortical cell is hooked up to, this array appears to be statistically distributed (Fig. 4B). There are some cells within each vertical column that appear to be excited from the whole receptive input field to this vertical array. These may be output neurons mainly in the deep layers or even inhibitory interneurons (17,67).

The good preservation of the neighbourhood relationship of afferent thalamocortical fibres on the one hand, and the lateral spread of intracortical branches on the other, is the basis of the well-known general principle of sensory cortical areas, the partial mutual overlap of afferent input points (70). This then leads to a continuous, overlapping representation of the topographical relationship of functional space as laid down in the respective afferent thalamic nucleus, which, in the case of a somatotopic organization of afferents in such a nucleus, results in a somatotopic organization of that cortical area (Fig. 4C). In cortical areas that receive their thalamic input from intrinsic thalamic nuclei, a somatotopy may not be so obvious anymore, but here, also the same projection principles hold, i.e., a preservation of the internal topography of the projection nucleus. This can be concluded from a recent anatomical analysis by Kuypers et al. (46) of the thalamocortical projection to the frontal cortex. If the internal topography of an intrinsic thalamic nucleus is somato- or retinotopic as in the case of some pulvinar nuclei, this retinotopy is also preserved up to the cortex (e.g., peristriate area of monkeys) and thus prevails throughout its depth (3). If direction of eye or limb movement would be represented in order in the

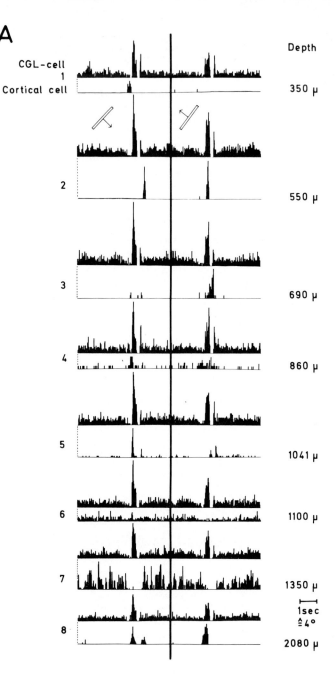

FIG. 4. Scatter of receptive field location in the visual cortex. **A:** Recording from one cell in the lateral geniculate body and from several cells successively in the visual cortex (area 17) of the cat. Poststimulus histograms show the responses of the various cells to a stimulus that moves back and forth across their receptive fields. Turn-around point of the stimulus is the thick center line. When the stimulus moves across the receptive field, a strong response is elicited in one or both movement directions. Whereas the CGL cell **(top record of each pair of records)** responds always when the stimulus moves across the same area of the visual field, the different cortical cells show variable response areas. **B:** Receptive fields of neurons recorded within a vertical penetration of the cortex are scattered around a mean value. For the parafoveal area the average scatter is ±0.81°, the range about the ±2°. Thus, cells located on top of each other within a vertical penetration of the cortex appear to be excited from retinal ganglion cells scattered over an area of the

B

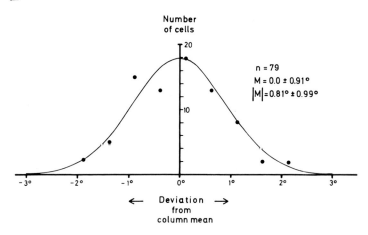

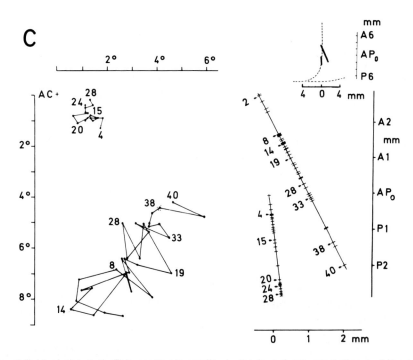

visual field of about 4°. This scatter is smaller in the foveal representation and larger in more peripheral representations of the visual field. (From ref. 17). **C:** Location of the receptive fields of neurons in area 17 which are recorded successively along two electrode tracks, which run approximately parallel to the cortical surface. The location of the electrode tracks is indicated by the sketch **(top right)** with Horsley-Clarke coordinates. Below, the same tracks are shown on a larger scale with the location of recorded units during each track marked by small lines. The recorded neurons are numbered in successive order; some numbers are indicated. **Left:** Location of the receptive fields of the units recorded along the straight tracks. The receptive fields progress in the visual field comparable to a random walk progression (**ordinates:** visual field coordinates relative to the area centralis, **AC**). Note the smaller magnification factor and, accordingly, the smaller scatter in the penetration nearer to the area centralis as compared to the more peripherally located. (From ref. 1.)

thalamic nucleus, this would also appear in the cortex in the same order. This may be behind the important observations of Hyvärinen and Poranen (43) and Mountcastle et al. (56) in the parietal cortex (areas 5 and 7), where small patches of cortex may respond quite specifically in conjunction with the execution of complex motor acts related to the extracorporal space. In area 5, the modality aspect of its somatosensory input is, of course, still quite obvious.

In the neocortex, the projections from separate but complementary sense organs may project into the same area. This is the case in the somatosensory cortex, for example, where afferents from deep and superficial mechano-receptors, or in the visual cortex, where afferents from the two eyes are projected into the same cortical area. These inputs from anatomically distinct but functionally related receptor systems are, to some extent, still separated in their cortical representation and thus form patches or stripes with a predominant or, over small distances, even exclusive input from only one or the other of the afferent sources. The best examples are the modality columns in the somatosensory cortex (55), and the ocularity stripes in the primary visual area 17 (38,39,48). These patches and stripes have, in the narrow direction, a diameter of less than 500 μm, i.e., a distance that is shorter than the reach of intracortical connections (see below), so that a somatotopic continuity of the separate modality or ocularity projections is still guaranteed. There are other systems that may have a similar peripheral origin but are used in a different functional context. Their cortical projection could then be completely separated such as in the case of the projection of Ia-afferents, which terminate separately from the projection area of the body surface.

The fact that neurons in all layers of the cortex may be excited by the same group of afferents has led to the "columnar hypothesis." According to how one looks at the system, one may be more impressed by the continuity of the thalamocortical projection with partial overlap of neighbouring thalamic volumes, or by the discreteness of the afferent input bundles (ocularity, deep versus superficial mechanoreception). The important aspect is that within a vertical penetration the neurons throughout the depth of the cortex appear to receive their main excitatory input from different individuals of the same, restricted group of thalamic projection cells. But if the columnar hypothesis means that a discrete group of cells within a cylinder or stripe of cortex 0.5 mm wide should be considered a separate functional unit and that the cortex is thus divided into separate functionally discrete columns, each assigned to a special purpose, the hypothesis becomes untenable (for further discussion of this aspect see refs. 12, 13, 72).

In addition to the thalamocortical projections, most areas of the cortex also receive afferent fibres from other cortical areas via association fibres, and these also ascend vertically through the cortex (30,45). The depth of their main termination is different from that of thalamocortical fibres, however, and seems to be typical for each type of association fibres. But here also, no principle differences in different cortical areas of the type of termination of callosal fibres, for example, has been discovered if an area receives callosal fibres at all. As can be judged from Golgi and degeneration pictures, the lateral spread and overlap of the intracortical branches of such fibres appears to be in principle the same as that of thalamocortical fibres.

The Intrinsic Connectivity of the Cortex

The Morphology of Dendrites

It is not clear to what extent the so-called *dendritic domain* determines the functional properties of cortical neurons. But the fact that the apical dendrites of pyramidal cells reach vertically up through several, or in the case of the large fifth and sixth layers of pyramidal cells, through all layers, indicates that the deeper pyramidal cells do not simply belong to one layer, but that they are functionally connected to afferent and intrinsic fibres terminating also in other layers. This aspect was pointed out by Sholl (65), Globus and Scheibel (29), and Garey (26) and has been recently again emphasized by Lund et al. (49), who concluded that pyramidal cells from the deeper layers "listen" to signals arriving also in the more superficial layers (51). The fact that the main output cells of the cortex in the fifth and sixth layers receive direct synaptic afferent input to their apical dendrites in the third and fourth layers made them, rightly, question the concept of a hierarchic signal analysis across the depth of the cortex.

The horizontal spread of apical and basal dendrites is occasionally taken as the morphological basis of cortical neuronal receptive fields, such as is the case in the retina (4,21). But since the excitatory thalamocortical input appears to be limited to only one or a few single fibres, the lateral spread of dendrites is not concerned with the shape of cortical excitatory receptive fields. In this context, it may be remembered that the length of dendritic branches is, to some extent, correlated with the size of the cell body and the latter with the thickness and length of its axon. Hence, the large pyramidal cells (Betz cells) in the fifth layer of the motor cortex. For this reason, one should consider also other functions for dendritic branches than just postsynaptic sites for summation of electrical signals arriving from afferent fibres. Such functions may be concerned also with metabolic needs of the cell and transmission of chemical signals.

Intracortical Fibre Connections

Golgi as well as degeneration studies indicate that most ascending or descending intracortical fibres take an oblique course. This is demonstrated by the degeneration pattern after small intracortical lesions in the chronically isolated cortex (15) (Fig. 5). Obliquely ascending fibres, apparently terminating in all layers, come almost exclusively from cells located in the middle parts of the cortex (corresponding about to layers III and upper V), while obliquely descending axons appear to be derived mainly from cells in the lower cortical layers. The obliquely ascending fibres terminate on their way up to the surface but some reach the first layer where they may spread over large distances (up to some millimeters). The obliquely descending fibres may get lost and possibly terminate in the fifth and sixth layers, but may turn horizontally and upward again in the sixth layer and in the subcortical white matter in order to come back into the adjacent cortex as short association or U-fibres. Although impressive in some Golgi preparations, vertically ascending intracortical fibres seem to be in the minority in degeneration pictures.

Horizontal fibres appear to arise throughout the whole of Gennari's stripe with a slight concentration in the inner and outer stripes of Baillarger, which

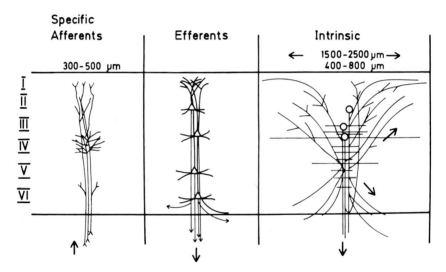

FIG. 5. Schematic representation of the principal fibre connections and their modular dimension in the cerebral cortex. Specific afferent fibres **(left column)** enter the cortex in a vertical direction, terminate at different levels of the cortex according to their origin and spread laterally over a limited distance essentially in their terminal zone (modular diameter, 300 to 500 μm). Associational, nonspecific, and aminergic fibres are not included. Efferent fibres **(middle)** leave the cortex from all layers except I in a strictly parallel manner often gathered in bundles, so that fibres leaving the cortex vertically are all derived from pyramidal cells piled up on top of each other throughout the whole thickness of the cortex. In the deeper layers, some fibres leave the vertical bundles to enter the white matter in an oblique direction (U-fibres, short association fibres). Intrinsic fibres **(right column)** show three dominant patterns: obliquely upward-going fibres, which arise from neurons within layers II and upper V and form a bouquet with a modular diameter of up to 1,500 to 2,500 μm before terminating in the upper layers or entering layer I; horizontal fibres originate mainly in the middle layers (III to V) and extend densely over a modular width of 400 to 800 μm, but a few fibres run for up to 3 mm; obliquely descending fibres leave the vertical efferent bundles in layers V and VI. (From ref. 15.)

in the cat are not very outstanding, however. In the monkey, the concentration of horizontal fibres in Baillarger's stripe is more outstanding (23). The horizontal spread of the oblique and horizontal fibres is less than 800 μm for the majority but may reach, in some single fibres, up to 2 to 3 mm. Such a cylinder with a diameter of about 1 mm would then be the domain of major intracortical connections and is, more or less symmetrically, arranged around any vertical line through the cortex. The intracortical fibre systems thus interconnect neighbouring cells in the cortex — and through that their afferent inputs — over distances of about 0.5 mm and across the cortical depth. There is no anatomical indication for distinct units or columns, but — like in the case of specific thalamocortical afferents — a network with continuous overlap of the locally arriving intracortical fibre systems.

What is the functional significance of these intracortical connections? It is often assumed that they might connect individual neurons in a selective manner and thus facilitate certain stimulus configurations (or features) and neglect or exclude others. With neurophysiological methods, only inhibitory actions of intracortical connections have been demonstrated so far (10,33,59). Postsynaptic excitation has been observed after antidromic stimulation of the pyramidal tract only in the motor cortex, thus suggesting recurrent excitation (see ref. 20). But in these experiments, stimulation of ascending fibres that are known to project into the motor cortex, by local current spread in the medulla, has not been excluded. It thus appears that *the intracortical network is essentially, if not exclusively, inhibitory*. This seems to be the same in all cortical areas, so that the effect of electrical afferent or direct cortical stimulation is always a short excitation of some followed by a longer inhibition of all neurons.

For the visual cortex, we arrive therefore at a model as shown in Fig. 6: the fuzzy representation of the visual field, with excitation from each ganglion cell to several cortical cells with a statistical overlap, is projected on a network with mutually overlapping inhibition. This principle can be generalized for other neocortical areas and has, in this laboratory, been found in all sensory and the motor areas. We thus came to the conclusion that conspicuous trigger features of cortical cells (e.g., orientation sensitivity of visual cells) results from the fact that certain stimulus configurations produce minimal inhibition rather than optimal excitation (18).

Efferent Organization

The new anatomical tracer methods now finally begin to throw some light on the details of *efferent organization* of cortical structures (for the visual cortex see refs. 28,34,35,50,53,62,68). From these new investigations the fact emerged that axons leaving the cortex for different destinations are derived from cells at different cortical depths i.e., from different layers (Fig. 7). There are some indications, at least in the visual cortex, that the

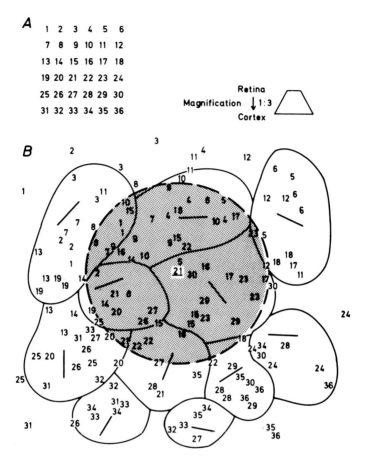

FIG. 6. Schematic representation of the projection from the retina to the visual cortex as an example of cortical representation of a sensory surface to the cortex and the intra-cortical functional connectivity. **A:** A matrix of retinal ganglion cells with numbers according to their position. It is, unrealistically, assumed that one retinal ganglion cell is in monoposition. It is, unrealistically, assumed that one retinal ganglion cell is in mono-synaptic contact with nine cortical cells (multiplication factor). **B:** Within the reach of branchings of geniculocortical fibres, each ganglion cell excites monosynapticly one cortical nerve cell. As a consequence, afferent inputs from nearby ganglion cells overlap considerably in random fashion, whereas across the whole projection field a retinotopic gradient is preserved. Intracortically, each ganglion cell is connected through intracortical inhibitory pathways to cells within a morphologically defined module. The inhibitory pool of any given cell (in this example cell **21**) may receive inhibition from cells with different, but nearby, receptive fields and with different functional properties, e.g., different orientation sensitivity. (From ref. 18.)

functional properties of cells projecting to subcortical target structures (i.e., the superior colliculus and the lateral geniculate body) are different from those projecting into the corpus callosum. Although the question remains of whether and to what extent systematic functional differences between different types of output cells exist, the situation on the output side appears to

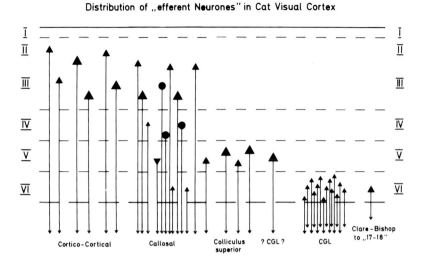

FIG. 7. Depth distribution of efferent neurons in the cat's visual cortex. **Triangles:** Pyramidal cells. **Circles:** Star cells. The sizes of the symbols indicate the relative sizes of the respective neurons. The destination of the axons is indicated below. The roman numerals indicate the cortical layers. Note that axons destined for the various target structures are derived from a restricted cortical layer except for callosal fibres which appear to originate from layers II to VI. Whereas the target structures are different for different cortical areas, the principle of depth distribution of efferent neurons appears to be general. (Compiled by D. Sanides using data from refs. 28,34,35,53,71.)

be comparable to that on the input side: Cells staggered on top of each other send their axons out of the cortex and have similar properties in certain dimensions, although statistically scattered around a mean.

The best example is the orientation sensitivity of cells in area 17 of the visual cortex: if one records many neurons simultaneously with a large microelectrode (multiunit recording), the same or nearly the same optimal orientation prevails throughout a vertical penetration (Fig. 8C). If one looks at individual cells, however, the optimal orientations vary considerably from cell to cell around the mean value with a range of up to 90°, and a standard deviation of ±15 to 25° (Fig. 8A and B). The mean orientations vary systematically along the cortical surface with a whole orientation cycle completed in about 1 mm [hypercolumn, Hubel and Wiesel (40,41), Albus (1,2)]. Thus, if one stimulates the visual system with gratings of one orientation, patches and stripes covering about 50% of area 17 will be more or less excited, due to the scatter and mutual overlap of the orientation sensitivities of neighbouring cells (47). This estimate, derived from experiments in cats, corresponds quite well with the width of stripes in area 17 produced by stimulation with parallel lines and anatomically demonstrated by autoradiographic labeling of the activated cells with radioactive deoxyglucose (Hubel and Wiesel, presentation at the American Neurosciences Meeting 1976 and personal communication).

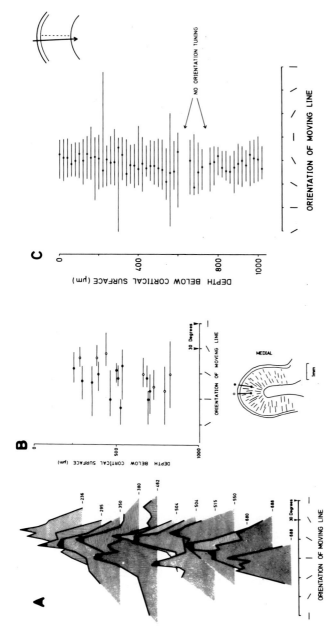

FIG. 8. Variability of optimal orientation in a vertical line through the visual cortex (area 17) of the cat. **A:** Units were recorded at various depths as indicated on the right-hand side beside the shaded areas. The shaded areas show the orientation tuning curves of the various cells with their optimal orientation marked as black peaks. **Abscissa:** Orientation of the moving stimulus. The total range of variability is about ±45°, i.e., a total of 90°. **B:** Two penetrations parallel to each other (**open and closed dots**). Shown are the optimal orientations of the different cells found during each penetration together with their "tuning half width," i.e., the orientation range, at which the response is above 50% of the maximum response in the optimal orientation. The optimal orientations represented in the two penetrations, which are about 500 μm apart, overlap. **C:** Determination of optimal orientation responses of mixed cell activities at different depths of the cortex as recorded with large microelectrodes. The scatter of optimal orientation is much smaller than that of single cells, but also the half width of orientation tuning is much wider. (From ref. 47.)

SOME GENERAL FUNCTIONAL PROPERTIES OF THE CORTICAL NETWORK

There is no reason to assume that the same principles of afferent–intrinsic–efferent organization do not apply also to the other neocortical areas not yet so well explored as the sensory areas. But if the general design of cortical connectivity shows the same principles, the *functional properties* should also be the same. To demonstrate this, the inputs to these cortical areas have to be stimulated appropriately. This is difficult and, to some extent, impossible, however, since the appropriate stimuli for the more complex thalamocortical and association systems are difficult to define and thus to simulate in an experiment. Recently, some major progress has been made in this direction by uncovering some functional properties of neurons in the frontal cortex (25) and in the parietal association areas 5 and 7 (43,56). A less satisfactory method is to use electrical stimulation of afferents, efferents, or intracortical systems.

Let me try to summarize some of the properties of the cerebral cortex that have been disclosed with electrophysiological methods, mainly recording of single unit activity, and that appear to be found in all areas so far investigated (see refs. 9,10,19,32,44).

(1) The spontaneous activity of cortical neurons is much lower than that of their thalamocortical afferents, but it is, essentially, driven activity and disappears after deafferentation.

(2) Electrical stimulation of thalamocortical afferents leads to primary, i.e., monosynaptic, excitation of more than 50%, possibly up to 70% of the cortical neurons within the domain of the stimulated afferents. The firing probability, i.e., the transmission of such monosynaptic excitation, varies considerably between various cells, however, which might indicate variable effectiveness of the excitatory input as well as of the inhibitory connections.

(3) The same electrical stimulus produces postsynaptic inhibition in all cortical cells. This postsynaptic inhibition is always disynaptic and, probably to a large extent, transmitted through recurrent collaterals of cortical nerve cells.

(4) The frequency up to which cortical neurons can be driven by electrical stimulation of their afferents is much lower (up to 20 to 30/sec, occasionally 50/sec), in contrast to a much higher driving frequency of thalamic or more peripheral neurons.

From these functional properties as derived from electrical stimulation, a number of nonlinear transmission properties of sensory cortices for physiological stimuli can be derived. These are:

(a) Simultaneous stimulation of a large sensory surface (e.g., diffuse light in the visual and pure tones in the auditory system) leads to no or only short phasic responses, since the afferent excitation breaks down due to mutual intracortical inhibition.

(b) Tonic, i.e., maintained activity, during a longer lasting sensory stimulus is largely if not completely suppressed, and cortical neurons respond preferentially if not exclusively to stimulus changes (transients) in time (on or off), or space (movement of the stimulus along the sensory surface).

(c) Repetitive stimulation, i.e., repetition of a signal, at a frequency of 5 to 20/sec gives better responses than single stimulation.

(d) Therefore, for many neurons in sensory projection areas, a combination of repetitive changes in space and time, i.e., repetitive movements along the sensory surface, are optimal stimuli. These may be moving objects in the visual field, recurrent movement along the skin, or temporally structured frequency as well as amplitude modulation in the auditory system.

If one analyses the specific trigger features of cortical cells with intracellular recording methods, it becomes obvious that inhibition plays a major role in the specification of these features. While the actual excitatory receptive field is small and restricted to one small area on the respective sensory surface such as the retina, the cochlea or the body surface, a larger stimulus must have such a spatiotemporal configuration that it keeps the inhibition to a cell from its inhibitory pool low in order to enable the excitatory input to reach the discharge threshold.

The cortical network thus can be considered as a nonlinear spatiotemporal filter that allows through only certain aspects of the signals transmitted to it through its thalamocortical afferents. This should be the case independently from the actual origin of the thalamocortical signals, i.e., whether they come from specific, somatotopically ordered relays or from intrinsic projection nuclei, which may already contain, in their internal topography, a highly complicated spatiotemporal transform of the environment.

Finally, adaptability must be considered an important property of the cortical network. This means the adaptation of certain filter characteristics or channels by repeated use, and the possible enhancement of others. Although not yet demonstrated convincingly with electrophysiological methods and certainly still obscure with respect to its mechanisms, this property of functional adaptation of cortical filtering to environmental and possibly also internal stimuli must be regarded as the basic condition of *memory*. While in early postnatal development this adaptation might lead to structural changes (27) and appears to enhance filters tuned to the applied stimulus, in adult life the suppression of filters by enhanced intracortical inhibition must also be taken into account as an important if not dominant mechanism of cortical memory functions (11,16).

CONCLUSIONS

This short (and certainly incomplete) review has demonstrated some general principles of structure and function of all neocortical areas as expressed in their afferent, intrinsic, and efferent organizations. General principles of structure concern aspects such as the generality of thalamocortical projections; the topographical organization of afferent inputs; the connectivity between single cortical neurons with a very restricted number of single afferent fibres; the distribution of intracortical connections; the depth distribution of output neurons; the reciprocal connections between each cortical field with its thalamic projection nucleus; and the afferent and efferent organization of callosal and of homolateral association fibres. On the functional side, I have pointed out the small excitatory convergence of specific afferent fibres in a high proportion of cortical cells; the primary excitatory action of cortical afferents; the predominantly if not exclusively inhibitory function of intracortical fibre systems; the phasic character of cortical responses; the property of cortical neurons to respond preferably to changes of stimulus fields in place and time (transients); the network structure of the neocortex; and the adaptability as a basis for memory function. In these and related aspects it is assumed that there are *no fundamental* differences between cortical areas.

In more general terms, the neocortex can be considered as a *cooperative network,* in which the activities of the individual elements interact with each other through inhibition. This gives the network the property of a nonlinear *filter,* which transfers, as a whole, transforms of a stimulus field. Individual elements of the network, as specific as their trigger features may appear to be, do not describe complex stimuli. This is done by the relationship of activities of individual elements of the network with each other, and only this combined activity describes the stimulus. One is reminded here of ideas of Gestalt psychology: the whole is more than its parts (see refs. 12,13).

The specific functional and morphological differences of the various cortical areas can be considered *unessential.* The "specific functions" of any cortical area are defined by the origin of its afferent, and the destination of its efferent connections. The afferents may convey activities directly from peripheral sense organs or only indirectly as selected intrinsic cerebral activities. The efferents may reach peripheral effectors directly or may only control intracerebral systems and thus influence behavior only indirectly. The thalamic and other subcortical inputs to the cortex may be brought into functional context with activities from other cortical areas via the intercortical association systems, and elaborate on them but by using the same principles again.

The neocortical network is thus only one link in the stream of activities from the thalamus and other afferent structures to the effectors. Viewing the cortex as such a link between input and output with defined, nonlinear, temporospatial filter characteristics, with feedback to its afferent structures and output to various cortical, subcortical, and peripheral target structures, assigns to the cortex a more relativistic function than it is usually given. It is not *the* final place of "recognition," "decision making," "programming," and whatever the terms may be which are used to entrust it with the "highest functions" of the nervous system. None of these functions are possible without the cortical link, but the neocortex *per se,* or any part of it, is not the seat of the soul or of any of these higher functions. If the cortical link of any specific functional system is lesioned, the whole function in which that system plays a role is also more or less disturbed *in that sense and only insofar as cortical localization of function is justified.* What is needed, at this point is further clarification and a clearer definition of the actual and general function of this cortical link along the lines indicated above.

In this general framework, the *morphological differentiation* of the various cortical areas can then also be considered unessential insofar as they are the consequence of the input and output connections of the cortex. Already Brodmann and Economo had realized that the morphological differences between cytoarchitectonic areas develop relatively late during ontogenesis, actually at a time at which the first thalamocortical afferents reach the cortex as we can infer from recent embryological studies (8,54,66). Apparently, specific morphological aspects of neurons in some cortical areas can easily be explained by circumstantial situations rather than by assuming a specific Bauplan: for example, individual neurons of the neocortex, having a common ontogenetic history, may develop certain rather specific morphological aspects due to circumstantial situations; the Betz cells of the motor cortex, for example, might become so big because their axons grow over such long distances before they reach a target area; or the density of cells in the koniocortex may be so high and their size relatively small because their thalamocortical afferents are more densely packed or appear at a different time of cortical maturation than thalamocortical afferents from intrinsic thalamic nuclei. The packing density of neurons in the different layers of the neocortex and thus the major morphological differences between the various "areas" may be considered to be a function of the developmental history and the quantity of its thalamic, cortical, and maybe other inputs. In this way, the afferent input and its output may mold, to some extent, the various parts of the neocortex in its morphological aspect without, however, changing its basic structural design. Of course, at present it cannot be excluded that the temporospatial signal structure of the different types of afferent inputs to various cortical fields might also mold to a limited degree the general internal functional structure of a given area (or even subarea, e.g., the representation area of the central versus the peripheral visual field). But data on this are lacking and, so far, only drastic procedures such as partial or complete sensory deprivation have been shown to alter certain input–output functions of the cortex, none of which make it necessary to postulate changes of the basic principles of operation of the respective areas.

The introductory remarks on the relationship between the evolution of the neocortex and the brain as a whole were made to indicate that the size of the neocortex should not be seen *per se* as the basis of higher functional capacity of a brain. The neocortex is only part of the circuits in the forebrain, in which the thalamocortical connections are essential. The quantitative increase of such circuits does not necessitate the application of new principles of connectivity. The increasing capacity of the machinery of the brain is due to the fact that more such circuits are introduced, some of them giving the system completely new capacities such as language. The situation is thus comparable to an increase of information loops in a computer program, each loop working, however, on the same principle. This does not exclude that some additional and new *general* functional and morphological principles of the neocortex might evolve parallel or as a consequence of the quantitative increase of such loops.

SUMMARY

Following a short review of the position on the significance of cortical cytoarchitectonic specificity, the thesis is put forward that there are fundamental similarities between various neocortical areas. The evidence in support of this thesis is shortly reviewed in pointing out the common afferent, intrinsic, and efferent organizational principles of the various cortical areas with special emphasis on the generality of thalamocortical circuits. Actual differences in morphology and function are unessential; i.e., they depend on the circuit in which a given cortical area is involved. The neocortex is a link in the chain of afferent-efferent signal processing, and can be understood as a cooperative network which acts as a nonlinear spatiotemporal filter with adaptive properties (memory) and transforms afferent signal flow. It is assumed that these filter properties are the same for all neocortical areas. The functional role of a circumscribed cortical area therefore depends on its position within a certain functional circuit and is defined by it. Destruction of that area disables performance of this function because an important link in its chain of execution is not functioning any more, or even interrupted completely. These functional deficiencies emphasize the important functional role of the cortex in executing higher nervous functions, but they do not indicate that the cortex is the "seat" of these functions. The functional significance of the general and fundamental filter properties of the cortex is only little understood, although such an understanding would be the basis for a general theory of the neocortex.

REFERENCES

The selection of papers quoted is to some extent subjective rather than a complete representation of work done in this field. The number of references to papers of the author may, therefore, seem disproportionally large, but this should not be confounded with his actual contributions. There is an economical element in it insofar as references to other and maybe earlier and more important publications are found in these papers. A representative sample of recent work, with ample bibliography, on the structure and function of the cerebral cortex can be found in the monograph: Afferent and intrinsic organization of laminated structures in the brain (O. Creutzfeldt, Ed.), *Exp. Brain Res.,* Suppl. 1 (1976).

1. Albus, K. (1975): A quantitative study of the projection area of the central and the paracentral visual field in area 17 of the cat. I. The precision of the topography. *Exp. Brain Res.,* 24:159–179.
2. Albus, K. (1975): A quantitative study of the projection area of the central and the paracentral visual field in area 17 of the cat. II. The spatial organization of the orientation domain. *Exp. Brain Res.,* 24:181–202.
3. Benevento, L., and Rezak, M. L. (1976): Cortical projections of inferior pulvinar and adjacent lateral pulvinar in Rhesus monkey. *Brain Res.,* 108:1–24.
4. Boycott, B. B., and Wässle, H. (1974): The morphological types of ganglion cells of the domestic cat's retina. *J. Physiol.,* 240:397–419.
5. Brodmann, K. (1909): *Vergleichende Lokalisationslehre der Grosshirnrinde in ihren prinzipien Dargestellt auf Grund des Zellenbaues.* Barth, Leipzig.
6. Campbell, A. W. (1905): *Histological Studies on the Localisation of Cerebral Function.* Cambridge University Press, Cambridge, Mass., 360 pp.
7. Colonnier, M. (1966): The structural design of the neocortex. In: *Brain and Conscious Experience,* edited by J. C. Eccles, pp. 1–23. Springer-Verlag, New York.
8. Cragg, B. G. (1974): Plasticity of synapses. *Br. Med. Bull.,* 30:141–145.
9. Creutzfeldt, O. D. (1970): Some principles of synaptic organization in the visual system. In: *Neuroscience 2. Study Program,* edited by F. O. Schmitt, pp. 630–647. Rockefeller University Press, New York.
10. Creutzfeldt, O. (1973): Synaptic organization of the cerebral cortex and its role in epilepsy. In: *Epilepsy, Its Phenomena in Man,* edited by M. A. B. Brazier. UCLA Forum in Medical Science, No. 17, pp. 11–27. Academic Press, New York.
11. Creutzfeldt, O. D. (1973): Some neurophysiological considerations concerning "memory." In: *Memory and Transfer of Information,* edited by H. P. Zippel, pp. 293–302. Plenum Press, New York.
12. Creutzfeldt, O. (1975): Some problems of cortical organization in the light of ideas of the classical "Hirnpathologie" and of modern neurophysiology. An Essay. In: *Cerebral Localization,* edited by K. J. Zülch, O. Creutzfeldt, and G. C. Galbraith, pp. 217–226. Springer-Verlag, New York.
13. Creutzfeldt, O. (1976): The brain as a functional entity. In: *Progress in Brain Research, Vol. 45,* edited by M. A. Corner and D. F. Swaab, pp. 451–462. Elsevier, Amsterdam.
14. Creutzfeldt, O. (1976): Thematic introduction: Definition and comparison of principles of functional organization of laminated structures in the brain. *Exp. Brain Res.,* Suppl. 1:12–17.
15. Creutzfeldt, O. D., Garey, L. J., Kuroda, R., and Wolff, J. R. (1977): The distribution of degenerating axons after small lesions in the intact and isolated visual cortex of the cat. *Exp. Brain Res.,* 27:419–440.
16. Creutzfeldt, O. D., and Heggelund, P. (1975): Neural plasticity in visual cortex of adult cats after exposure to visual patterns. *Science,* 188:1025–1027.
17. Creutzfeldt, O., Innocenti, G. M., and Brooks, D. (1974): Vertical organization in the visual cortex (area 17) in the cat. *Exp. Brain Res.,* 21:315–336.
18. Creutzfeldt, O. D., Kuhnt, U., and Benevento, L. A. (1974): An intracellular analysis of visual cortical neurones to moving stimuli: Responses in a cooperative neuronal network. *Exp. Brain Res.,* 21:251–272.
19. Creutzfeldt, O., Lux, H. D., Watanabe, S. (1966): Electrophysiology of cortical nerve cells. In: *The Thalamus,* edited by D. P. Purpura, and M. D. Yahr, pp. 209–235. Columbia University Press, New York.
20. Creutzfeldt, O., Maekawa, K., and Hösli, L. (1969): Forms of spontaneous and evoked postsynaptic potentials of cortical nerve cells. In: *Progress in Brain Research, Vol. 31, Mechanisms of Synaptic Transmission,* edited by K. Akert and P. G. Weiser, pp. 265–273. Elsevier, Amsterdam.

21. Creutzfeldt, O. D., Sakmann, B., Scheich, H., and Korn, A. (1970): Sensitivity distribution and spatial summation within receptive-field center of retinal on-center ganglion cells and transfer function of the retina. *J. Neurophysiol.,* 33:654–671.
22. Economo, C. von (1927): *Zellaufbau der Großhirnrinde des Menschen,* Springer-Verlag, Berlin.
23. Fisken, R. A., Garey, L. J., and Powell, T. P. S. (1975): The intrinsic association and commissural connections of area 17 of the visual cortex. *Philos. Trans. R. Soc. Lond. [Biol.],* 272:487–536.
24. Flechsig, P. (1896): *Gehirn und Seele,* 2nd ed. Veil und Compagnie, Leipzig, 112 pp.
25. Fuster, J. M. (1973): Unit activity in prefrontal cortex during delayed response performance: Neuronal correlates of transient memory. *J. Neurophysiol.,* 36:61–78.
26. Garey, L. J. (1976): Synaptic organization of afferent fibres and intrinsic circuits in the neocortex. In: *Handbook of Electroencephalography and Clinical Neurophysiology, Vol. 2A,* edited by A. Rémond, pp. 57–85. Elsevier, Amsterdam.
27. Garey, L. J. (1976): Morphological evidence for plasticity in the visual thalamo-cortical system of the cat. *Exp. Brain Res.,* Suppl. 1:264–266.
28. Gilbert, C. D., and Kelly, J. P. (1975): The projections of cells in different layers of the cat's visual cortex. *J. Comp. Neurol.,* 163:81–105.
29. Globus, A., and Scheibel, A. B. (1967): Synaptic loci on visual cortical neurons of the rabbit: the Specific afferent radiation. *Exp. Neurol.,* 18:116–131.
30. Grant, G., Landgren, S., and Silfvenius, H. (1975): Columnar distribution of U-fibres from the postcruciate cerebral projection area of the cat's group I muscle afferents. *Exp. Brain Res.,* 24:57–74.
31. Hassler, R. (1959): Anatomy of the thalamus. In: *Introduction to Stereotaxis with an Atlas of the Human Brain, Vol. 1,* edited by G. Schaltenbrand, and P. Bailey, pp. 230–290. Grune & Stratton, New York.
32. Hellweg, F. C., Schultz, W., and Creutzfeldt, O. D. (1977): Extracellular and intracellular recordings from the cat's cortical whisker projection area: Thalamo-cortical response transformation. *J. Neurophysiol. (in press).*
33. Hess, R., Negishi, K., and Creutzfeldt, O. (1975): The horizontal spread of intracortical inhibition in the visual cortex. *Exp. Brain Res.,* 22:415–419.
34. Holländer, H. (1974): On the origin of the corticotectal projections in the cat. *Exp. Brain Res.,* 21:433–439.
35. Holländer, H. (1976): On the origin of corticofugal projections in the visual system. *Exp. Brain Res.,* Suppl. 1:301–304.
36. Hubel, D. H., and Wiesel, T. N. (1962): Receptive fields, binocular interaction and functional architecture in the cat's visual cortex. *J. Physiol.,* 160:106–154.
37. Hubel, D., and Wiesel, T. (1965): Receptive fields and functional architecture of two nonstriate visual areas (18 and 19) of the cat. *J. Neurophysiol.,* 28:229–289.
38. Hubel, D. H., and Wiesel, T. N. (1969): Anatomical demonstration of columns in the monkey striate cortex. *Nature,* 221:747–750.
39. Hubel, D. H., and Wiesel, T. N. (1972): Laminar and columnar distribution of geniculocortical fibers in the macaque monkey. *J. Comp. Neurol.,* 146:421–450.
40. Hubel, D., and Wiesel, T. (1974a): Sequence, regularity and geometry of orientation columns in the monkey striate cortex. *J. Comp. Neurol.,* 158:267–294.
41. Hubel, D., and Wiesel, T. (1974b): Uniformity of monkey striate cortex: A parallel relationship between field size, scatter, and magnification factor. *J. Comp. Neurol.,* 158:295–306.
42. Hubel, D. H., Wiesel, T. N., and LeVay, S. (1976): Columnar organization of area 17 in normal and monocularly deprived macaque monkeys. *Exp. Brain Res.,* Suppl. 1:356–361.
43. Hyvärinen, J., and Poranen, A. (1974): Function of the parietal associative area 7 as revealed from cellular discharges in alert monkeys. *Brain,* 97:673–692.
44. Ito, M., Sanides, D., and Creutzfeldt, O. D. (1977): A study of binocular convergence in cat visual cortex neurons. *Exp. Brain Res.,* 28:21–36.
45. Jones, E. G. (1976): Commissural, cortico-cortical and thalamic "columns" in the somatic sensory cortex of primates. *Exp. Brain Res.,* Suppl. 1:309–316.
46. Kuypers et al., (1977) *(in press).*
47. Lee, B. B., Albus, K., Heggelund, P., Hulme, M. J., and Creutzfeldt, O. D. (1977): The depth distribution of optimal stimulus orientations for neurones in cat area 17. *Exp. Brain Res.* 27:301–314.

48. LeVay, S., Hubel, D. H., and Wiesel, T. N. (1975): The pattern of ocular dominance columns in macaque visual cortex revealed by a reduced silver stain. *J. Comp. Neurol.,* 159:559–567.
49. Lund, J. S., and Brothe, R. G. (1975a): Interlaminar connections and pyramidal neuron organization in the visual cortex, area 17, of the macaque monkey. *J. Comp. Neurol.,* 159:305–334.
50. Lund, J. S., Lund, A. E., Hendrickson, A. E., Bunt, A. M., and Fuchs, A. F. (1975): The origin of efferent pathways from the primary visual cortex, area 17, of the macaque monkey as shown by retrograde transport of horseradish peroxidase. *J. Comp. Neurol.,* 164:287–304.
51. Lund, J. S. (1976): Laminar organisation of the primary visual cortex, area 17, of the macaque monkey. *Exp. Brain Res.,* Suppl. 1:288–291.
52. Macchi, G., and Rinvik, E. (1976): Thalamo-Telencephalic Circuits: A neuroanatomical Survey. In: *Handbook of Electroencephalography and Clinical Neurophysiology, Vol. 2A,* edited by A. Rémond, pp. 86–159. Elsevier, Amsterdam.
53. Magalhaes-Castro, H. H., Saraiva, P. E. S., and Magalhaes-Castro, B. (1975): Identification of corticotectal cells of the visual cortex of cats by means of horseradish peroxidase. *Brain Res.,* 83:474–479.
54. Marin-Padiha, M. (1970): Prenatal and early nostnatal development of human cerebral cortex. *Brain Res.,* 23:167–183.
55. Mountcastle, V. B. (1957): Modality and topographic properties of single neurons of cat's somatic sensory cortex. *J. Neurophysiol.,* 20:408–434.
56. Mountcastle, V. B., Lynch, J. C., Georgopoulos, A., Sakata, M., and Acuna, C. (1975): Posterior parietal association cortex of monkey: Command functions for operations within extracorporal space. *J. Neurophysiol.,* 38:871–908.
57. Peters, A. (1976): Projection of lateral geniculate nucleus to area 17 of the rat cerebral cortex. *Exp. Brain Res.,* Suppl. 1:296–300.
58. Powell, T. P. S., and Mountcastle, V. B. (1959): Some aspects of the functional organization of the cortex of the postcentral gyrus of the monkey: A correlation of findings obtained in a single unit analysis with cytoarchitecture. *Johns Hopkins Hosp. Bull.,* 105:133–162.
59. Renaud, L. P., and Kelly, J. S. (1974): Identification of possible inhibitory neurons in the pericruciate cortex of the cat. *Brain Res.,* 79:9–28.
60. Rolls, E. T., and Cowey, A. (1970): Topography of the retina and striate cortex and its relationship to visual acuity in rhesus monkeys and squirrel monkeys. *Exp. Brain Res.,* 10:298–310.
61. Sanderson, K. J. (1971): Visual field projection columns and magnification factors in the lateral geniculate nucleus of the cat. *Exp. Brain Res.,* 13:159–177.
62. Sanides, D., and Donate-Oliver, F. (1977): Identification and localization of some relay cells in cat visual cortex (*this volume*).
63. Sanides, F. (1972): Representation in the cerebral cortex and its areal lamination patterns. In: *The Structure and Function of Nervous Tissue,* edited by G. H. Bourne, pp. 329–453. Academic Press, New York.
64. Schultz, W., Galbraith, G. C., Gottschaldt, K. M., and Creutzfeldt, O. D. (1976): A comparison of primary afferent and cortical neurone activity coding sinus hair movements in the cat. *Exp. Brain Res.,* 24:365–381.
65. Sholl, D. A. (1956): *The Organization of the Cerebral Cortex.* Methuen, London, 125 pp.
66. Sidman, R. L., and Rakic P. (1973): Neuronal migration, with special reference to developing human brain: A review. *Brain Res.,* 62:1–35.
67. Singer, W., Tretter, F., and Cynader, M. (1975): Organization of cat striate cortex: A correlation of receptive field properties with afferent and efferent connections. *J. Neurophysiol.,* 38:1080–1098.
68. Spatz, W. B. (1976): The laminar distribution of cortical neurons projecting onto the visual area MT: A study with horseradish peroxidase in the marmoset callithrix. *Exp. Brain Res.,* Suppl. 1:305–308.
69. Szentágothai, J. (1973): Synaptology of the visual cortex. In: *Handbook of Sensory Physiology, Vol. VII/3, B,* edited by H. Autrum, R. Jung, W. R. Loewenstein, D. M. Mackay, and H. L. Teuber, pp. 269–324. Springer-Verlag, Berlin.
70. Talbot, S. A., and Marshall, W. H. (1941): Physiological studies on neural mechanisms of visual localization and discrimination. *Am. J. Ophthalmol.,* 24:1255–1263.

71. Tömbol, T., Hadju, F., and Somogyi, G. (1975): Identification of the Golgi picture of the layer VI cortico-geniculate projection neurons. *Exp. Brain Res.*, 24:107–110.
72. Towe, A. L. (1975): Notes on the hypothesis of columnar organization in somatosensory cerebral cortex. *Brain Behav. Evol.*, 11:16–47.
73. Tsumoto, T., Creutzfeldt, O. D., and Legéndy, C. R. (1977): Functional organization of the corticofugal system from visual cortex to lateral geniculate nucleus in the cat. *J. Neurophysiol. (in press)*.
74. Vogt, O. (1903): Zur anatomischen Gliederung des Cortex cerebri. *J. Psychol. Neurol.*, 2:160–180.
75. Vogt, C., and Vogt, O. (1926): Die vergleichend-architektonische und die vergleichend-reizphysiologische Felderung der Großhirnrinde unter besonderer Berücksichtigung der menschlichen. *Naturwissenschaften*, 14:1190–1194.
76. Valverde, F. (1967): Apical dendritic spines of the visual cortex and light deprivation in the mouse. *Exp. Brain Res.*, 3:337–352.
77. Walker, A. E. (1938): *The Primate Thalamus*. University of Chicago Press, Chicago, 321 pp.
78. Walker, A. E. (1959): Normal and pathological physiology of the thalamus. In: *Introduction to Stereotaxis with an Atlas of the Human Brain, Vol. 1*, edited by G. Schaltenbrand and P. Bailey. Grune & Stratton, New York.
79. Wernicke, C. (1874): *Der aphasische Symptomenkomplex*. Cohn and Weigert, Breslau, 72 pp.
80. Wilson, J. R., and Sherman, M. S. (1976): Receptive field characteristics of neurons in cat striate cortex: Changes with visual field eccentricity. *J. Neurophysiol.*, 39:512–533.
81. Wundt, W. (1896): *Grundriss der Psychologie*. Alfred Kröner Verlag, Leipzig (quoted from 12th ed., p. 252, Leipzig, 1914).

Architectonics of the Cerebral Cortex,
edited by M. A. B. Brazier and H. Petsche.
Raven Press, New York © 1978.

Complex Functional Properties of Cortical Whisker Cells

F. C. Hellweg

*Max Planck-Institut für biophysikalische Chemie, 3400 Göttingen,
Federal Republic of Germany*

Electrophysiological investigations of the more central nuclei of the visual (5) as well as of the auditory system (1) have shown that single cells may respond particularly well to certain complex stimulus constellations. The aim of this work was to show whether or not such cells also occur in the somatosensory system. Therefore, the classic psychophysical stimulus parameters, like velocity, amplitude, etc., were not simply varied, but in addition more complicated or complex stimulus conditions were set up. Such an approach has not been used in the somatosensory system research before, even though it has been reported that stimulus motion on primate skin seems to be especially encoded (11). In order to avoid effects of anaesthetics, chronic preparations without any medication were used. However, for comparison of cortical responses with those of subcortical structures, recordings from anesthetized animals are mainly available (7–9, 13, but see also ref. 3).

METHODS

The experimental cats were prepared for the chronic recording under deep pentobarbital anaesthesia. A metal headholder was screwed and cemented to the head, and a small trephine hole was drilled to gain access to the cortical whisker projection area. This hole could be closed while the animal was recovering from the surgery (usually 1 or 2 days). In the actual recording sessions, the cats sat in a hammock, while the glass-coated tungsten electrodes (1–10 $M\Omega$ resistance at 1,000 Hz AC) were transdurally inserted into the cortex. For stimulation, an electromechanical transducer without feedback was used (10). The actual mechanical movement applied to single vibrissae could be monitored with phototransistors.

RESULTS

Ramp-Shaped Mechanical Displacements

This kind of stimulus was used as a standard to explore initial basic response properties of single cortical cells. In anaesthetized animals, responses

385

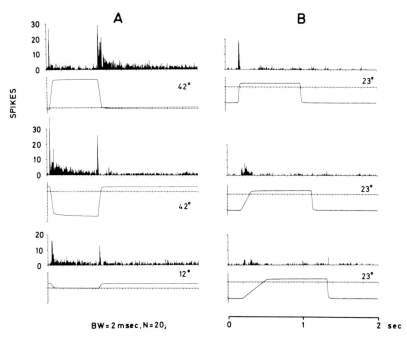

FIG. 1. Two types of responses of cortical cells after ramp-shaped mechanical displacement of a single vibrissa. As in all the other figures, the peristimulus time histogram is given, averaged from 20 stimulus presentations, and the mechanical stimulus is indicated below, including the angle of maximum displacement. **A:** Cell with a relatively pronounced tonic response component. Note the poor dynamic range and the directional sensitivity of this cell. **B:** Cell with response discharges throughout the movement part of the stimulus (phasic summator response). Note some postexcitatory discharge suppression at all three movement velocities.

to this stimulus have been described (4), and, in principle, similar discharge patterns occurred in the unanaesthetized cat. One common finding was, for instance, that a relatively small number of cells had an enhanced firing rate throughout the steady part of the stimulus. In only 11 out of 66 cells in the awake cat was any tonic firing activity found. This proportion is a little larger than in the anaesthetized animal but much smaller than the proportion of tonic firing cells at more peripheral stations of the vibrissae system (2,12). Also, in cortical cells this response was less intense and adapted faster than in thalamocortical fibers, for instance (compare Figs. 1A and 3A). Of all 66 cortical cells investigated, six responded characteristically only during the movement part of the stimulus with a rate proportional to the movement velocity (Fig. 1B). This discharge pattern has been described for more peripheral neurons as phasic summator response (8) and can be found also at the thalamic level (Fig. 3B). Particularly in the cortex of anaesthetized animals, however, this response pattern is found rarely; it may be that postexcitatory inhibition cuts this response into separate discharge peaks

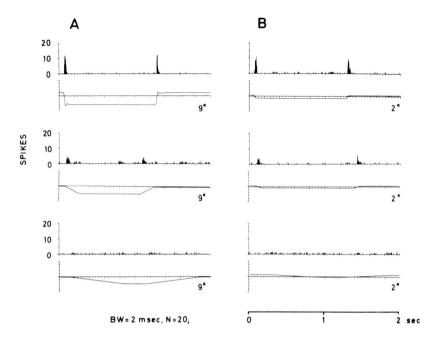

FIG. 2. Cortical cell with a phasic response. Three different stimulus velocities at two different amplitudes **(A, B)** were applied. Note that the cellular response depends only on the displacement velocity and not on the amplitude.

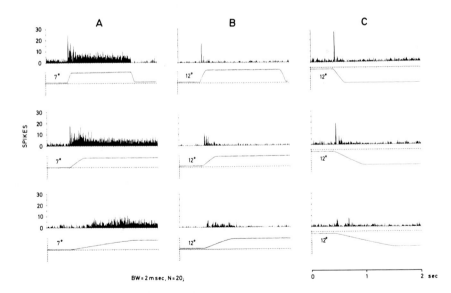

FIG. 3. Discharges of three different thalamocortical fibers recorded in the anaesthetized cat. **A:** Unit with slowly adapting tonic activity (compare with Fig. 1A). **B:** Fiber with a response only during the movement part of the stimulus (phasic summator response). **C:** Thalamocortical fiber with a phasic response. (From ref. 4.)

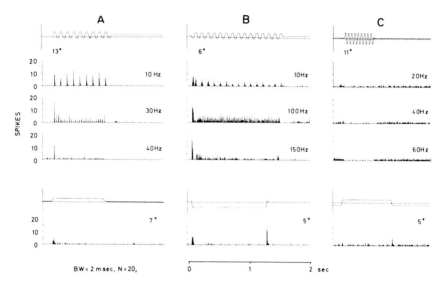

FIG. 4. Responses of three different cortical cells after repetitive sinusoidal whisker displacements at different frequencies. For each cell the response to a ramp-shaped stimulus is also given (bottom trace). **A:** Cell with a low following frequency, as was typically found in the cortex. The threshold of this cell to follow repetitive stimulation lies between 30 Hz and 40 Hz. **B:** Specimen of a cortical cell with a particularly high following frequency. At 100 Hz, the response is not greatly reduced, as compared with the response at 10 Hz stimulation frequency, but at 150 Hz the amount of discharges decreases considerably. **C:** Cell with tonic inhibition during stimulation. Note that this cell has some background activity but only a weak response to the ramp stimulus.

(4). Such postexcitatory discharge suppression can also sometimes be seen in unanaesthetized cats (for instance, in the cell of Fig. 1B).

Most cortical cells in anaesthetized (4) as well as in unanaesthetized animals (49 out of 66 cells in the present study) responded only phasically at "on" or "off" set of the stimulus. The reliability and the number of discharges usually depended only on the movement velocity and not on the amplitude of displacement (Fig. 2A and B). This type of response could be recorded also from several subcortical nuclei in the vibrissae system (Fig. 3C) (8,13), but the percentage of phasic responses in the cortex is particularly high. Among the cortical cells, different velocity thresholds were found.

Sinusoidal Repetitive Stimulation of Vibrissae

After having recorded the cell's responses to ramp stimuli, single vibrissae were moved sinusoidally using the same electromechanical device. Most cells, like the one shown in Fig. 4A, had a recovery cycle of about 30 to 40 msec. This means that responses to the second and following

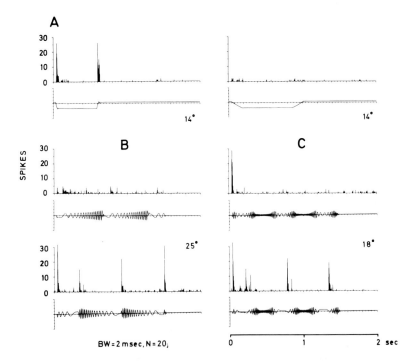

FIG. 5. Cortical cell responding to complex mechanical stimulation. **A:** Ramp-shaped displacements elicit a phasic response with velocity threshold. **B:** Frequency-modulated mechanical movement, between 0 and 100 Hz, sweeping upward (upper record) or downward (lower record). The cell responded only in the second case, probably to some abrupt transients in the stimulus. **C:** Frequency-modulated mechanical stimulus, sinusoidally modulated between 18 and 100 Hz (upper record) and 0 and 100 Hz (lower record). It also seems as if under these conditions the cell responds only to sudden transients, if they occur after a period of mechanical silence.

stimuli were strongly reduced, if these stimuli occurred within 30 to 40 msec after the preceding one. Three cells had a recovery cycle of about 10 msec. Even though these cells, like the one shown in Fig. 4B, did not faithfully respond to each stimulus cycle every time (Fig. 4B, at 100 Hz), several peaks representing time-locked responses can be recognized in the PSTH. Two of the 66 cells, which did not clearly respond to a ramp stimulus, were inhibited by repetitive mechanical stimulation (Fig. 4C). Almost all the cells responding to sinusoidal whisker displacement showed a continually decreasing number of spikes per stimulus cycle and decreasing overall discharge activity at higher stimulation frequencies. Four cortical cells, however, had noncontinuous stimulus-frequency-response functions. They either responded or were inhibited within a very small frequency range. It is interesting to note in this context that peripheral receptors of sinus hairs can follow much higher frequencies of stimulation than cortical cells (6). A detailed comparison of cortical with subcortical response properties after this type of stimulation, however, would require experimental data from other sensory nuclei in the vibrissae system as well.

Complex Mechanical Stimulation

When more complex functions (amplitude-modulated or frequency-modulated sinusoidal, triangular, or square functions) were fed into the electromechanical transducer, corresponding complex movements of the single sinus hair resulted. Since the transducer system had certain frequency characteristics, but no feedback control, a pure frequency-modulated input function was always transduced into a frequency- and amplitude-modulated mechanical movement (Fig. 5, stimulus trace). In Fig. 5A, responses of a cortical cell to such complex movements are shown. Responses in Fig. 5A after ramp-shaped stimulation characterize the cell as a phasic responder with velocity threshold. In Fig. 5B, a sinusoid was frequency-modulated, sweeping either upward (top) or downward (bottom). The cell responded only in the second case at the abrupt change from low to high frequencies. In Fig. 5C, responses of the same cell are shown, with the frequency of stimulation being modulated sinusoidally between 18 and 100 Hz (top) and 0 and 100 Hz (bottom). Only in the second case does each transient in the mechanical stimulus from very low to higher frequencies elicit a response.

DISCUSSION

Responses of cortical cells were investigated after ramp-shaped and—for the first time—more complex mechanical displacements applied to single sinus hairs. In the awake cat, which was used in the present investigation, practically all cells were responsive to mechanical stimulation, but not exclusively to a single parameter. Characteristic types of responses were seen among cortical cells (tonic, phasic summator, and phasic) but transient forms also existed. Most cells responded to ramp-shaped mechanical displacements only with a phasic discharge, the intensity of which was a function of displacement velocity. After sinusoidal repetitive stimulation, cortical cells usually showed irregular, but to some degree, stimulus-locked responses at stimulation frequencies of up to about 40 Hz, in exceptional cases of up to 100 Hz; in a few cells firing activity was suppressed by this stimulation.

Cellular responses to more complex stimuli can be as complex as the stimulus itself. The test of the cell in Fig. 5A with ramp-shaped stimulus, for instance, reveals a phasic response with velocity threshold. Much more could not be found out in such a stimulus situation anyway. After complex mechanical stimulation, however (Fig. 5B and C), the response cannot be described simply by velocity thresholds. Apart from the onset response at the very beginning, the cell apparently was best driven by particular transients in the stimulus, which occurred in a certain context. Not the velocity-amplitude parameter in itself was important, but also the recent history, the stimulus situation preceding that particular velocity-amplitude parameter. Therefore, the ramp-shaped stimulus as such is insufficient for the analysis of more elaborate functional response properties of cortical cells; responses to repetitive stimulation as well as to more complex stimuli also have to be taken into account.

Since under natural physiological conditions a continuously changing mechanical input reaches the vibrissae receptors, larger ensembles of cortical cells with such elaborate responses may be essential for coding and analyzing the Gestalt of particular stimulus parameter combinations by the central vibrissae system.

REFERENCES

1. Feher, O., and Whitfield, I. C. (1965): Auditory cortical units which respond to complex tonal stimuli. *J. Physiol.,* 182:39.
2. Gottschaldt, K.-M., Iggo, A., Young, D. W. (1973): Functional characteristics of mechanoreceptors in sinus hair follicles of the cat. *J. Physiol., (Lond.),* 235:287–315.
3. Hayward, J. N. (1975): Response of ventrobasal thalamic cells to hair displacement on the face of the waking monkey. *J. Physiol. (Lond.),* 250:385–407.
4. Hellweg, F. C., Schultz, W., and Creutzfeldt, O. (1977): Extracellular and intracellular recordings from the cat's cortical whisker projection area: Thalamocortical response transformation. *J. Neurophysiol.,* 40:463–479.
5. Hubel, D., and Wiesel, T. N. (1968): Receptive fields and functional architecture of monkey striate cortex. *J. Physiol. (Lond.),* 195:215–243.
6. Nier, K. (1975): Stabilization phenomena in synchronous neural activity of vibrissae receptors. In: *The Somatosensory System,* edited by H. H. Kornhuber, pp. 204–207. Thieme, Stuttgart.
7. Schultz, W., Galbraith, G. C., Gottschaldt, K.-M., and Creutzfeldt, O. D. (1976): A comparison of primary afferent and cortical unit activity coding sinus hair movements in the cat. *Exp. Brain. Res.,* 24:365–381.
8. Shipley, M. T. (1974): Response characteristics of single units in the rat's trigeminal nuclei to vibrissae displacements. *J. Neurophysiol.,* 37:73–90.
9. Waite, P. M. E. (1973): The responses of cells in the rat thalamus to mechanical movements of the whiskers. *J. Physiol. (Lond.),* 228:541–561.
10. Werner, G., and Mountcastle, V. B. (1965): Neural activity in mechanoreceptive afferents: Stimulus response relations, Weber functions and information transmission. *J. Neurophysiol.,* 28:359–397.
11. Whitsel, B. L., Roppolo, J. R., and Werner, G. (1972): Cortical information processing of stimulus motion on primate skin. *J. Neurophysiol.,* 35:691–718.
12. Young, D. W. (1975): Some properties of neurones in the spinal trigeminal nucleus responding to movements of the vibrissae. *J. Physiol. (Lond.),* 244:75–76.
13. Zucker, E., and Welker, W. I. (1969): Coding of somatic sensory input by vibrissae neurones in the rat's trigeminal ganglion. *Brain Res.,* 12:138–156.

Architectonics of the Cerebral Cortex,
edited by M. A. B. Brazier and H. Petsche.
Raven Press, New York © 1978.

Some Electrophysiological Data About Neocortical Association Areas

J. Scherrer and Y. Burnod

Laboratoire de Physiologie, Pitié-Salpêtrière, F-75634 Paris Cedex 13, France

What we now know about association areas originates from the convergence of different approaches. Clinicians have observed in patients disturbances related to lesions in such areas. Anatomists have described their architectonics: among them Constantin von Economo produced the most remarkable data on this subject. Classical neurophysiologists and experimental psychologists performing ablation and stimulation experiments on association areas demonstrated changes in perception, performance, or behavior due to this type of approach. Finally, electrophysiological techniques have also brought forth important facts concerning the role of neocortical association areas in different mammalia. This chapter tries to summarize briefly and synthetize data in this last field.

Cortical electrophysiological investigations started officially nearly half a century ago when Berger (3) described the electroencephalogram. However, several studies anticipated this discovery. It may be interesting to underline that one of the first attempts to obtain an electrical response on the brain was performed in Vienna by Fleischl von Marxow in 1890 (quoted by Brazier, ref. 4) several years before von Economo started his medical career in the same city.

Very schematically, two types of electrophysiological approaches can be used: the recording of spontaneous electrocortical activity under different conditions and registration of the evoked electrical activity. The latter technique produced the most important experimental data. This chapter will consider the following points:

1. Electrophysiological investigations using the evoked electrical phenomena.

2. Those using the spontaneous electrical activity.

3. Some data obtained during ontogenesis and phylogenesis.

4. What is known about electrophysiology of association cortex in humans.

EVOKED ELECTRICAL ACTIVITY IN ASSOCIATION AREAS

Two different approaches are used. The first considers global statistical responses of neuronal populations (field potential type of cortical responses) following the stimulation of an afferent system. Usually the stimulus is strong and primitive (flash, click, electrical stimulation of nerve or skin). This type of investigation may be performed under general anesthesia, since it is aimed at demonstrating the arrival of sensory messages at the cortical level.

In the second approach, unitary neuronal activity is recorded. Afferent stimulation is frequently much more elaborate, no general anesthesia being used. The second approach has yielded important data concerning the way the cortex handles sensory information.

Arrival of Afferent Messages at the Cortical Level

Before its application to association areas, the field potential technique was used for topographical studies of the cortical primary projection areas. Following the pioneering work during the late 1930s, many authors investigated evoked potentials with surface electrodes. In the early 1950s, it became possible to establish maps showing in different animals, usually under barbiturate anesthesia, the neocortical regions responding to somesthetic, auditory, or visual stimuli.

As a general rule, for a given afferent system, two primary receiving areas were described (for instance S-I and S-II for somesthesia), both demonstrating short latency stable responses. The two primary regions show a definite topographical organization: area I has a broader cortical extension than area II. On a map showing these different cortical afferent regions and the motor area, some territories remain free (Fig. 1). For the electrophysiologist, these regions are extraprimary and in fact coincide with what the anatomists usually consider as association areas. So the simplest and perhaps the least misleading conception of association areas should be to consider them as occupying cortical territories outside primary sensory and motor areas. However, the definition of a primary area might sometimes be less simple than expected. (For example, in the cat, response in the auditory area A-II has a much longer latency and a higher variability than A-I: Is it still a primary area?)

A comparison of cortical maps obtained in different animals demonstrates that in the first approximation the relative surface of extraprimary areas increases with phylogenetic evolution as shown in Fig. 1.

The fact that sensory impulses may also reach extraprimary areas was well established about 20 years ago by several research groups working on the cat under chloralose anesthesia. Under this condition, as seen by Amassian (2), Albe Fessard and Fessard (1), and Thomson et al. (21),

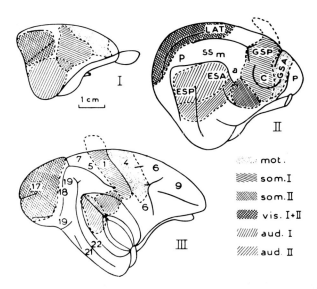

FIG. 1. Sensory motor and association areas in rabbit **(I)**, cat **(II)**, and monkey **(III)**. For the cat, the following gyri are mentioned: proreus **(p)**; anterior and posterior sigmoïd **(GSA, GSP)**; coronal **(C)**; lateral **(LAT)**; suprasylvian anterior, medial, posterior **(SS a, m, P)**; and ectosylvian anterior and posterior **(ESA, ESP)**. For the monkey, architectonic areas according to Brodmann (from Buser, 1957) and data obtained by Woolsey and Fairman, Rose and Woolsey, Ruch, and Dell were used.

large evoked potentials are recorded in extraprimary territories (Fig. 2). They have a longer latency than those registered in primary areas. The responses persist even after suppression of the primary afferent areas equally well for somesthetic as for visual or auditory stimuli. Extraprimary areas in the cat (middle suprasylvian, anterior marginal, pericruciate) are

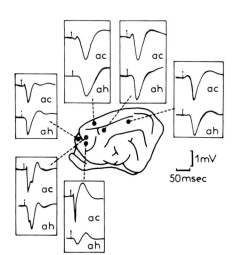

FIG. 2. Responses evoked in cat under chloralose by electrical stimulation of the controlateral **(ac)** and homolateral **(ah)** forepaw. (From ref. 1.)

responsive to stimulation of various sensory modalities (auditory, somatic, visual). It is not clear, however, whether there are definite localized extra-primary association foci or whether the topographical distribution of these responses is more diffuse. The relatively short latency association responses obtained under chloralose (see Buser and Bignall, ref. 5) may pass through thalamic projection nuclei, primary cortical areas, and thalamic association nuclei. The longer latency responses recorded under chloralose are postulated to be mediated by a common polysensory afferent system (nonspecific thalamus).

Responses under chloralose anesthesia are open to criticism. It is well known that chloralose has a strong synchronizing effect that may considerably modify neuronal events. So the experiment aiming to demonstrate the arrival of afferent messages in cortical association areas had to be duplicated without anesthesia. Results obtained under chloralose were confirmed (6). However, under these conditions, primary evoked potentials appear much more labile and of lower amplitude. The latencies of association responses are longer than those of the primary projection areas. Very sensitive to the level of vigilance as shown by Meulders (14), their amplitude diminishes during arousal and increases in the quiet animal or during slow wave sleep. The responses disappear following the administration of a small dose of barbiturates, whereas the cortical evoked potentials in the primary areas are especially well seen during barbiturate anesthesia. The question is still unsettled as to whether there exists a preferential topography of these association responses according to the type of stimulation. Figure 3, published by Buser and Bignall (5) summarizing different results, shows some topographical differences for somesthetic, auditory, and visual stimulations with many overlapping regions. In primary visual areas there are also cross-modality responses to somatic and auditory stimuli.

According to Hirsch et al. (9), who used the transcortical recording technique to eliminate electrical diffusion, the "association" responses for a given somesthetic stimulation are definitely present not only in all the extraprimary explored areas, but also in motor and primary auditory and visual ones (Fig. 4). The rather long latency (20 to 40 msec) of these "association" responses may vary from one region to another.

The association cortex of the cat has been recently reinvestigated by Robertson et al. (16) with selective microelectrodes under chloralose, as well as in unanesthetized cats. Most of the recorded neurons in the suprasylvian area respond to the three types of stimulation, somesthetic, visual, and auditory, equally well under chloralose anesthesia as without any general anesthesia. Thus, in the cat, for peripheral stimuli, an intermodal convergence is well established. However, to see this phenomenon, it seems necessary to use a rather intense afferent stimulation. The abovementioned experimental procedure confirms that the motor cortex receives afferent inputs as is the case for association areas. The neurons in the motor areas

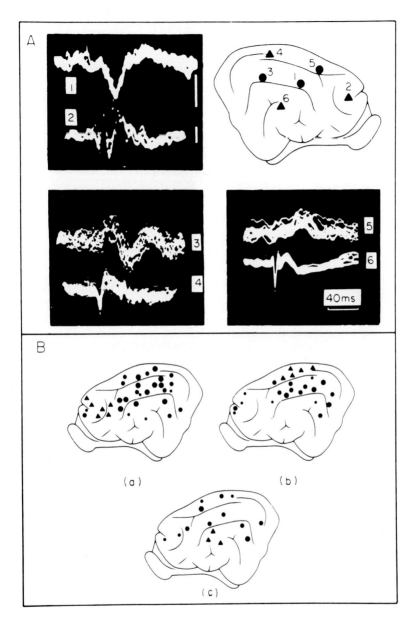

FIG. 3. A: Extraprimary responses recorded for somesthetic **(1),** visual **(3),** and auditory **(5)** stimulations, with primary corresponding responses **(2,4, and 6)** in an immobilized cat. **B:** Distribution of extraprimary somatic **(a),** visual **(b),** and auditory **(c)** responses. (From ref. 5.)

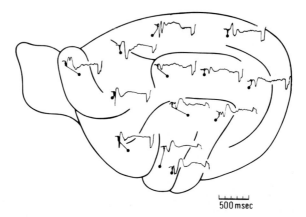

500 msec

FIG. 4. Cortical averaged responses to ipsilateral-forepaw electrical stimulation in an immobilized cat. Transcortical electrodes. **Arrow:** Shock artifact. Calibration at the end of the sweep. (From ref. 9.)

respond to photic, auditory, and somesthetic inputs with intermodal convergence in contrast to cells in close adjacent areas (S-I and S-II) which respond only to somesthetic inputs and not to other modalities.

How Association Areas Handle Afferent Signals

Using unitary neuronal activity and elaborate stimulation, an important amount of data concerning central integration of afferent messages has been obtained during the past 15 years. Integration already takes place in the sensory network at the spinal, brainstem, thalamic, and eventually retinal levels. At the cortical level, important integrative phenomena have been described in the primary sensory areas not only in the visual system but also in the auditory one.

Two examples may be given. In the primary visual area, neurons fire for a precise geometrical combination of visual punctate stimuli, and this combination may imply a temporal order relation (10). In the primary auditory area in squirrel, monkey, and macaque, specific responses to vocalization of their own species have been observed (23).

At the present time, there are also a good number of publications dealing with neuronal activity in association areas, related to sensory input, spontaneous or learned behavior. We shall consider here only some of the available data related to the parietal cortex: those obtained in the monkey by unitary recording in areas 5 and 7. The experimental procedure implies a precise and often a multiple somatic stimulation. The animal may be immobilized but is more commonly freely moving. In the latter case, neuronal activity is frequently registered during the performance of a learned task.

If more schematization is permitted than several authors of this type of investigation, such as Sakata et al. (17), Mountcastle et al. (15), and Hyvarinen et al. (11), have undertaken, the outcome would be that three particular properties can be attributed to neuronal activity in extraprimary parietal areas.

(1) Extraprimary parietal neurons have a definite tendency to fire or change their firing rate for combined somatic stimulations. For example, the following are especially efficient: passive movement of two joints, simultaneous directional skin stimulation and joint displacement, bilateral contact interaction between two limbs, etc. Figure 5, published by Sakata et al. (17) is a good example of such interactions. A more complex interaction is demonstrated by the fact that neurons fire more during active than passive joint rotations. However, in the parietal cortex of the monkey, intermodal convergence is rare.

(2) An afferent message does not always have the same significance, and this fact can be reflected in neuronal activity, so a cutaneous vibratory stimulus gives a more prominent discharge in some parietal association neurons, particularly if it was previously tied to a signal indicating a reward rather than if to one without reward. This type of signal-reward relation, also seen in motor cortex, seems to be absent from the primary sensory area. In the opposite way, neurons located in parietal association and in motor cortex areas do not follow each cycle of a vibratory stimulus as do neurons in the primary area. Figure 6, using results obtained by Hyvarinen et al. (11), definitely shows the phenomena described above.

(3) The third property of association neurons was well analyzed by Mountcastle et al. (15). In a freely moving animal, some neurons, more frequently recorded in area 7 than in area 5, seem to be related to the "conception" of a movement or of a posture. So a neuronal discharge is tied to the goal of a movement rather than to its mechanical characteristics. For

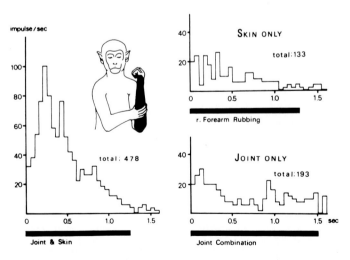

FIG. 5. Histograms showing responses of a cortical neuron in area 5 in an immobilized monkey to shoulder adduction. Enhancement by skin contact. (From ref. 17.)

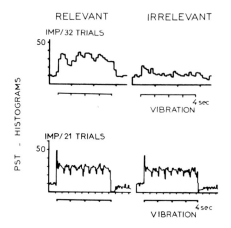

FIG. 6. Histograms demonstrating the neuronal discharge related to somesthetic stimuli (vibration), which previously were followed or not by a reward (relevant and irrelevant). Relevance changes the neuronal discharge only in the association area. (From ref. 11.)

instance, firing corresponds to the projection of the anterior limb, aiming to catch some interesting object, independently of the geometrical pattern of the movement or of the muscles used to perform the motion. Figure 7, published by Mountcastle et al. (15), demonstrates this fact. The three properties schematized above for areas 5 and 7 are certainly not restricted to parietal association areas. In fact, related characteristics are found in other extraprimary cortical regions.

SPONTANEOUS ELECTRICAL ACTIVITY IN ASSOCIATION AREAS

Since Berger (3), it was known that the EEG differs in the occipital and frontal regions. As early as 1932, an experimental attempt was made by

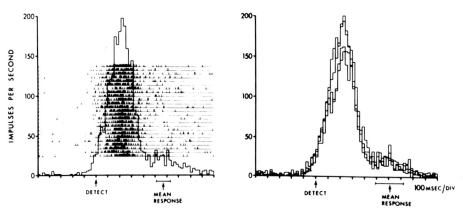

FIG. 7. Histogram showing discharge of a parietal association neuron occurring between the time of signal detection and the motor response. Variations in the motor responses (and also in sensory input) do not modify the discharge pattern: in four different conditions the traces are identical (from ref. 15.)

Kornmüller (12) to relate electrocortical activity to architectonics. However, technical difficulties left this type of study unsuccessful until recently. For such an investigation, a precise localization and a statistical approach to the EEG phenomena are necessary in order for it to be possible to demonstrate in the cat a definite difference in the spontaneous electrical activity of primary sensory and extraprimary areas (7). The precise topographical localization is obtained by using simultaneously in several discrete neocortical regions transcortical electrodes that permit one to record simultaneously wave type activity and concomitant discharges. The statistical approach is performed by a pattern-recognition device so that the same type of cortical wave can be analyzed and averaged. Using this technique, it appears that in the cat definite differences exist in the spontaneous activity of various cortical regions, mainly for the surface-negative wave (7,18). This wave, which lasts from 0.1 to 0.3 sec, is concomitant with a decrease or even a suppression of neuronal cortical firing. Probably related to a somatic hyperpolarization, the surface-negative wave is recorded during drowsiness and sleep; in fact, slow-wave sleep may be considered as a succession of surface-negative waves. A statistical study of the surface-negative waves demonstrates that their amplitude is far more pronounced in the extraprimary areas (suprasylvian gyrus, for instance) than in sensory primary areas (Fig. 8). Similarly, whereas in the association areas a complete firing suppression might be observed during the surface-negative wave, in the primary areas only a diminution of unitary activity takes place. To sum up, inhibition of neuronal firing is deeper in association areas.

A related type of observation is made when the cortical extension of the

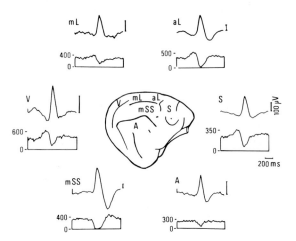

FIG. 8. Averaging of surface-negative waves **(upper trace)** and simultaneously neuronal discharge **(lower trace)** performed successively for different cortical leads during a period of slow-wave sleep in the cat. Higher wave amplitude and total suppression of spike discharge in associative areas. (From ref. 7.)

surface-negative wave is studied. During slow-wave sleep, the surface occupied by a given surface-negative wave is not always the same. When the
extension is restricted, the wave is mainly localized in the suprasylvian
gyrus, i.e., in an association area. When the wave extends, the primary sensory somesthetic and auditory areas are less involved than other territories
(Fig. 9). It is likely that the extension of the surface-negative wave is related to the depth of the slow-wave sleep. If this is true, the conclusion would
be that cortical sleep starts first in association areas and predominates thereafter in the same regions. This should be compared with the fact that recruiting responses evoked by thalamic stimulation are more prominent in extraprimary areas (20).

ELECTROCORTICAL DATA OBTAINED DURING ONTOGENESIS AND PHYLOGENESIS

Ontogenesis

Much classic anatomical work demonstrates that association areas mature
later than primary areas. An indirect electrophysiological approach to this
problem is already found in papers devoted to maturation of evoked potentials in afferent primary areas. A topical investigation produced interesting data about unitary responses in cat association cortex during development (13). Under chloralose anesthesia, the first responses appear in the
suprasylvian gyrus on the 8th postnatal day. On the 50th day, unitary responses are of the same type as in the adult animal (Fig. 10). In the primary
sensory areas, the same type of responses appear earlier. So the somesthe-

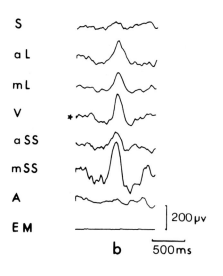

FIG. 9. Averaging of surface-negative
waves performed simultaneously in seven
different cortical areas. Later stage of
slow-wave sleep. The wave extends
mainly to extra primary areas. S-I **(S)**,
anterior and medial lateral gyrus **(a
L, mL)**, V-I **(V)**, anterior and medial
suprasylvian gyrus **(a SS, a SS)**, A-I
(A), and eye movements **(EM)**. (From
ref. 7.)

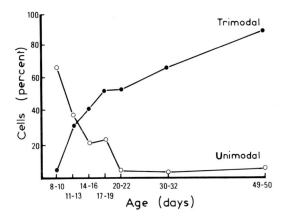

FIG. 10. Increase with age in percentage of cells that respond to auditory visual and somesthetic stimuli (trimodal neurons) in the posterior-middle suprasylvian gyrus. Cat: chloralose anesthesia. (From ref. 13.)

tic responses are already present in the first postnatal days. The sequence in which responses appear in the suprasylvian association area is the following: first visual responses, then auditory and finally the somesthetic ones. This order differs from the sequence demonstrated in the cortical primary projection areas where somesthetic responses appear first and visual ones are the last. An interesting fact is that in the newborn animal, the responses in primary and association areas are labile and have a long recovery cycle; these properties disappear with maturation in primary areas and persist in association areas.

Phylogenesis

The usual and probably most correct assumption is that what we call cortical association areas appear and develop in more evolved species. Figure 1 already demonstrates this fact. However, a point should be stressed: complex behavioral patterns are observed in species in which most or even the totality of the neocortex is occupied by the sensory projection and motor areas. This fact implies that in these species very complicated neuronal operations are handled in these areas. In more highly evolved species, many complex operations are shared between projection and association areas. Some complex operations are probably transferred to association areas. How association areas develop during evolution is unknown. Two hypotheses may be considered: one is that in some phyla in which projection areas already exist, association areas progressively develop in some newly formed cortical regions. Another possibility is that in an undifferentiated cortical network, aimed at receiving and handling afferent messages, the

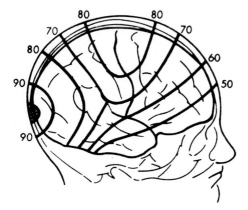

FIG. 11. Isopotential map for a long-latency positive component (P 200) of the visually evoked response. Such a distribution indicates a participation of associative areas in the cortical response. (From ref. 22.)

primary areas, mainly characterized by a rapid arrival of incoming messages, develop progressively. So primary areas could be considered phylogenetically to be younger. The data observed by Diamond and Hall (8) in the hedgehog, the tree shrew, and the squirrel could fit the latter hypothesis. The abovementioned authors wonder if the development of association areas is not a characteristic of some biological niches, which is a rather stimulating hypothesis.

SOME ELECTROPHYSIOLOGICAL DATA ON ASSOCIATION CORTEX IN HUMAN

Evoked potentials have been registered in the human subject for more than 20 years. With some exceptions, the recordings have been performed on the scalp. So localization of the electrocortical phenomenon is not precise. Usually, it is accepted that the early part of the response is located in the primary area, whereas the delayed one spreads to a larger area. Isopotential lines studied by Vaughan (22) during the visual response indicate clearly that a larger surface than the primary visual areas is involved in the late response (Fig. 11). According to the same author, the extension is even more conspicuous in the stimulus-deleted responses (19). Averaged evoked potentials, time-locked to regularly presented visual and auditory stimuli, are recorded. As mentioned above, the electrical generator corresponds to primary areas for the shorter latency responses and to association areas for the longer latency waves. However, when a stimulus is randomly deleted, the corresponding potential originates even for its first component from association areas, with a more powerful contribution than in evoked potential. Its second component is unspecific and is maximal in the parietal region. So it appears that in the human as in the animal an afferent stimulation produces simultaneously an early focal response and a long-latency, more diffuse potential change, which mainly interests association regions.

REFERENCES

1. Albe Fessard, D., and Fessard, A. (1963): Thalamic integrations and their consequences at the telencephalic level. In: *Progress in Brain Research, Vol. I*, edited by G. Moruzzi, A. Fessard, and H. H. Jasper, pp. 115–148. Elsevier, Amsterdam.

2. Amassian, V. E. (1954): Studies on organization of a somesthetic association area including a single unit analysis. *J. Neurophysiol.*, 17:39–58.

3. Berger, H. (1929): Uber das Electrenkephalogramm des Menschen. *Arch. J. Psychiatry*, 87:527–570.

4. Brazier, M. A. B. (1959): The historical development of neurophysiology. In: *Neurophyslology, Vol. I*, edited by J. Field, H. W. Magoun, and V. E. Hall, pp. 1–58. American Physiological Society, Washington, D.C.

5. Buser, P., and Bignall K. E. (1967): Nonprimary sensory projections on the cat neocortex. *Int. Rev. Neurobiol.*, 10:111–165.

6. Buser, P., and Borenstein, P. (1959): Réponses somesthesiques, visuelles et auditives recueillies au niveau de cortex associatif suprasylvian chez le chat curarisé non anesthesié. *Electroenceph. Clin. Neurophysiol.*, 11:285–301.

7. Calvet, J., Fourment, A., and Thieffry, M. (1973): Electrical activity in neocortical projection and association areas during slow wave sleep. *Brain Res.*, 52:173–187.

8. Diamond, I. T., and Hall, W. C. (1969): Evolution of neocortex. *Science*, 164:251–262.

9. Hirsch, J. F., Anderson, R. E., Calvet, J., and Scherrer, J. (1961): Short and long latency cortical responses to somesthetic stimulation in the cat. *Exp. Neurol.*, 4:562–583.

10. Hubel, D., and Wiesel, T. (1968): Receptive fields and functional architecture of monkey striate cortex. *J. Physiol. (Lond.)*, 195:215–243.

11. Hyvarinen, J., Poranen A., and Jokinen, Y. (1974): Central sensory activities between sensory input and motor output. In: *The Neurosciences, 3rd Study Program*, edited by F. O. Schmitt, and F. G. Worden, pp. 311–318. MIT Press, Cambridge, Mass.

12. Kormüller, A. E. (1932): Architecktonische Localisation bioelectrischer Erscheinungen auf Grosshirnrinde. I. Mitteilung: Untersuchungen am Kanichen bei Augenbelichtung. *J. Psychol. Neurol.*, 44:447–459.

13. Mayers, K. S., Robertson, R. T., Rubel, E. W., and Thompson, R. F. (1971): Development of polysensory responses in association cortex of kitten. *Science*, 171:1038–1040.

14. Meulders, H. (1962): *Etude Comparative de la Physiologie des Voies Sensorielles Primaries et des Voies Associatives*. Bruxelles Arscia et Paris, Maloine.

15. Mountcastle, V. B., Lynch, J. C., Georgopoulos, A., Sakata, H., and Acuna, C. (1975): Posterior parietal association cortex of the monkey: Command functions for operations within extrapersonal space. *J. Neurophysiol.*, 38:871–908.

16. Robertson, R. J., Mayers, K. S. Teyler, T. J., Bettinger, L. A., Birsch, H., Davis, J. L., Phillips, D. S., and Thompson, R. F. (1975): Unit activity in posterior association cortex of cat. *J. Neurophysiol.*, 38:780–794.

17. Sakata, H, Takaoka, Y., Kawarasaki, A., and Shibutani, H. (1973): Somato-sensory properties of neurons in the superior parietal cortex (area 5) of the rhesus monkey. *Brain Res.*, 64:85–102

18. Scherrer., J., and Calvet, J. (1972): Normal and epileptic synchronization at the cortical level in the animal. In: *Synchronization of EEG Activity in Epilepsies*, edited by H. Petsche, and M. A. B. Brazier, pp. 113–132. Springer-Verlag, Wien.

19. Simson, R., Vaughan, H. G., and Ritter, W. (1976): The scalp topography of potentials associated with missing visual stimuli. *Electroenceph. Clin. Neurophysiol.*, 40:33–42.

20. Starzl, T. E., and Magoun, H. W. (1951): Diffuse thalamic projection system in monkey. *J. Neurophysiol.*, 14:133–146.

21. Thomson, R. F., Johnson, R. H., and Hoopes, J. J. (1963): Organization of auditory, somatic, sensory and visual projections to association fields of cerebral cortex in the cat. *J. Neurophysiol.*, 26:343–364.

22. Vaughan, H. G. (1968): The relationships of brain activity to scalp recordings. In: *Average Evoked Potentials*, edited by E. Donchin, and D. Lindsley; NASA, Washington, D.C.

23. Wollberg, Z., and Newman, J. D. (1972): Auditory cortex of squirrel monkey: Response pattern of single cells to specific vocalization. *Science*, 175:212–114.

Architectonics of the Cerebral Cortex,
edited by M. A. B. Brazier and H. Petsche.
Raven Press, New York © 1978.

Electrocortical Activity in Association Versus Projection Areas During Active Wakefulness and Paradoxical Sleep

J. Calvet

*Laboratoire de Recherches Neurophysiologiques de l'Association Claude Bernard
EPHE et INSERM, Hôpital de la Salpêtrière, 75013 Paris, France*

As was reported by Dr. J. Scherrer, the electrical phenomena specific to slow-wave sleep in the cat, i.e., the negative-surface slow waves, usually found in all cortical areas, have three specific properties when recorded in the suprasylvian gyrus, ordinarily considered as an association area:

1. Their amplitude is much greater than in primary areas.
2. They are accompanied by almost complete arrest of unitary discharges.
3. They start about 50 msec before the waves in the primary area.

In addition to these characteristics of their electrical patterns in slow-wave sleep, the association areas have further specific electrical properties when compared with the projection areas during active wakefulness, on the one hand, and during paradoxical sleep on the other. The following discussion will, therefore, compare the properties of an already described (1) electrical pattern, i.e., the positive-surface slow wave, in these two states and usually recorded in all cortical areas.

Figure 1 shows averages of these waves simultaneously recorded from six different areas by transcortical electrode couples. (For slow-wave recognition and averaging, see ref. 2.) During active wakefulness, (Fig. 1, W) the two different association areas (mSS and aL), from which the waves have been recognized and averaged, are rather well synchronized with those of the visual primary areas (V and mL), but not at all with the other association areas. In contrast, during paradoxical sleep (Fig. 1, P) the positive-surface waves have a greater amplitude and an obviously wider topographic extension: they occur simultaneously, not only in primary visual but also in all association areas.

Figure 2 points out the discrepancies between these two kinds of areas and concerns their unit firing patterns. The unitary discharges recorded from a primary visual (V) and from an association area (suprasylvian: mSS) are correlated with each other and are compared in two different states: active wakefulness (W) and paradoxical sleep (P). It appears from these regression

407

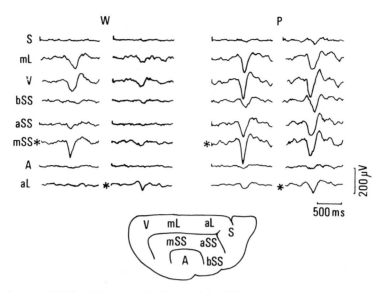

Fig. 1. Averaged EEG activity, recorded from eight different cortical areas of a chronically prepared cat when positive-surface slow waves occur in pilot leads (*): either medial suprasylvian cortex **(mSS)** or lateral anterior cortex **(aL)** during 31 sec of wakefulness **(W)** and of paradoxical sleep **(P)**. From left to right: average of 24 waves, 23 waves, 28 waves and 17 waves. **S**, somesthetic; **mL,** mediolateral; **V,** primary visual cortex; **bSS,** basal suprasylvian; **aSS,** anterior suprasylvian; and **A,** primary auditory cortex. Cortical surface positivity downward. Notice that, except for the pilot leads (*), the other association areas are more silent during wakefulness than they are during paradoxical sleep (Fourment A., Thieffry M., and Calvet J., *in preparation*).

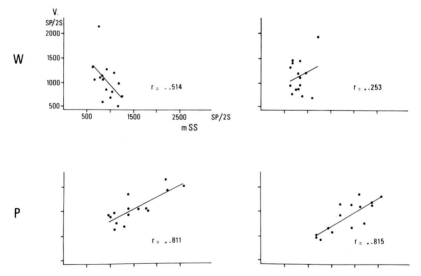

FIG. 2. Four regression diagrams between multiunit discharges recorded from primary visual cortex **(V)** and associative medial suprasylvian cortex **(mSS)** in two different states of active wakefulness **(W,** upper left and right) and of paradoxical sleep **(P,** lower left and right) during four periods of 30 sec (Fourment A., Thieffry, M., and Calvet, J., *in preparation*). Note the constant and strongly positive correlation between the discharges of the two areas during paradoxical sleep.

diagrams that no constant correlation exists between the level of discharges of the two areas studied during active wakefulness, while the correlation remains strongly positive and significant during paradoxical sleep.

To sum up, *slow-wave sleep* appears to be a strong synchronization of the negative-surface slow waves, with a maximum in association areas. The unitary discharges, *especially from these association areas,* reflect, during this kind of sleep, the importance of synchronization: a great number of neurons ceases to fire together during the occurrence of these waves.

The positive-surface slow waves of the *paradoxical phase of sleep* are also highly synchronized, since they spread over to most association areas and are concomitant with electrical events in the primary visual cortex.

On the contrary, during *active wakefulness,* both positive slow waves and unitary discharges occur much more independently and randomly in the different areas. The association cortex is active only from time to time and is synchronized only occasionally with the primary visual area.

REFERENCES

1. Calvet, J., Calvet, M. C., and Langlois, J. M. (1965): Diffuse cortical activation waves during so-called desynchronized EEG patterns. *J. Neurophysiol.,* 28:893–907.
2. Calvet, J., Fourment, A., and Thieffry, M. (1973): Electrical activity in neocortical projection and association areas during slow wave sleep. *Brain Res.,* 52:173–187.

Architectonics of the Cerebral Cortex,
edited by M. A. B. Brazier and H. Petsche.
Raven Press, New York © 1978.

Projection and Association Levels of Cortical Integration

O. S. Adrianov

*Brain Research Institute, U.S.S.R. Academy of Medical Sciences,
Moscow, U.S.S.R.*

The problem of levels or stages of integration suggests first the concept of degree and specificity of the structural and functional organization of cerebral systems participating in the formation of adaptive human or animal reactions.

Isolated levels or systems of integration are ruled out, since it is well known that the brain activity is ensured by their intricate interaction. Thus, the task of the investigator is to study this interaction.

The principle of regulation of the structure and function of the brain constitutes the basic principle of cerebral organization which should be extended to various systems and levels of the brain. We are especially pleased to emphasize that von Economo (21) was one of the outstanding founders of studies of regulation of brain structure. We are marking the centenary of his birth this year. Economo made an invaluable contribution to studies of the architectonics of cortical formations.

This report deals with projection and association levels of integration. Meynert and Flechsig were among the first to give an idea of these levels. However, it was not until recently that new, abundant, and original data has appeared on specificity and integration in the organization and, primarily, on a close interaction of these levels. We have focused our attention on the problem of cortical integration, although the latter, as is quite clear, cannot be separated from other levels of the brain. It is no mere chance that a necessity has arisen lately to distinguish special thalamotelencephalic association systems of integration.

It is expedient to start considering the problem of brain levels or systems with some definitions.

Projection (sensory) systems (PS), called analyzers by Pavlov, appeared in early stages of evolution. They are known to be adapted to perceiving, analyzing, and dynamically processing excitation of one particular sensory modality or submodalities.

Association (intersensory or interanalyzer) systems (AS) originated much later in the course of evolution. Being underdeveloped in lower mammals, they are more clearly pronounced in subprimates, whereas it is in primates and especially in man that they are differentiated to the greatest degree. AS are levels of integration situated mainly within the forebrain and ensuring primarily the synthesis (convergence) of nonprimary, earlier integrated excitations. The processes of multisensory (sensori-sensory) integration are of paramount importance for AS. These processes underlie complicated forms of perception, gnosis, and constructive activity (in man, speech also). Thalamoparietal, thalamofrontal, and thalamotemporal systems can be regarded as primarily association systems.

It is also necessary to distinguish integrative trigger systems (ITS). Cortical levels of these systems are represented first of all by the motor and orbital regions. ITS neurons are related predominantly to the processes of sensori-biological convergence of afferent influences, i.e., to the integration of sensory stimuli with various alimentary (interoceptive), nociceptive, or proprioceptive stimuli.

Such interaction makes it possible for efferent excitations to be formed in ITS and arrive at the efferent apparatus of the spinal cord and brainstem and, thus, to effect a motor adaptive reaction.

According to classic studies, the source of afferentation of cortical projection areas is, in sensory systems, located at the diencephalic level (thalamic relay nuclei), while that of association systems can be found in thalamic association structures. Recent neuromorphological and neurophysiological findings, however, significantly amend these assumptions.

These findings made it possible for us to formulate (7) the principle of spatial and temporal dispersion of afferent excitations of one particular modality. These excitations are conducted through several channels. This fact makes it possible for a signal to be treated in different systems of the brain, including the association and integrative trigger ones.

Figure 1 demonstrates the distribution of excitations originating from the retina. This diagram is based on our own findings and those found in the literature describing morphological and functional connections of the visual system with various limbic structures, neocortical association, and integrative trigger areas.

The analysis of our morphophysiological findings (6) provides support for the existence of fairly distinct connections of thalamic relay nuclei with the parietal and motor regions of the neocortex (Fig. 1). Such inputs to the parietal association cortex are organized in the cat according to the so-called "nonspecific" type. Axonal terminals are distributed in an even manner over the cortex and ascend to the parietal region from thalamic relay nuclei—the posterior ventral (12) and the lateral geniculate body (11). At the same time, the main afferent terminals of thalamic relay nuclei are known to be concentrated in cortical projection regions, predominantly in layer IV and the lower sublayer of layer III (Fig. 2).

The observed peculiarities of the organization of specific afferents, like the nonspecific ones outside the primary sensory zones, are of particular

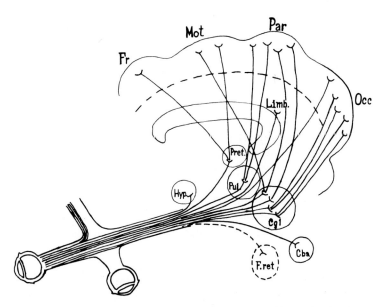

FIG. 1. Diagram of "dispersion" of visual excitations in different brain structures. **Fr**, frontal; **Mot**, motor; **Par**, parietal; **Occ**, occipital; **Limb**, limbic regions of the neocortex; **Hyp**, hypothalamus; **P**, pulvinar; **Pret**, pretectum; **Cgl**, corpus geniculatum laterale (lateral geniculate body); **Fret**, brainstem reticular formation; and **Cba**, anterior bigeminal body.

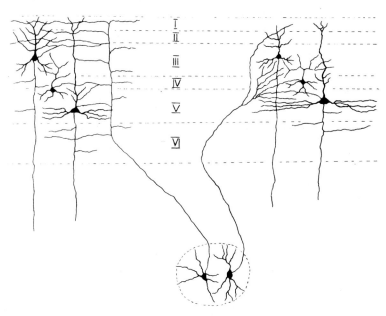

FIG. 2. Schema to illustrate the differences in layer distribution of specific afferents of the posterior ventral thalamic nucleus to the projection somatic **(b)** and associative parietal **(a)** regions of the cat brain.

interest in studies of the so-called early components of association responses (ECAR) recorded in the parietal region in response to specific somatic (41) and visual stimuli (40,41) (Fig. 3). Noteworthy is the absence of phase inversion of the responses as the electrode passes through the association cortex (Fig. 4). At the same time, a distinct inversion of primary responses is observed in the projection cortex. These physiological observations can be related to the morphological peculiarities described above. The scattered type of fiber terminations arising from thalamic relay nuclei to reach the parietal association cortex is likely to be responsible to a great measure for a higher threshold of sensitivity of ECAR to neurotropic drugs than that observed in the primary response (13).

As far back as 1953 Liang and Pouly (34) demonstrated the connection of the posterior ventral thalamic nucleus to the parietal cortex in monkey. Artemenko and Mamonez (14) point to a direct connection between the posterior ventral thalamic nucleus and area 5 of the suprasylvian gyrus of the cat.

Direct inputs from thalamic relay nuclei to the motor cortex have been described by Poljakova (42) in our laboratory as well as by Ogawa (39). Their observations have been supported by morphological findings (45). On the other hand, in some studies, including our own (11), direct afferent inputs have been found to exist arising from the thalamic association nuclei to the visual projection cortex. However, the organization of these inputs differs from that of the inputs of the main geniculostriate pathway.

All these findings point to another most important principle of the or-

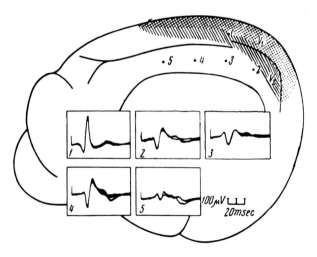

FIG. 3. Evoked potentials to light stimulation in projection (points 1 and 2) and parietal associative (points 3 to 5) cat cortical regions. (From ref. 40.)

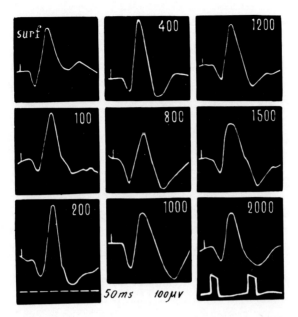

FIG. 4. The absence of ECAR inversion as the electrode passes through the cortex. (From ref. 41.)

ganization of various afferent excitations, namely the principle of overlapping of their projections at the cortical level.

Cytoarchitectonic studies also support this view. They testify to the existence of so-called transitory cortical areas exhibiting features of neighboring fields. This was suggested by Brodmann as early as 1909 (19). Von Economo (21) emphasized this transition by dividing the human cortex into numerous areas and designating them by letters.

The outstanding Soviet neurologist, Filimonov (23), proposed the theory of so-called intermediate formations. According to this theory, genetically different cortical regions—the neocortex, archicortex, and palaeocortex—are separated from one another by transitory periarchicortical and peripalaeocortical formations.

In our studies (8), transitory formations have been distinguished and described in detail both within the neocortex and on its border to the entorhinal cortex in dog (Fig. 5). For example, in the dog, area OP (area occipito-parietalis) shows architectonic features of the neighboring visual (O_2) and parietal (P) areas. Somatosensory areas Pc_1 and Pc_3 gradually go over into the motor cortex and elsewhere. To some degree such transition is typical of the parietal and other cortical regions in cat.

These findings are supported by studies of the functional organization of the parietal cortical region. The functional heterogeneity of the parietal association cortex has been demonstrated not only in our studies but also

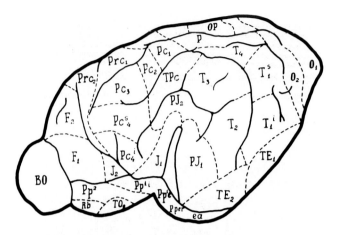

FIG. 5. Map of cytoarchitectonic areas of the dog brain. (From ref. 8.)

in those of Narikashvili and Timchenko (37), Batuyev et al. (15), Kazakov et al. (28), and others. As a matter of fact, neurons of the posterior aspects of the parietal region respond primarily to visual stimuli, while those of the anterior parts react mainly to somatic ones. Parietal cortical neurons exhibit a high degree of convergence (17). Sixty percent of neurons were found to respond to complex sensory stimulation in cat (14).

All the above findings made it possible for us to show graphically the possibility, in principle, of interrelations between various types of vertically organized influences arriving at projection and interprojection (association) neocortical zones. According to the diagram (Fig. 6), while transiting from one structure to another, the correlation of different types of afferent influences should change in accordance with the functional hierarchy of this structure. Naturally, this diagram takes no account of quantitative values of such interrelations.

We think that motivational influences are manifested first of all on the cortical level of AS and ITS. It has been demonstrated by our co-worker Shugalev (44) that, during the conditioning of the instrumental alimentary reflex to light in cat, alimentary motivational influences resulted in greater excitation of neurons of the parietal association cortex than those of the visual region.

Thus, both in primates and subprimates, the parietal association cortex is specialized in a fairly complex manner. This assumption is supported by the results of behavioral experiments. Neurons of area 7 of the monkey's cortex incorporate fairly complex receptive areas (26). In dog, the posterior aspects of the parietal region are also related to complicated forms of the visual perception. According to Prazdnikova's findings (43), these structures are associated with the standard mechanism of recognition of visual signals differing in shape.

Primary projective zone „A"   Secondary projective zone „A"   Interprojective (associative) zone   Secondary projective zone „B"   Primary projective zone „B"

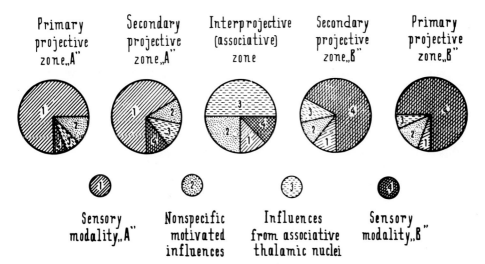

Sensory modality „A"   Nonspecific motivated influences   Influences from associative thalamic nuclei   Sensory modality „B"

FIG. 6. Diagram of the principal interrelations of different types of afferentation in the projection and interprojection cortical zones.

Following removal of the parietal cortical region, the time of conditioned running of the dog to the positive signal depends upon the number of figures presented simultaneously in combination with this stimulus (two, four, and eight images), but not accompanied by food reinforcement; whereas before the operation the time of running did not depend on the number of negative stimuli. It is noteworthy that in Prazdnikova's experiments destruction of nonprimary visual areas (areas 18 and 19) resulted in disturbances of the standard type of response to the simpler visual stimuli, i.e., when the positive signal differed from the differentiated ones in its magnitude, or in lines of different orientation.

In studies carried out in our laboratory (35), the parietal cortex has been demonstrated to play an important role in processes of discrimination of a positive consecutive heteromodal complex from its components in dog.

A very important and previously unknown peculiarity of interrelations between projection auditory and parietal association regions of the neocortex has recently been found by our co-worker, N. Popova. She has recorded potentials evoked by acoustic stimuli in the dog's cerebral cortex during the elaboration of the conditioned avoidance reflex and has come to the conclusion that, judging by evoked responses, the function of an ablated auditory zone is compensated by the parietal association region of the cortex. At the same time, in intact dogs, the conditioning of an avoidance response to sound is effected predominantly by specific auditory and sensorimotor regions of the neocortex.

The principle of correlation and interaction of vertically (subcorticocortical) and horizontally (intercortical) organized pathways of excitation conduction is very important for the analysis of mechanisms of organization of cerebral function.

Although the routes of propagation of excitation from one part of the cortex to another have been studied for a long time, the problem is far from solved.

Classics of association psychology advocated the idea of a predominantly horizontal propagation both inter- and intracortically. The discovery of the ascending activating influence of the brainstem reticular formation on the cortex suggested a predominantly vertical arrangement of integration processes and seemed to underline the concept of the importance of horizontal connections for processes of cortical zone interaction. However, the role of intercortical connections in integration has recently been attracting great neuroscientific attention once again.

Well known is the fact that in the course of evolution a distinct increase and complexity of intercortical connections is observed as well as a progressive development of long-fiber association systems. This process is reflected functionally, since the deficit in behavior resulting from the cutting of association connections has been found to be greater in monkeys than in dogs. However, we were able to demonstrate in dogs (1–4,7) that neopalliotomy (the disconnection of the frontal halves of the hemispheres from the posterior ones when the cortex and white matter are cut down to the lateral ventricle) has varying effects on different forms of conditioned reflexes. The neopalliotomy resulted in minor disturbances of alimentary motor conditioned reflexes (e.g., running to the foodtray). At the same time, motor avoidance (electrocutaneous stimulation of the paw) and salivatory motor-conditioned reflexes were impaired to a much greater degree and for longer periods.

A similar observation was made by our co-worker Nekludova (38) in rhesus monkeys. The neopalliotomy resulted in a severe deficit in instrumental alimentary motor-conditioned reflexes, while running to the food tray was maintained immediately after the operation. Disturbances of local forms of the conditioned reflex and disintegration of mechanisms of sensory interaction following the operation were pronounced in monkeys to a greater degree than in dogs. The disturbances of visual-motor coordination were most vividly pronounced in monkeys.

The disconnection of the hemispheres in monkeys was also accompanied by changes in different forms of behavior: a considerable decrease was observed in emotional tones, exploratory activity, and play reflexes.

According to some studies (16,20,31,32), systems of intercortical connections between widely spaced cortical regions and areas are developed to a much greater extent in primates, especially in man, than in carnivores. In Fig. 7, findings are presented obtained in studies of the cortical association connections carried out in dog by Marchi, Nauta, and Fink-Heimer methods (5,7) and the method of fiber division in the rhesus monkey (38).

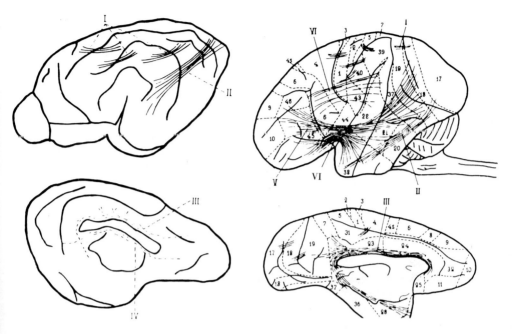

FIG. 7. Schema of the associative intercortical connections in dogs (A) and monkeys (B). **I,** short "U"-shaped fibers; **II,** occipitotemporal fascicle; **III,** cingulate band; **IV,** subcallosal fascicle; **V,** frontooccipital fascicle; and **VI,** arcuate fascicle.

While studying direct degeneration in the monkey's brain by the method of Nauta, Jones (27) came to the interesting conclusion that there existed a definite sequence and, from our point of view, an original "hierarchy" of association connections of each cortical sensory representation. For each sensory modality, Jones singled out particular transmission chains in the complex of structures interconnected by association pathways.

Association systems of the cerebrum are involved in ensuring the function of the "horizontally organized" interaction of various cortical areas. This interaction is based on common dynamogenic influences of some cortical structures on others and, probably, on the "exchange" of some streams of excitations fairly specific in their modality, and on their integration.

The importance of horizontal connection systems for intercortical integration has been recently established in acute experiments performed by our co-worker Poljakova on cat. Cooling of the visual cortical region resulted in a fairly rapid decrease in the amplitude of the evoked potential in the parietal cortex, while cooling of the latter resulted in changes of the excitability of the visual projection cortex. The analysis of temporal parameters of these changes makes it possible to suggest that they are accomplished not only by connections of these regions via subcortical structures and in particular via the posterior lateral thalamic nucleus but, primarily, by inter-cortical connections.

Original studies made by Khananshvili (30) and his co-workers testify to the possibility of transcortical transmission of excitations. They have studied functions of a neuronally isolated cortex, when the cortex and the underlying white matter have been surgically isolated from the basal ganglia and the diencephalon.

Bignall (18) suggested that the temporofrontal system of connections in monkey could be involved in the transmission of acoustic information to the frontal cortex, as it is projected to the same parts of the latter, from which evoked potentials to acoustic stimulation were registered.

Summing up the data found in the relevant literature and the results of our studies of the role of various pathways in the integration of brain processes, different possibilities of propagation and integration of excitation in the higher parts of the brain (cortex–cortex, subcortical structures–cortex, cortex–subcortical structures–cortex) can be regarded as proved.

All the above facts made it possible for us to propose (7) the idea of a "gradual but incomplete substitution" of specific excitations, during their consecutive transition from some to other structures, for the types of excitation characteristic of these structures (Fig. 8).

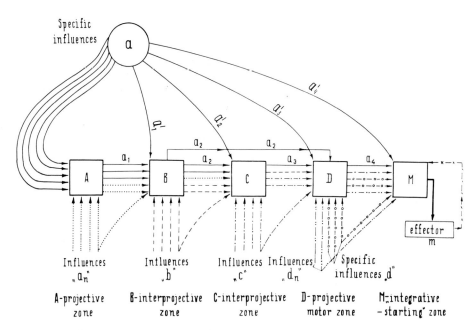

FIG. 8. Schema of "gradual but incomplete substitution" of specific excitations. Explanation in the text.

Peripheral influences (a) arriving at the cortical projection zone A are assumed to preserve their modality specificity during their spread through a number of synapses in different cortical areas up to the integrative trigger structure M. However, informative value of type "a" influences decreases in intermediate cortical structures ("interprojection zones" B, C, D, etc.), since these structures have their own specific type of peripheral influences (type b, c, d, etc.). Specificity of type "a" influence can be preserved in structure M provided $M_a > 0$, where "a" is the informative value of specific influences in the projection structure A. Preservation of the informative value of type "a" influences (a_1, a_2, a_3, a_4 . . .) spreading along the horizontal systems of connections is assisted by specific influences of the same modality ($á_1, á_2, á_3, á_4$, etc.) running through vertical channels of connections to corresponding intermediate structure B, C, D, etc. These influences are likely to sum with influences a_1, a_2, a_3 . . . and, furthermore, owing to the fairly short latency, the vertically transmitted type $á_1$ influences can provide some functional tuning of neurons of intermediate structures to the perception of type a_1, a_2, etc., influences, i.e., reduce the threshold of response of these neurons to these excitations. It is understood that in other situations there can be other interrelations. In the case of a behavioral response m (movement) evoked by the stimulus "a" or secretion in structure D, a predominantly sensory kinesthetic area of the particular integrative trigger (motor) structure, we shall observe convergence of influences a_3 and $á_3$ primarily with afferent peripheral influences of type d specific for this structure and, probably, with influences of "nonspecific" type d_n and influences produced by other structures. This convergence will be manifested in the integrative trigger structure M as well. The efferent messages formed here will reach the effector and produce a reaction m.

This hypothesis can be extended to vertically organized multineuronal forms of interaction.

Our hypothesis is supported by the results of clinical research. In this respect, studies of syndromes of "disconnection" of association connections in man made by Geschwind (25) are of particular interest.

The development of association neocortical connections is an integral part of the general process of progressive development of the forebrain. Wiener (46) said: "Progress makes not only new possibilities for the future but also new restrictions." At our institute, Filimonov (24) found divergent development of the neo- and paleocortex. In studies carried out at the Laboratory of Cytoarchitectonics of our institute (29) this tendency formed the basis of the assumption of divergent development of most and least evolved brain formations: e.g., in primates an increase is observed in the share held by phylogenetically new cortical areas, namely the inferior parietal, temporal, and frontal ones, with relative stability of the precentral region and a reduction of the limbic and occipital regions. This process is particularly characteristic of the human brain (Table 1).

TABLE 1. *The surface of the neocortical regions in man, monkeys, and apes in percent of the surface of the whole cortex*

Neocortical regions	Marmoset	Baboon hamadryad	Orangoutang	Chimpanzee	Man
Occipital	24.0	—	21.5	—	12.0
Inferior parietal	0.4	0.4	2.7	2.6	7.7
Limbic	4.2	3.8	3.0	3.1	2.1
Temporal	17.0	—	18.6	18.0	23.0
Precentral	8.3	6.8	7.6	7.6	8.4
Frontal	—	12.2	13.7	14.5	24.4

Naturally, development of the neocortex and association system in particular is accompanied by the appearance of qualitatively new functional possibilities of the brain. Nevertheless, we can assert that cortical association regions (both posterior–parietal–temporal and anterior–frontal ones) are characterized by a certain stability of their leading function in animals and man. We have already seen that the parietal cortical region is distinguished by the analysis and integration of complicated forms of sensory messages and excitations of different modalities and, on this basis, formation of simultaneous and consecutive complexes of sensory perceptions (afferent behavior programs). The frontal neocortical region is mainly concerned with the analysis and integration of complex forms of motor activity involved in the planning of reactions and mostly prognostication of behavior in new conditions.

Here are some findings obtained during many years of our studies of the function of the frontal region carried out in cooperation with the laboratory of physiology and genetics of behavior of the Moscow State University (9,10,36). Some functions of the frontal cortical region were studied in animals. This part of the cortex is developed in man most intensively and accounts for almost one-fourth of the surface of the neocortex. It is known from clinical practice that lesions to the frontal region, along with other disturbances, deprive the lesioned person of the ability to foresee the course of events and to evolve a program of behavior on the basis of the prognosis of his future activity. Similar disturbances were observed in such relatively lowly organized animals as cat and dog following operations on the frontal region (Fig. 9). The purpose of the study was to elucidate the effect of ablating the frontal cortex on the capacity of dogs and cats for elementary prognostication of the direction of a moving food stimulus disappearing from the visual field [after Krushinsky's extrapolation reflex (ER)]. In operated cats, ER changes were recorded in a simple variant of the experiment when the animals were making their way toward the feeding trough in a direction parallel to its movement behind a nontransparent screen. Particularly distinct and significant disturbances were revealed in

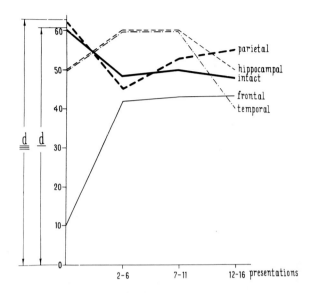

FIG. 9. The dynamics of the decision of extrapolatory task by dogs after ablation of different cortical zones. **Ordinate:** Percent of correct answers. **Abscissa:** Cue presentation. (From ref. 10.)

the dogs, which, after the operation, were given a complicated problem variant, without preliminary experience: the animal was to move in the direction opposite to that of the movement of the food. At the same time, the capacity for solving an extrapolation problem by means of conditioned learning was not impaired. A hypothesis is proposed that ablation of the frontal cortex may result in disjoining two types of reflex activity, extrapolation and conditioned ones. In these animals the frontal region is three to seven times smaller than in man. In cat and dog it accounts, respectively, for only 3 and 7% of the neocortex. Nevertheless, its destruction results in disturbances of the mechanism ensuring the animal's adequate behavior in new conditions.

Elucidation of general mechanisms of disturbances of this ability in man and animals contributes to a better understanding, from the biological point of view, of the formation and structural organization of one of the most important manifestations of the mental activity of the man—foresight, as a basis of high psychic functions.

Our recent studies carried out in cooperation with Urmancheyeva and Panina (Institute of Experimental Pathology and Therapy, USSR Academy of Medical Sciences) testify to a sufficiently distinct functional differentiation in the dorsolateral frontal cortex of the baboon. Noteworthy is the fact that the frontal cortex has been found to be differentiated according to areas. Thus, removal of area 10, exhibiting a tendency to increase in primates, results in the most severe disturbances in behavior as well as in a stable hyperactivity. In such monkeys the solution of different types of extrapolation problems was found to be significantly impaired, whereas the extirpation of area 9 had practically no effect on the high level of solving extrapolation problems of various complexities. Highly significant differences in the character and degree of disturbances of other forms of higher nervous activity were observed in monkeys during selective removal of areas 9, 10, and 47 of the frontal cortical region.

These and other findings support von Economo's words: "It is probable that each area has a special physiologic function, significance of which is not yet known, but the effect of the activity between them represents what we call a cerebral function. At the present time we must leave alone this speculation as to the physiologic significance of each area. . . but we may correlate our anatomical knowledge with our physiological experiences" (22).

The rapid development of neurology makes it possible to regard the data on functional differentiation of both projection and association neocortical regions no more as mere speculation.

REFERENCES

1. Adrianov, O. S. (1960): Motor avoidance conditioned reflexes in dogs after disconnection of cortical ends of analysers (in Russian). *Zh. Vyssh. Nerv. Deait.,* 10:377–385.
2. Adrianov, O. S. (1960): Integration of analysers in the elaboration of motor food conditioned reflexes (in Russian). *Zh. Vyssh. Nerv. Deiat.,* 10:851–859.
3. Adrianov, O. S. (1962): The influence of neopalliotomy on different components of food condition reflex in dogs (in Russian). *Zh. Vyssh. Nerv. Deiat.,* 12:835–843.
4. Adrianov, O. S. (1966): On the structural premises of the conditioned closure. In: *Evolution of the Forebrain,* edited by R. Hassler and H. Stephan, pp. 338–345. Thieme, Stuttgart.
5. Adrianov, O. S. (1970): On the structural organization of closure brain activity (in Russian). In: *Rukovodstvo po Physiologii, Physiologia Vysshei Nervnoi Deaitellnosti, Part 1, Nauka,* pp. 40–74. Moscow.
6. Adrianov, O. S. (1974): On thalamic projections of the cat parietal cortex (in Russian). *Zh. Vyssh. Nerv. Deiat.,* 24:596–605.
7. Adrianov, O. S. (1976): On the principles of organization of brain integrative activity (in Russian). *Medizina (Moscow),* 280 pp.
8. Adrianov, O. S., Mering, T. A. (1959): *Atlas of the Dog's Brain* (in Russian). Medgiz, Moscow, 237 pp. See also: E. Domino (ed.) (1964): *Atlas of the Canine Brain,* Ann Arbor, Mich., 349 pp.
9. Adrianov, O. S., Molodkina, L. N. (1971): Complicated form of extrapolatory reflex in dogs after prefrontal lobectomy (in Russian). *Zh. Vyssh. Nerv. Deait.,* 21:914–921.
10. Adrianov, O. S., Molodkina, L. N. (1972): Decision of the extrapolatory task by dogs before and after prefrontal lobectomy (in Russian). *Zh. Vyssh. Nerv. Deait.,* 22:726–734.
11. Adrianov, O. S., Orlova, T. V., and Shugalev, N. P. (1973): Characteristics of responses in the cat parietal and visual cortical areas to photic stimuli of different biological significance (in Russian). *Zh. Vyssh. Nerv. Deait.,* 23:1003–1010.
12. Adrianov, O. S., Poljakova, A. G. (1972): The peculiarities of connection of the ventrobasal complex of the thalamus with the parietal and somatosensory cortical regions in cat (in Russian). *Zh. Vyssh. Nerv. Deait.,* 22:1039–1045.
13. Adrianov, O. S., Poljakova, A. G., Orlov, B. N., and Gelashvili, D. B. (1975): The influence of neurotropic factors on the evoked potentials of associative and projective neocortical regions of the cat (in Russian). *Zh. Vyssh. Nerv. Deait.,* 25:1035–1043.
14. Artemenko, D. P., Mamonez, T. M. (1972): Neuronal reactions in cat to different stimuli (in Russian). *Neurophysiologia,* 4:375–383.

15. Batuyev, A. S., Vasiljeva, L. A., Kulikov, G. A., Keliaev, V. G., Pirogov, A. A., and Tairov, O. P. (1969): Comparative analysis of the nature of associative evoked potentials in frontal and parietal cortical regions (in Russian). Vsesouz, symposium. *"Electric. Reakt. Kori Golov. Mozga na Afferent Razdrazhenia."* Kiev, 10.
16. Bechterev, V. M. (1899): *Die Leitungsbahnen im Gehirn und Rückenmark.* Leipzig, Georgi, 692 pp.
17. Bental, E., Bihari, B. (1963): Evoked activity of single neurons in sensory association cortex of the cat. *J. Neurophysiol.,* 26:207–214.
18. Bignall, K. E. (1969): Bilateral temporofrontal projections in the squirrel monkey: Origin, distribution and pathways. *Brain Res.,* 13:319–327.
19. Brodmann, K. (1909): *Vergletchende Lokalisationslehre der Grosshirnrinde.* Leipzig, Barth, 324 pp.
20. Dzugaeva, S. B. (1975): The pathways of human brain (in Russian). *Medizina (Moscow),* 255 pp.
21. Economo, von C. (1927): *Zellaufbau der Grosshirnrinde des Menschen.* Springer-Verlag, Berlin, 145 pp.
22. Economo, von C. (1930): Cytoarchitectony and progressive cerebration. *Psychiatr. Q.,* 4:142–150.
23. Filimonov, I. N. (1949): *The Comparative Anatomy of Mammalian Cortex* (in Russian). Medgiz, Moscow, 158 pp.
24. Filimonov, I. N. (1963): *The Comparative Anatomy of Reptilian Brain* (in Russian). Akademia Nauk USSR, Moscow, 242 pp.
25. Geschwind, N. (1965): Disconnexion syndromes in animals and man. *Brain,* 88:237–294.
26. Hyvärinen, J. (1973): Functional properties of cells in the parietal somatosensory and association cortices of the monkey. *Acta Physiol. Scand.,* Suppl. 89, 396:36.
27. Jones, E. G. (1969): Interrelationships of parieto-temporal and frontal cortex in the rhesus monkey. *Brain Res.,* 13:412–415.
28. Kasakov, V. N., Ismestjev, V. A., Perchurova, V. D. (1972): Neuronal and focal reactions of parietal associative cortex to different peripheral stimuli (in Russian). *Neurophysiologia,* 4:358–367.
29. Kesarev, V. S., Bogolepova, I. N., Trikova, O. V. (1974): On the structural criterion of evolutional complication of human brain. In: *Functional-Structural Basis of System Activity and Mechanism of Brain Plasticity* (in Russian). Trudi Instituta Mozga Amn USSR, Moscow, 111, pp. 423–428.
30. Khananshvili, M. M., Zarkeshen, A. G., and Silakov, V. L. (1971): Conditioning of single unit activity by intracortical electric stimulation of neuronal-isolated cortex (in Russian). *Sechenov, Physiological Journal of the USSR,* 57:490–496.
31. Kononova, E. P. (1926): *Anatomy and Physiology of Occipital Lobes* (in Russian). Ist Moscow State University, Moscow, 146 pp.
32. Krieg, W. J. S. (1949): Connections of the cerebral cortex. 11. The macaque. A. Topography. *J. Comp. Neurol.,* 91:1–39.
33. Krushinski, L. V. (1958): Extrapolatory reflexes as an elementary basis of rational activity in animal (in Russian). *Dokl. AN USSR,* 121:762–765.
34. Liang, C. K., Pouly, K. (1953): The "association cortex" of *Macaca mulatta.* A review of recent contributions to its anatomy and functions. *Brain,* 76:625–677.
35. Mering, T. A., Muchin, E. I. (1976): Conditioned reflex on the "pure time" and on the present stimuli after extirpation of parietal cortical region (in Russian). *Zh. Vyssh. Nerv. Deait.* (*in press*).
36. Molodkina, L. N., Adrianov, O. S. (1966): Concerning the effect of lobectomy on the ability of animals to solve elementary logical problems. XVIII International Congress of Psychology, Moscow, Part 10:121–124.
37. Narikashvili, S. P., Timchenko, A. S. (1967): About differences of cortical associative responses to different peripheral stimuli (in Russian). *Physiolog. Zh. USSR,* 53:1322–1330.
38. Nekludova, E. S. (1965): Peculiarities of conditioned reflex activity of the monkeys after disconnection of cortical ends of analyzers (in Russian). *Trudi Instituta Experimental. Patol. Therapii AMN USSR, Suchumi:* 26–29.
39. Ogawa, T. (1975): Visual input to the cat's motor cortex. *J. Physiol. Soc. Jpn.,* 37:369–370.

40. Orlova, T. V. (1971): Evoked responses to visual stimuli in the projection and associative (parietal) areas of the cerebral cortex in cat (in Russian). *Zh. Vyssh. Nerv. Deait.*, 21:597–602.
41. Poljakova, A. G. (1972): The origin of the early component of the evoked response in the associative cortex of the cat. *Electroencephal. Clin. Neurophysiol.*, 32:129–138.
42. Poljakova, A. G. (1974): The comparative analysis of the early evoked responses in motor and parietal regions (in Russian).*Zh. Vyssh. Nerv. Deiat.*, 24:138–146.
43. Prazdnikova, N. V. (1973): Three types of recognition of visual images in animals (in Russian). In: *"11 Symposium Physiol. Sensor. Systems — "Physiol. of vision,"* Leningrad, pp. 89–90.
44. Shugalev, N. P. (1972): Evoked responses in cat brain to photic stimuli electing a food procuring conditioned reflex (in Russian). *Zh. Vyssh. Nerv. Deait.*, 22:962–968.
45. Totibadze, N. K., Pirtskhalaishvili, M. S. (1972): Some new data on the direct cortical projection of the lateral geniculate body in cats (in Russian). In: *Sovrem. Problemi Deiat. i Sroeenia Centr. Nerv. System,* "Metsniereba," Tbilisi; pp. 223–229.
46. Wiener, N. (1954): *The Human Use of Human Beings: Cybernetics and Society.* Eyre & Spottiswood, London, 199 pp.

Architectonics of the Cerebral Cortex,
edited by M. A. B. Brazier and H. Petsche.
Raven Press, New York © 1978.

Electrophysiological Study of Experimental Epileptogenesis in Various Neocortical Structures During Postnatal Ontogenesis in Rabbit

D. Volanschi

Institute of Neurology and Psychiatry of the Academy of Medical Sciences, Bucharest, Romania

Electrophysiological data concerning epileptogenesis during ontogeny in various animal species, accumulated over the past 25 years, have shown that a particular brain structure possesses a different epileptogenic reactivity across successive ontogenetic stages, depending on the degree of maturation of the neurons and of their connections; on the other hand, this reactivity may differ from structure to structure in the same ontogenetic stage (2–4,7,8,12,13,19–22).

The cause of such differences can only be understood by correlating them with the morphohistological, physiological, and biochemical characteristics of the brain in various ontogenetic stages (5,6,9–11,14,17,18,21).

In previous studies (19–21) we approached the electrophysiological characteristics of the penicillin-induced neocortical focus in cats versus kittens, and we attempted to correlate them with the morphohistological data available in the literature and also with some histo- and biochemical aspects.

We shall report here on the results obtained by studying the penicillin focus in various neocortical areas of young and adult rabbits. Interpretation of surface graphoelements in terms of electrogenesis is easier to perform in a lissencephalic than in a gyrencephalic animal.

Some tentative correlations of electrophysiological patterns with available morphohistological, physiological, and biochemical information will also be made.

We investigated 89 rabbits grouped into following postnatal age groups: 1 to 3 days, 5 days, 1 week, 2 weeks, 3 weeks, 1 month, and adults.

METHODS

Local procaine anaesthesia for surgical procedures, immobilization with gallamine, and artificial ventilation were used in acute experiments. In each animal, bone flaps were removed to permit approach to the four neocortical areas selected for investigation. We chose four areas shown in Rose's (16) cytoarchitectonic atlas of the rabbit brain as the precentral granular (Prae. gr.), precentral agranular (Praec. agr.), retrosplenial (Rsg. beta), and striate (Str.) ones. The dura mater was opened and electrocorticograms were recorded from these areas by means of Ag-AgCl ball electrodes, the reference electrode being placed on the frontal or occipital bone (Fig. 1). After recording the spontaneous electrocorticogram, a 4-sq-mm piece of filter paper soaked with a total dose of 400 IU of potassium penicillin in aqueous solution was applied to one neocortical area, and recording of the local tracing as well as of those from the remaining three areas continued for at least 1 hr. For each age group, penicillin was applied to the same area in at least four animals. The electrocorticograms were recorded on an eight-channel Schwarzer machine. For each area, two recordings were concomitantly obtained using two time constants, i.e., 1 and 0.3.

The electrocorticograms were studied with reference to the following aspects: latency of the first interictal discharge; 1-hr evolution of the interictal discharges (morphology, frequency); time location of the first seizure; seizure characteristics; and seizure recurrence.

The following comparisons were made: for the same area, the patterns corresponding to each age group; for the same age group, the patterns corresponding to the various neocortical areas.

RESULTS

Figure 1 shows the electrode locations in the four neocortical areas and the smallest individual latency of the first occurring focal interictal discharges and focal seizures, comparatively in the four areas in each group studied. In the succeeding figures also, the data refer to the most reactive animals per age group and area.

Figure 2 shows the evolution of the interictal discharge frequency and of the electrical seizures per age group and per neocortical area studied over the 1-hr testing after penicillin application. The curves represent the average incidence per minute of interictal discharges over successive 5-min periods. The occurrence of seizures is marked by squares.

Figures 3 to 6 represent the penicillin focus evolution in one of the areas investigated across the seven age groups.

Figure 7 summarizes the general characteristics of the fully developed interictal discharge comparatively in the four areas investigated across the seven age groups.

It appears from Figs. 1 to 7 that for the first 3 postnatal days interictal discharges were not recordable in any area over the 1-hr testing time.

Five days following birth the single area in which penicillin application resulted in occurrence of interictal discharges was the Prae. gr. area (Figs. 1 to 7). The shortest latency of the first occurring discharge was extremely

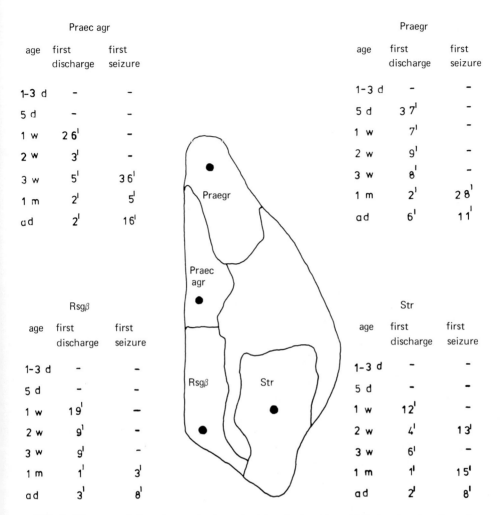

Praec agr

age	first discharge	first seizure
1-3 d	–	–
5 d	–	–
1 w	2 6^I	–
2 w	3^I	–
3 w	5^I	3 6^I
1 m	2^I	5^I
ad	2^I	1 6^I

Praegr

age	first discharge	first seizure
1-3 d	–	–
5 d	3 7^I	–
1 w	7^I	–
2 w	9^I	–
3 w	8^I	–
1 m	2^I	2 8^I
ad	6^I	1 1^I

Rsgβ

age	first discharge	first seizure
1-3 d	–	–
5 d	–	–
1 w	1 9^I	–
2 w	9^I	–
3 w	9^I	–
1 m	1^I	3^I
ad	3^I	8^I

Str

age	first discharge	first seizure
1-3 d	–	–
5 d	–	–
1 w	1 2^I	–
2 w	4^I	1 3^I
3 w	6^I	–
1 m	1^I	1 5^I
ad	2^I	8^I

FIG. 1. Diagram of dorsal aspect of cerebral hemisphere in rabbit showing location of electrodes on the four cytoarchitectonic areas explored; minimum individual values of the latencies of the first interictal discharge and of the first seizure per area and per age group.

high (37 min). The interictal discharge morphology was that of a monophasic, surface-negative or biphasic initially surface-negative slow wave; the shortest duration of the negative wave could reach 800 msec, and the shortest duration of the discharge as a whole was 2 sec or even more (at time constant 1). The maximum amplitude of this slow discharge never exceeded 110 μV. The shortest interval between two discharges was 2 sec. A third, slower, surface-negative component was recorded, mostly using a long time constant. At no time were repetitive discharges noted in the form of electrical seizure followed by silence.

One week following birth, interictal discharges were present in all the

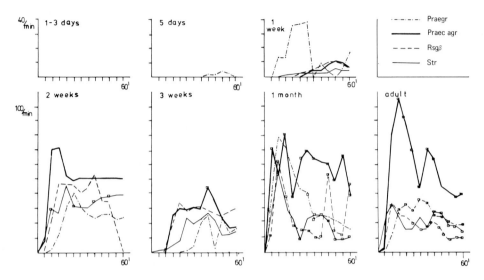

FIG. 2. Interictal discharge incidence and seizure occurrence over 1-hr testing after penicillin application in the most reactive animal per age group and area. Average rate per minute of interictal discharge occurrence during successive 5-min periods. Seizure occurrence during a 5-min period is marked by a square. **Ordinate:** Average rate per minute of interictal discharge occurrence. **Abscissa:** Time divided into 5-min periods.

areas investigated (Figs. 1 to 7), the earliest ones (7 min) occurring in the Prae. gr. area (Figs. 1 to 3), the only area responsive also before the age of 1 week, and the latest ones (26 min) in the Praec. agr. area (Figs. 1, 2, and 4). In every area the interictal discharge morphology was the same: slow and ample waves, bi- or triphasic, with early surface-negative component (Fig. 7). The highest amplitude recorded did not exceed 230 μV. The initial negative component did not exceed 600 msec. The shortest interval between two discharges was 2 sec. Not even at 7 days were seizures recorded in the form of fast repetitive discharges followed by electrical silence. As for the interictal discharge frequency, there was a clear peak in the Prae. gr. area (Figs. 2 and 7).

Two weeks after birth, the shortest latency of the first interictal discharge was less than 10 min in all areas, the lowest (3 min) now being recorded in the Praec. agr. area (Figs. 1, 2, and 4). A marked frequency increase of the interictal discharges was evident in every area studied, the peak having moved from the Prae. gr. (1 week) to the Praec. agr. area (Fig. 2).

At 2 weeks, the initial surface negativity of the 1-week interictal discharges was replaced by positivity, either at the very first discharge (Figs. 4 and 5) or, as was more common, at the next ones (Figs. 3 and 6). The fully developed discharge had a spike-and-wave morphology (Fig. 7). Its comparatively slow negative spike (120 to 130 msec) temporarily interrupted the initial positive deflection. The spike amplitude could reach 1 mV. The

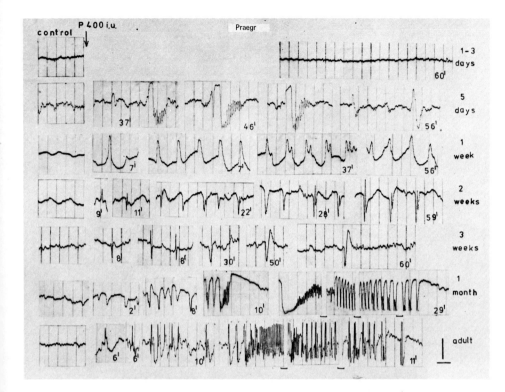

FIG. 3. Comparative development of penicillin focus in the Prae. gr. area in the most re-active animal per age group during a period of 1 hr following penicillin application. Electrocorticographic recordings with reference electrode on the nasal bone. Time location in minutes of significant graphoelements occurrence is shown by figure on respective electrocorticographic segment. In this and following figures, negativity is upward. Calibration: **Horizontal bar,** 1 sec; **vertical bar,** 50 μV for 1 to 3 and 5 days, 100 μV for 1 week, 500 μV for 2 weeks and 3 weeks, and 1 mV for 1 month and adult groups.

minimum interval between two discharges could be less than 1 sec. Longer periods of such accelerated discharge rhythms were recorded in the Praec. agr. area (Fig. 4). In the Str. area seizure-like 3 to 5/sec high-voltage waves were recorded for periods of 10 to 15 sec (Fig. 6).

Three weeks from birth the incidence of interictal discharges was lower than at 2 weeks in all areas (Fig. 2). At this age, it was only in the Praec. agr. area that the comparatively small amount of penicillin applied produced seizure patterns (Fig. 2), developing from the increasingly numerous positive afterdischarges incident upon the negative wave of the interictal discharge (Fig. 4). The frequency of the seizure discharges never exceeded 4 counts/sec.

One month following birth, the shortest latency of the first interictal discharge had decreased to 2 min and even less in every area (Figs. 1 and 3 to

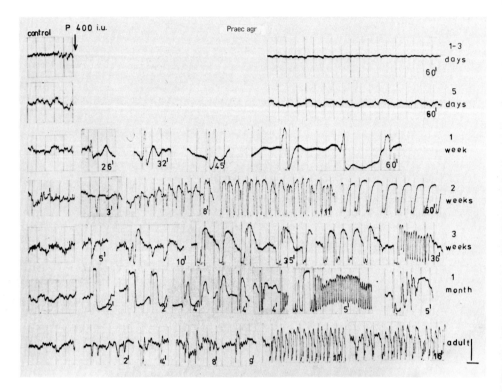

FIG. 4. Praec. agr. area. See legend to Fig. 3.

6). The general pattern of the interictal discharge did not differ from that obtained at 2 weeks, except for the occurrence also of the polyspike-and-wave morphology. The duration of the spike-and-wave complex and of its various components showed a decrease tendency. The maximum amplitude of discharges exceeded 2 mV, as a rule. The maximum frequency of discharge was higher than before, in all areas (Fig. 2); periods of rapidly succeeding interictal discharges became longer, and in all areas true focal electrical tonic-clonic seizures were also recorded (Figs. 3, 4, 5, and 6). The maximum discharge frequency during the tonic phase of the seizure was 9 to 14/sec. The earliest occurring (Figs. 1 and 2) and the most frequently recurring seizures were noted in the Praec. agr and Rsg. beta areas (15 and 10 during 1 hr, respectively). The longest seizures lasted more than 200 sec in all areas except the Prae. gr. one.

In the adult rabbit, the first interictal discharge was occurring within 2 to 6 min, with minimum latency in the Praec. agr. and Str. areas (Fig. 1). Interictal discharges were faster, the duration of the various components of the spike- or polyspike-and-wave complex being lower than in the antecedent groups (Figs. 7 and 8). The maximum amplitude of spikes was upward

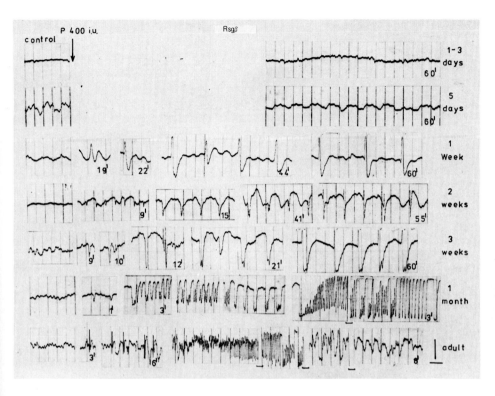

FIG. 5. Rsg. beta area. See legend to Fig. 3.

to 2 mV; the incidence of the interictal discharges was much superior in the Praec. agr. area to that recorded in the remaining areas where the maximum interictal discharge incidence was lower than in 1-month-old animals, and rather close to one another (Fig. 2). The earliest occurring seizures were recorded in the Str. and Rsg. beta areas. Over the 1-hr testing period, they recurred in all areas at least eight times, the highest incidence being noted in the Praec. agr. (16 seizures during 1 hr). The maximum duration of the seizures exceeded in all areas 140 sec.

A close examination of the tracings permitted to distinguish in adult rabbits a relatively specific succession of interictal discharges as a function of the area (Fig. 9). The Prae. gr. area was characterized by grouping of three to five interictal discharges separated by intervals of a few seconds. In the Praec. agr. area, an irregular succession of spike-and-wave complexes was characteristic, very frequently the succeeding discharge occurring within a very short interval and interrupting the negative slow wave of the antecedent discharge. In the Rsg. beta area, the discharge frequency was as irregular as, although lower than, in the Praec. agr. area. In the Str. area, there was

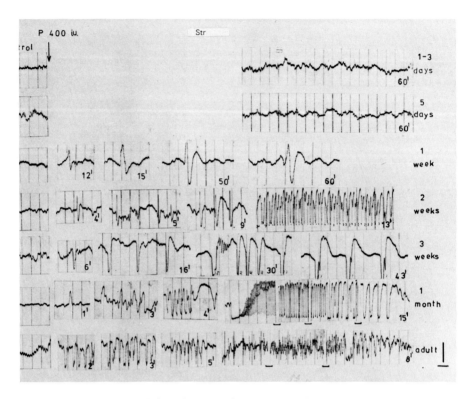

FIG. 6. Str. area. See legend to Fig. 3.

a grouping tendency of a few discharges with gradual transition from spike-and-wave to polyspike-and-wave patterns.

The general electrocorticographic appearance of the seizure, once it had set in, as well as its duration indicated no area specificity.

DISCUSSION

According to the information available in the literature (2,9,17) regarding the rabbit up to the 3rd postnatal day, the neuronal division is practically completed, since the number of neurons is 95% of the adult one. The cerebral cortex is thin and the density of neurons is great. Neurons are comparatively small, numerous neuroblasts are bipolar, and the perinuclear cytoplasm is detectable only in deep layers. The electroencephalogram during this period shows in every area solely high-frequency oscillations of low amplitude interrupted by silent periods of irregular slow waves (1 to 2.5/sec). Between the 3rd and 15th postnatal days, the first period of pallium growth takes place. In this phase, cell growth and development and branching of axons and dendrites occur. At first, between the 3rd and 10th postnatal days apical

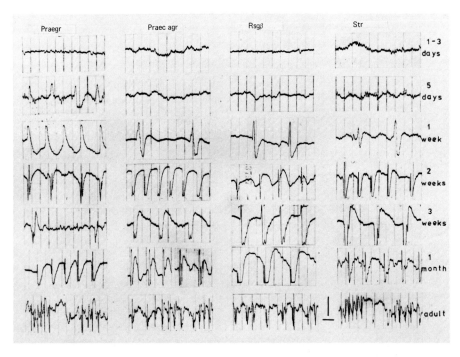

FIG. 7. General pattern of the interictal fully developed discharge comparatively in the four areas investigated across the seven age groups. Electrocorticographic recordings with reference electrode on the nasal bone. Calibration: **Horizontal bar,** 1 sec; **vertical bar,** 50 μV for 1 to 3 and 5 days, 100 μV for 1 week, 500 μV for 2 weeks and 3 weeks; and 1 mV for 1 month and adult groups.

dendrites develop, which reach only as far as the axonal plexus of the plexiform layer. The cerebral cortex is still thin and its neurons are very dense. After 10 days an outgrowth of the fibers in all directions takes place, starting from the deep layers. Basal and apical dendrites develop and the pyramidal cell axons are now possible to impregnate with silver. Between the 8th and 15th days, the electroencephalogram modifies itself, assuming its mature appearance (characterized by the occurrence of spindles at 12 to 15/sec). Maturation of EEG begins in frontal areas, at 10 days the pattern of the motor area being still immature.

The second postnatal period of pallium growth occurs between the 18th and 50th day. The ratio of specific growth of the pallium is significantly lower in the second postnatal period. Further development of dendritic plexuses is taking place now, more particularly in the deep layers, and cortex myelination begins. At 20 days, the cortical cytoarchitectonics look very similar to the mature structure, and the cerebral cortex reaches its ultimate thickness at this period. Up to 30 days, there is an incessant growth of the dendritic plexus, chiefly in the superficial layers. The spreading depression

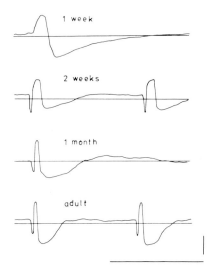

FIG. 8. Comparative aspects of fully developed interictal discharge in the Praec. agr. area at 1 week, 2 weeks, 1 month, and adult rabbit. Electrocorticographic recordings with reference electrode on the nasal bone. Time constant-1. Calibration: **Horizontal bar,** 2 sec for 1 week group; 1 sec for the remaining three groups; **vertical bar,** 50 μV for 1 week; 100 μV for 2 weeks; 1 mV for 1 month and adult rabbits.

is elicitable by potassium chloride application or DC only after the age of 3 weeks, the rate of propagation being in 24- to 30-day-old rabbits the same as in adults (2). Slow potential changes and increase in the impedance of the cerebral cortex accompany the occurrence of spreading depression.

After 55 days from birth there is no gain in palleal weight.

Our data show that during completion of neuronal division until the 3rd postnatal day, the neocortical structure is unable to develop any electrical epileptogenic activity on application of about 100 IU of potassium penicillin per square millimeter of surface. Overall neocortical epileptogenic immaturity is paralleled by overall spontaneous electrocorticographic tracing immaturity. Interictal discharges start occurring only on the 5th postnatal day in the precentral agranular area (frontal cortex), growing more frequent on the 7th day, while the remaining areas, still silent at 5 days, start firing slow discharges at 7 days only, paralleling EEG maturation at first in the frontal and then in the remaining areas. The biphasic, initially surface-negative character of the interictal discharge on the 5th and 7th postnatal days, first period of pallium growth, suggests, considering also the morpho-histological information, that at this stage the postsynaptic epileptogenic activity in the rabbit's neocortical neurons is generated in the superficial neuropil, at the apical dendrite level. The succeeding positive component probably corresponds especially with the propagation of depolarization in the depth of the cortex to cell bodies and proximal parts of apical dendrites. Surface postsynaptic hyperpolarization phenomena may also be considered, as the interictal potential reflects extracellularly a wide and complex summation of EPSPs and IPSPs (15). The late appearance of the first discharges, their low frequency and the slowness of their different components are due to the functional peculiarities of the immature neocortical neurons and of

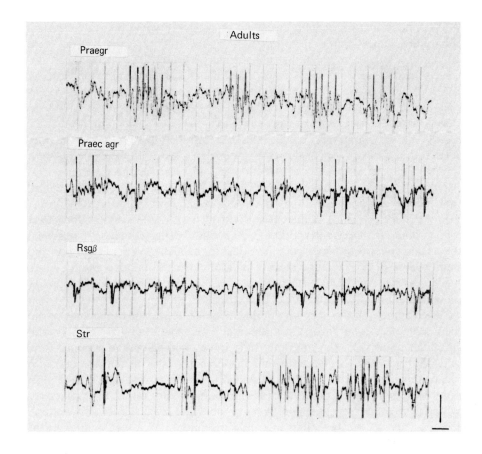

FIG. 9. Comparative sequences of fully developed interictal discharges in the four areas explored in adult rabbit. Electrocorticographic recording with reference electrode on the nasal bone. Calibration: **Horizontal bar,** 1 sec; **vertical bar,** 1 mV.

their connections. Their high threshold of excitability and their great fatigability were demonstrated in kittens by Purpura et al. (14) and Crighel et al. (6). PSPs evoked in immature neocortical neurons differ from those observed in adults. EPSPs have a slow rise time and are extremely long lasting. IPSPs are also of very long duration. These characteristics are also accountable by delayed enzymatic inactivation of synaptic transmitters (15). In kittens again, it was shown that the slow interictal penicillin discharges evoked in the neocortex correspond, on intracellular recordings, to depolarization shifts of longer duration and greater variability than in the adult animal. That no afterdischarge phenomena and no passage from interictal discharges to a self-sustained seizure were noted may be, to a certain extent, explained by the poor development of axon collaterals, internuncial neurons, intracortical horizontal connections, and also of some corticosubcortical connections. Consequently, intracortical and corticosubcortical neuronal chains and reverberating circuits involved in the mechanism of initiation and maintenance of the epileptic seizure in adults are still undeveloped.

The growth since the 10th postnatal day of the basilar dendrites, axon collaterals, and apical dendritic collaterals, starting from the deep layers, i.e., the development of the deep neuropil and consequently the prevalence of the deep seat of generation of the discharge, can explain why from this stage the initial polarity of the interictal fully developed discharge becomes surface positive. The discharges occurring first may still be surface negative because of the immediate action of penicillin at the surface. In Bishop's (2) study on neocortical strychnine spike in the postnatal rabbit, the spikes recorded during the first postnatal week were slow, biphasic, initially surface negative, just as the penicillin interictal discharge. At 2 weeks after birth, the strychnine spike assumes a triphasic character, initially surface positive, just as the penicillin discharge again. A morphology reversal in the same way was noted in rabbit between the 11th and 21st postnatal days on the evoked response in the visual cortex (9). Noteworthy is the stereotyped configuration of the immature cortex evoked activity, elicited by physiological and pathological agents.

As for the surface-negative spike of the penicillin spike-and-wave interictal discharge, it is possible that its generation involves postsynaptic depolarization in the superficial layers and propagation to the surface of the depolarization initiated in the deep layers. According to Ajmone Marsan (1), the penicillin effect is an enhancement of neuronal excitatory influences and a blocking of the inhibitory ones. The higher degree of functional maturation of the neurons, the lowering of the threshold of excitability, and the decrease of fatigability (6,9) account for the earlier appearance of the discharges and for the shorter duration and raised frequency. The still-reduced degree of maturation of intracortical and corticosubcortical connections may account for the reduced tendency to afterdischarges and to transition from the interictal discharges to self-sustained seizures.

The higher epileptogenic capacity of the Praec. agr. area as compared to the other three areas, noted at 2 weeks after birth, points to a more advanced maturation of the motor neocortex, to which new motor acquisitions correspond at this age behaviorally also. The capacity of the Str. area for developing short seizures at 2 weeks of age is paralleled by visual cortex maturation which occurs concomitantly with eye opening at 10 days. An initially surface-positive phase of the visual cortical response was noted on the 12th postnatal day, as well as a further progressive amplifying of this phase (9).

Rather unaccountable seems to be the relative frequency decrease of interictal discharges in all the areas studied at the age of 3 weeks. From physiological evidence, it emerges that spreading depression in rabbit neocortex can be induced for the first time at this age only (17). In its determinism, a specific part is played by apical dendrite development. In this stage of maturation, certain inhibitory mechanisms may be incriminated, likely to reduce the frequency of interictal discharge and the seizure development tendency also.

At the age of 1 month the morphohistological development of the brain reaches the stage permitting passage from focal neocortical interictal discharges to self-sustained seizures beginning with fast repetitive oscillations which pass into high-voltage slow waves and are concluded by electrical silence. The mechanism of epileptic synchronization approximates the complexity characterizing the mature brain, based on highly developed superficial dendritic plexuses, basilar dendrites, axon collaterals of pyramidal cells, internuncial neurons, and synaptic spines. Among the four areas of the neocortex studied, the motor one retains the highest epileptogenic capacity that will persist in the adult too.

Undoubtedly, the relatively specific succession of the interictal discharges in the various neocortical areas studied depends on the local cytoarchitecture as well as on the vertical corticothalamocortical connections of the given area. Our present data permit no discussion of the role played by subcortical structures. These are known to progressively generate secondary oscillations which play a significant part in the development and arrest of the focal seizure.

The general characteristics of the postnatal evolution of the penicillin neocortical focus in rabbit reported here are identical to those found in a previous study in cat (21); they are therefore likely to suggest similar development of neocortical epileptogenic mechanisms in both species.

As already mentioned above, the epileptogenic functional immaturity of the neocortical structures in early postnatal stages has not only morphohistological but also biochemical and histochemical correlates. An example of this are the data concerning the development of the alkaline and acid phosphatase in the immature and mature neocortex in cat (21). In agreement with Bishop's (2) data in rabbit, we failed to find any significant differences in alkaline phosphatase reaction between immature and mature neocortex.

On the contrary, the acid phosphatase reaction showed wide differences. In kittens versus cats, the reaction was somewhat weaker at the cell-body level, four times weaker at the neuropil level, and exceedingly weak in the white matter. Certain authors consider the acid phosphatase, found in a larger amount than the alkaline one in the adult brain, to be of greater importance for the metabolic function of the nerve cell. The poor development of the acid phosphatase at the neuropil and white-matter levels in the immature neocortex should be kept in mind when the interpretation of differences in epileptogenesis between immature and mature neocortex is attempted.

REFERENCES

1. Ajmone-Marsan, C. (1969): Acute effects of topical epileptogenic agents. In: *Basic Mechanisms of the Epilepsies,* edited by H. H. Jasper, A. A. Ward, and A. Pope. Little, Brown, Boston.
2. Bishop, E. J. (1950): The strychnine spike as a physiological indicator of cortical maturation in the postnatal rabbit. *Electroenceph. Clin. Neurophysiol.,* 2:309–315.
3. Cadilhac, J., Passouant Fontaine, T., Mihailovic, L., and Passouant, P. (1960): L'épilepsie expérimentale du chaton en fonction de l'âge. Etude corticale et sous-corticale. *Pathol. Biol. (Paris),* 8:1571–1581.
4. Caveness, W. F., Nielsen, K. C., Yakovlev, P. I., and Adams, R. D. (1962): Studies of epilepsy during the maturation of the monkey. *Epilepsia (Amsterdam),* 3:137–150.
5. Caveness, W. F. (1969): Ontogeny of focal seizures. In: *Basic Mechanisms of the Epilepsies,* edited by H. H. Jasper, A. A. Ward, and A. Pope. Little, Brown, Boston.
6. Crighel, E., Sotirescu, N., and Marcovici, N. (1965): Reactivity of the cat immature neocortex to direct stimulation. *Rev. Roum. Neurol.,* 2:45–52.
7. Crighel, E. (1971): Experimental data concerning the epileptic activity in immature kittens. *Rev. Roum. Neurol.,* 8:47–53.
8. French, J. D., Gernandt, B. E., and Livingston, R. B. (1956): Regional differences in seizure susceptibility in monkey cortex. *Arch. Neurol. Psychiatry,* 75:260–274.
9. Hunt, W. E., and Goldring, S. (1951): Maturation of evoked response of the visual cortex in the postnatal rabbit. *Electroenceph. Clin. Neurophysiol.,* 3:465–471.
10. Marinescu, G., and Kreindler, A. (1935): *Des Réflexes Conditionnels. Etudes de Physiologie Normale et Pathologique.* Felix Alcan, Paris.
11. Nobak, C. R., and Purpura, D. P. (1961): Postnatal ontogenesis of cat neocortex. *J. Comp. Neurol.,* 117:291–308.
12. Passouant, P., Cadilhac, J., Ribstein, M., Passouant-Fontaine, T., and Mihalovic, L. (1960): *Epilepsie et Maturation Cérébrale,* Report at the XVIIth Congress of the Association des Pédiatres de Langue Française, Montpellier, 12–14 Oct. 1959, edited by Centre d'Electroencéphalographie des Hôpitaux de Montpellier, 82 pp.
13. Prince, D. A., and Gutnik, M. (1971): Cellular activities in epileptogenic foci of immature cortex. *Proc. Internat. Union Physiol. Sci.,* 9:460 (*Abstract*).
14. Purpura, D. P., Carmichael, M. W., and Housepian, E. M. (1960): Physiological and anatomical studies on development of superficial axodendritic synaptic pathways in neocortex. *Exp. Neurol.,* 2:324–347.
15. Purpura, D. P. (1969): Stability and seizure susceptibility of immature brain. In: *Basic Mechanisms of the Epilepsies,* edited by H. H. Jasper, A. A. Ward, and A. Pope., Little, Brown, Boston.
16. Rose, M. (1931): Cytoarchitektonischer Atlas der Grosshirnrinde des Kaninchens. *J. Psychol. Neurol.,* 43:353–440.
17. Schadé, J. P. (1959): Maturational aspects of EEG and spreading depression in rabbits. *J. Neurophysiol.,* 22:245–257.
18. Scherrer, J., and Oeconomos, D. (1955): Réponses évoquées corticales somesthésiques

des mammifères adultes et nouveau-nés. In: *Les Grandes Activités du Lobe Temporal*, edited by D. Albe-Fessard et. al., pp. 249–268. Masson, Paris.

19. Volanschi, D. (1960): Cercetări experimentale asupra reactivității convulsivante a creierului imatur (in Romanian). *St. Cerc. Neurol.,* 5:505–515.
20. Volanschi, D., Sterescu, N., Voiculet, N., and Leca Mioara (1961): Studiul comparativ al capacității convulsivante a creierului imatur și matur. Cercetări cu P^{32} (in Romanian). *St. Cerc. Neurol.,* 6:291–302.
21. Volanschi, D. (1972): Experimental research on the ontogenetic development of the mechanism of epileptic synchronization. Comparative study on the immature and mature brain. In: *Synchronization of EEG Activity in Epilepsies,* edited by H. Petsche and M. A. B. Brazier., pp. 189–203. Springer-Verlag, Wien.
22. Yakovlev, P. I. (1962): Maturation of cortical substrata of epileptic events. *World Neurol.,* 3:299–315.

Architectonics of the Cerebral Cortex,
edited by M. A. B. Brazier and H. Petsche.
Raven Press, New York © 1978.

Cortical Architectonics: General and Areal

Valentino Braitenberg

*Max Planck-Institut für Biologische Kybernetik,
Tübingen, Federal Republic of Germany*

The most significant development since the time of von Economo is the shift of emphasis from the brain considered as a collection of cells to the brain considered as a network of fibers, from the neuropathologist's view of the brain to that of the computer engineer; in short, from Nissl pictures to wiring diagrams. Of course, Golgi preparations, which are almost wiring diagrams, had already been invented, but the work of Cajal (7) was largely ignored by those neuroanatomists who called their work "architectonics." They would occasionally use Weigert preparations, which also show fibers, but only for macroscopical purposes, since myelin stains are disappointing at higher magnification and are hardly apt to conjure a picture of the filigrane nature of the neuropil as we see it today.

Thus, architectonics 50 years ago was little more than the recognition of the different histological "styles" of cortical areas in Nissl and Weigert preparations viewed at low magnification, with the goal of putting them in relation to the different "styles" of the neurological symptoms which are produced by the destruction of these areas. Nobody, at that time, would even seriously ask the question of a possible *causal* connection between the style of the wiring and the type of performance. Wiring, computation, logic, messages, signals, storage, and retrieval of information were concepts which had either not been formulated yet or belonged to domains far removed from neuroanatomy.

The question is now: what sense can we make out of "architectonics" when we interpret the structural differences of the areas as indicating variations of a common computing scheme, locally applied to different tasks? The answer can only be tentative, since before we can hope to do "areal architectonics" we must try to solve the problems of "general architectonics" of the cortex. This paper is intended as a contribution to speculations on the nature of the generalized cortical machinery, with some anatomical data from the mouse cortex to support those ideas which are at variance with current views.

THE BIG QUESTIONS

The great success of single neuron recording in response to sensory stimulation should not obscure the remaining difficulties in our understanding of the cerebral cortex. Here are some:

(1) Activities of single neurons in sensory regions are correlated with partial *features* of the relevant situations in the input (e.g., moving objects, animals, places), not with the things themselves. Similarly, activities of individual motor neurons are correlated with very partial aspects of the motor response. Therefore, things in the input must be represented by *sets* of neurons and motor responses by different sets. The way we respond to specific situations by means of specific motor responses must be defined in the brain by sets of fibers connecting sets of input neurons to sets of output neurons. We don't even know how this could be done theoretically without getting involved in exorbitantly complicated schemes, let alone how it is actually done in the brain.

(2) It is easy to recognize a histological (e.g., Golgi) preparation as being cortex rather than cerebellum or tectum. It is much more difficult to tell whether it is human or bovine, motor, sensory, or associative cortex. The typical wiring of the cortex, which is invariant irrespective of local functional specialization, must be the substrate of a special kind of operation which is typical for the cortical level. We have difficulties in trying to imagine a kind of computation which makes equally good sense in sensory, motor, language-related, and other areas of the brain, in man, in the cow, in the mouse, or in the alligator. Theoretical schemes that have been proposed for the function of the cerebral cortex and similar schemes proposed (sometimes by the same author) for the cerebellar cortex or for other pieces of grey substance look much less different than the corresponding histological preparations. Apparently we have not really understood why the brain is articulated in many suborgans with different wiring and, in particular, we have no explanation why the histology of the cortex is what it is.

(3) There is a strong suspicion that memory is layed down in the cortex in the form of an ongoing modification of the pattern of internal connections. We do not know which parts of the synaptic apparatus are involved in this, nor do we know whether such a scheme is sufficient to account for all aspects of memory and, especially, what the mechanisms of inscription and retrieval of this memory are. All we know is that certain structures at the margin of the cortical sheet must be intact for new memory traces to be accepted.

Work in our laboratory in recent years was related to question (2) and to some extent (see also Schüz, *this volume*) to question (3). The aim is also to set the scene for theoretical approaches to the big question, (1).

A MODEL CORTEX: MUS MUSCULUS

The mouse has a small cortex, containing about $^1/_{1,000}$ of the neurons of the human cortex. The variety of neurons in it [like in the cortices of other rodents (7)] is less pronounced than in larger mammals. Still, the main types of neurons in the mouse cortex are the same as in other animals and also the layering of the cortex is essentially similar. Also, a definite areal variation both of the arrangement and of the shape of neurons can be observed in the mouse, so that we can expect to be able to study in this simple model cortex the most impressive feature of larger cortices, the local variation, related to functional specialization, of a unitary wiring scheme.

The account I am presenting here is based on the study of several series of sections stained with the Nissl, Heidenhein Woelke (for myelin), and Bodian technique and of 157 Golgi preparations, prepared with the modification proposed by Colonnier (8). Electron microscopy was done on material fixed in glutaraldehyde and stained with osmium, uranium, and lead.

SIZE, SHAPE, AND LIMITS

Each cerebral hemisphere of the mouse has roughly the shape of a truncated cone, with the narrow end pointing forward. The cortex covers the dorsal, lateral, posterior, and part of the basal aspect of the cone. The limits of the cortex are well defined almost everywhere by layers of white substance that separate it from adjoining grey structures, except for a somewhat uncertain transition between the basal frontal olfactory cortex and the septal nuclei on one hand and the continuity of the cortical grey substance with that of the striatum via the amygdala on the other.

In the terminology I adopt here, the hippocampus belongs to the cortex and so does the olfactory nucleus because both contain a majority of neurons of the "pyramidal cell" type, clearly oriented in a cortex-like array continuous with the rest of the cortex. On the other hand, the amygdala does not belong to the cortex because in it the cortical array is lost, nor does the fascia dentata because the layer of its (nonpyramidal) neurons is nowhere continuous with any of the cortical layers but is rather oriented at right angles to the plane of the cortex. A similarly detached band of grey substance, the induseum griseum, less conspicuous than the fascia dentata, accompanies the margin of the cortical hemisphere outside of the hippocampal region. The neurons of the induseum, like those of the fascia dentata, are different from pyramidal cells because their dendrites leave the cell bodies all within a conical region, with no dendrites going in the opposite direction. It is worth noting that (almost) all neurons of the frog pallium are of this morphological type, even if I do not want to suggest that the extra band of atypical cortex at the margin of the higher vertebrate pallium (the fascia dentata and the induseum griseum) is a residuum of an earlier, less successful cortex.

The surface of the mouse cortex is about 1 cm^2 on each side. The thickness is between 0.7 and 0.8 mm in our Golgi preparations, which show less shrinkage than the paraffin series.

TYPES OF NEURONS

Most of our Golgi preparations gave excellent results in the sense that each contained at least 100 well-stained cortical neurons. By this I mean complete staining of dendrites and of a well-ramified intracortical axonal tree (Fig. 1). Axons leaving the cortex could usually not be followed to their destination because of the insufficient thickness of our preparations (100 to 120 μm), nor was an attempt made to follow intracortical axons or dendrites from one section into neighboring sections. However, under the supposition of a spherical (stellate cells, basal dendrites) or cylindrical (apical dendrites of pyramidal cells) symmetry of the ramification, the portion of the neuron contained in one section could be used to extrapolate the parts that were cut off. This is possible especially if the neuron is well centered in the section and oriented parallel to it.

This large material, an estimated 10,000 neurons, several hundreds of which were well oriented in the section, sufficed to confirm the traditional classification of cortical neurons in three main types. A discussion of each follows.

Pyramidal Cells (Fig. 2a–c)

These are characterized by: (a) an apical dendrite reaching the first layer, (b) an average of from 1.5 to 2.8 spines per micron dendritic length (27), (c) an axon leaving the cortex at the base, after a straight vertical course, (d) relatively straight axon collaterals, which may in turn have relatively straight branches of the second order.

The total length of the dendritic arborization of pyramidal cells in the mouse cortex is about 3 or 4 mm, that of the intracortical axon ramification about the same or slightly more. The values for the neuron of Fig. 2a are: dendrites, 3,200 μm; axons, 2,700 μm. For Fig. 2b they are: dendrites, 4,000 μm; axons, 4,700 μm. For Fig. 2c they are: dendrites, 3,100 μm; axons, 6,000 μm. These values were obtained by measuring the projected length of the fibers on camera lucida drawings enlarged 1,000 times and by applying a correction by a factor $\pi/2$ to account for the different orientations of the segments measured. In fact, under the supposition that all orientations are equally probable, the average shortening equals the average of the cosine for all angles α between 0 and $\pi/2$ ($\alpha = 0$ when the fiber is parallel to the section)

$$\frac{1}{\pi/2} \int_0^{\pi/2} \cos \alpha \, d \, \alpha = \frac{2}{\pi}$$

A further correction factor $4/3 \times r/d$ (= volume of the sphere with radius r/volume of the cylinder with radius r and height d) was applied under the

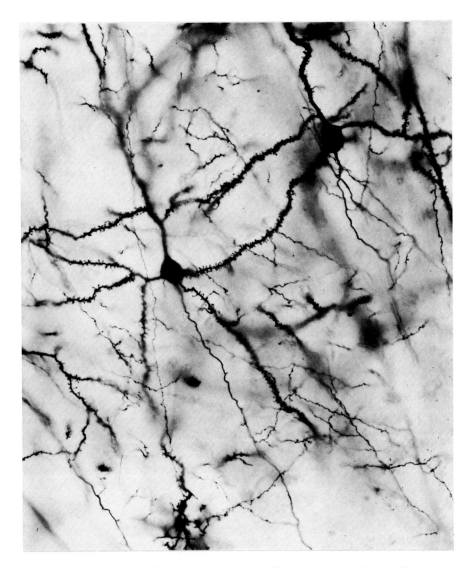

FIG. 1. Some pyramidal cells of the mouse cortex. Example of a satisfactory Golgi stain.

assumption that the total ramification was contained in a sphere of radius r when the segments measured were contained in a circular region with diameter 2r in a section of thickness d.

The first correction tends to fall short of the real value since segments almost perpendicular to the plane of the drawing would be overlooked in the measurements. On the contrary, the second correction is strictly justified only when the density of the ramifications is constant throughout the spheri-

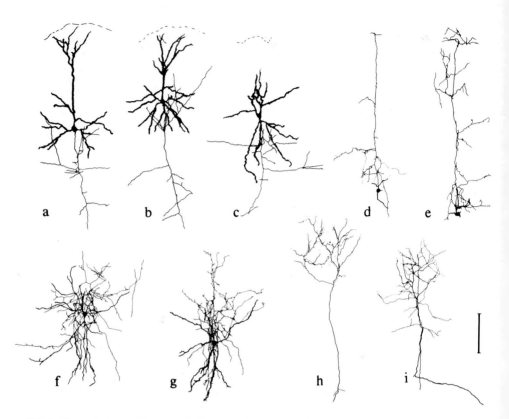

FIG. 2. The main types of neuronal elements of the cortex. Camera lucida drawings, mouse. The bar on the right indicates 100 μm. **a–c:** Pyramidal cells. **c:** From the lower part of the hemisphere, where the arrangement of the neurons becomes similar to that in the "allocortex." **d, e:** Martinotti cells. **f, g:** Stellate cells. **h, i:** Afferent fibers ("specific afferents"). In **i** two fibers have telodendria which occupy almost exactly the same territory. The measurements of the dendritic and axonal lengths of these elements are mentioned in the text.

cal (or cylindrical) region and tends to exaggerate the value with star-shaped ramifications.

Martinotti Cells

No transition is possible between the preceding type and the Martinotti cells, since these are (a) characterized by an axon which runs as straight vertically upward as the axons of the pyramidal cells run downward. The terminal ramification of the axon, no matter at what height the cell body is situated, is in the first layer. (b) The collateral branches of the axon are strangely scraggy, irregularly bent, and frequently have very short, as if abortive branches. (c) The dendrites carry sparse, stubby spines, no more than about 0.3 spines per micron length.

The dendrites on Fig. 2d and e, like those of all other Martinotti cells which we found in our frontal sections, are incomplete in the sense that they leave the section on both sides. This made us suspect that they may have a preferential anteroposterior orientation. Indeed, the two Martinotti cells which we found in our (less numerous) horizontal series showed impressive dendritic ramifications, with a total dendritic length 2,000 μm in one case and 2,500 in the other. It is possible that the branches of the axon in the first layer are also oriented, and therefore much reduced in length on our frontal sections, but this could not be checked on sections with different orientation. With this caveat, the axonal tree in the cases of Fig. 2d and e measured 3,200 and 4,400 μm, respectively.

Stellate Cells

The absence of transitions is less convincing between stellate cells and Martinotti cells than between pyramidal cells and the other types. Still, common type of stellate cells can be well defined by the following character-istics: (a) dendrites arranged radially around the cell body; (b) no spines; (c) axonal tree with no definite axial orientation, contained in a roughly spherical region.

The total length of the dendritic tree in the specimen of Fig. 2f was 6,700 μm, that of the axonal tree 17,000 μm. The neuron of Fig. 2g measured 4,500 μm and 10,200 μm, respectively.

Afferent Fibers

Some fibers coming from the white substance, with terminal arborizations within the cortex were occasionally stained. Besides very loosely ramified fibers, for which the complete extent of their distribution could not be as-sessed, the well-known dense arborizations at or slightly above the half height level of the cortex were often present (Fig. 2h and i). In Fig. 2i two such arborizations seem to share the same territory. The total length of the fiber h is 5,600 μm, that of the other two fibers is 4,000 and 3,700 μm.

DIFFERENCES IN AXONAL DENSITY

Each pyramidal, Martinotti, and stellate cell contributes several milli-meters of axonal fibers to the intracortical fiber population, the stellate cell holding the record with 17 mm of axonal ramification. When comparing this value with the values for the other neuronal types, it must be remembered that the axon of pyramidal cells, as illustrated in Fig. 2 is certainly incom-plete, since its extracortical continuation and the part of the axon peripheral to its reentry into the cortex are missing. The Martinotti cell is probably incomplete, since the spread of its collaterals in the first layer of the cortex may be much wider than shown on the drawings. Thus, it is possible that for all types the total axonal length is close to 10 mm.

There is, however, a difference in the *density* of the axonal ramification produced by the three neuronal types. The pyramidal cell distributes its relatively long, straight, and unbranched collaterals in the widest territory, producing a very low density of axons per volume. The Martinotti cell has a denser ramification, as can be seen on the picture, and the stellate cell has its great length of fibers concentrated in the smallest territory. The afferent arborizations have a density about equal to that of the stellate cells.

COMPLETENESS OF THE CLASSIFICATION

It is my contention that the distinction of pyramidal cells, Martinotti cells, and stellate cells covers almost all cortical neurons in the mouse. This is at variance with Lorente de Nó's (21) account of the mouse and even more so with various descriptions of the cortex of other animals. I could always convince myself that a pyramidal cell with an apical dendrite not reaching the first layer, corresponding to Lorente de Nó's "short pyramidal cell," had in reality an apical dendrite cut by an oblique section, nor could I find any of Sholl's (28) stellate cells with axons leaving the cortex. Also, we never found a pyramidal cell with an axon stained down to the bottom of the cortex that did not have a continuation of the axon into the white substance.

The exceptions I have to admit are localized to a very exceptional part of the cortex, the "barrel field" of Woolsey and van der Loos (31). There, within the barrels, some neurons can be found (29) which by their spiny dendrites and by their descending axon would be classified as pyramidal, while the asymmetrical spread of their dendrites and axon collaterals and especially the lack of an apical dendrite does not fit this definition. It is possible that our Golgis have accidentally failed to reveal some other aberrant types of neurons, but it is not likely unless the aberrant types are very rare, or unless we want to attribute to the method a specific selectivity for pyramidal, Martinotti, and stellate cells as defined here.

CELL COUNTS

The number of neuronal cell bodies per unit volume varies a great deal with the region and especially with the depth of the cortex. The first layer is almost without neural cell bodies. The density of neural cell bodies in layers II to VI, measured in Nissl preparations and corrected for shrinkage varies between 1 and 2.5. $10^5/mm^3$. The correction was applied only for the difference in shrinkage between the Golgi and the Nissl preparations, while no attempt was made to refer the cell density to the unfixed brain. This explains in part the discrepancy between these values and those reported earlier by

Cragg (9), which were slightly below $10^5/mm^3$. The number of cortical neurons in both hemispheres must be close to 2.10^7. The number of non-neuronal nuclei, as far as one can tell from their appearance in our Nissl preparations, is about one-third that of neuronal nuclei, in accordance with a figure given by Friede (10).

The differential cell count of the three neural types is practically impossible, since the criteria available in Nissl pictures are insufficient. A very rough estimate can be made on the basis of the supposition that the band of somewhat smaller cell bodies between the upper and the lower pyramidal layer is made entirely of stellate cells, and that some (say, half) of the neurons of the lowermost layer are Martinotti cells. It turns out, then, that two-thirds or three-quarters of all cortical neurons are pyramidal cells, in some places possibly even more.

TOTAL AXONAL DENSITY

Out of the values for the neuronal density and for the axonal length contributed by each neuron we are able to calculate the total axonal density, the sum of the lengths of all axonal branches present in 1 mm^3 of gray matter. With 2.10^5 neurons/mm^3 and a more or less conservative estimate of 5 to 10 mm per neuron, we get 1 or 2.10^6 mm axon/mm^3, 1 or 2 km of axons in every cubic millimeter of cortex. If we imagine the fibers arranged in a cubic lattice, this value would correspond to a unitary mesh of a size between 1 and 2 μm. Consequently, on electron microscopical pictures of the mouse cortex one expects to find, on an average, one cross section and two long sections of axons on every square with a side of 1 or 2 μm.

A check on electron micrographs of the first layer confirms the order of magnitude, although an estimate obtained on the basis of measurements and counts of profiles which could be recognized as axons (either positively or by exclusion, if they could not be diagnosed as either dendritic, dendritic spines, or glia) was slightly higher, about 4.10^6 mm axon/mm^3. This may reflect the well-known difficulty (25) of distinguishing the finer processes of dendrites and axons. Also, it is quite likely that layer I contains relatively more axonal terminations than any of the other layers.

COMPARISON OF AXONAL AND SYNAPTIC DENSITY

It is easy to convince oneself that the order of magnitude 10^6 mm of fibers in 1 mm^3 of cortical tissue is not an exaggeration by checking it against the number of synapses in the cortex (see ref. 27). If 10^9 μm of axons are to be presynaptic to 10^9 synapses, each axon must enter a synapse on average every micron of its course. The old illustrations of axons making small numbers of "terminal bouton"—type of synapses with other neurons are highly unrealistic. The vast majority of synapses in the cortex must be "en passant."

For a comparison of the density of synapses with the density of dendritic spines, which is also of the same order of magnitude, see Schüz (ref. 26).

DENDRITIC DENSITY

The dendrites are shorter than the axons in all three major neuronal types. We may estimate the total dendritic density as about half that of the total axonal density, 0.5 to 1.10^6 mm/mm^3. This would make the frequency of synapses on dendrites even higher than that on axons, about two synapses every micron of dendritic length.

However, for the pyramidal cells, the most numerous neuronal type, this crowding of synapses is avoided because of the presence of many dendritic spines. If we add the length of all spines to the length of the dendrites, the total length of the dendritic tree of a pyramidal cell becomes about three times that without spines. The total length of the spines by themselves is about equal to that of the axons. This may be an explanation for the spiny conformation of pyramidal cell dendrites: an expedient to produce, by means of a peculiar pattern of ramification, a great total length of very thin fibers without incurring the limitations of decremental conduction in dendrites.

RELATIVE AXONAL DENSITY

For a quantitative appraisal of the coupling of neurons within the cortex it is important to know to what proportion of the total local synaptic population any one particular neuron contributes axonal terminations.

This is, of course, a function of the density of the axonal tree. In the central part of its axonal field, where the branches are densest, a stellate cell provides an estimated $^1/_{1,000}$ of the local axonal population. On the other hand, the loose tree of the axon collaterals of a pyramidal cell occupies a large region within which it provides only one part in 10,000 or even in 100,000 of the axons.

The length, lack of branches, and straight course of the axon collaterals of pyramidal cells, which are responsible for this low density, have the following interesting consequence. It is not very likely that an axon collateral of a pyramidal cell entering the dendritic territory of another pyramidal cell be connected to it more than once, except perhaps in the case that it happens to run exactly parallel to one of the dendrites. The network of axon collaterals seems to be constructed in such a way as to guarantee the greatest possible number of synaptic neighbours for each cell.

It is interesting to observe that the fibers carrying input to the cortex also have relatively low-density terminal ramifications. The densest, the "specific thalamic" afferents to the fourth cortical layer, at least in the mouse do not go much beyond a relative density of $^1/_{1,000}$. Already in the input, the excitation is not point-like, but spread over regions containing the processes of thousands of neurons.

This suggests that in the cortex no neuron and no fiber has the power to determine by itself the events within the region of its termination. Everything happens on the background of excitation and inhibition contributed by elements spread over wide regions of the cortex.

CORTICOCORTICAL CONNECTIONS

The subcortical white substance in the mouse is about 0.1 mm thick, one-seventh or one-eighth the thickness of the cortex. The corresponding value in man cannot be measured directly because of the convoluted layout of the human cortex. It may, however, be calculated approximately from its volume which, when spread out evenly over a flattened cortex, corresponds to a thickness of a few millimeters, about the same as the thickness of the cortical gray substance. Does the difference in the quantity of the corticocortical connections between mouse and man reflect a difference in the computational power of the two brains?

The subcortical white substance in the mouse is mostly composed of fibers running parallel to the plane of the cortex. In Golgi preparations these are easily recognized as axons of pyramidal cells. The separation of neighbouring fibers, as measured in Bodian preparations, is about 0.7 μm. From this the total length of fibers in the white substance of one hemisphere can be calculated as about 2.10^7 mm. If half of the cortical neurons are "associational" pyramidal cells, in the sense that they send an axon into the white substance which enters the cortex again in a different place, the average length of their subcortical trajectory turns out to be about 4 mm. This is compatible with the idea of a complete set of connections between every small region of the cortex and every other such region. In fact, it can be shown that such a scheme in a round cortex would require fibers of an average length about equal to one-half the diameter of the cortex.[1]

A similar quantitative reasoning applied to the white substance of man yields an average length of corticocortical connections of a few centimeters. Again, this is not far from what one would expect in a complete set of corticocortical connections. Hence, the principle in mouse and in man turns out to be about the same.

It is important to realize that both in the mouse and in man the number of corticocortical connections is much larger than that of cortical afferent and efferent fibers. Even the thalamus, which provides the numerically prevalent set of inputs to the cortex, in both species has only about 1% of the number

---

[1] To be precise, for a round cortex of radius r the average length of the connections is: $[(16/3\pi) - (8/9)r]$. Dr. Günther Palm's help is gratefully acknowledged.

of neurons of the cortex. Thalamic afferents, specific and aspecific, cannot be more than 1% of the afferents which enter any region of the cortex, mostly issued from other cortical regions.

The cortex is largely a reflexive machine, working on its own output.

SQUARE ROOT COMPARTMENTS

Corticocortical connections are certainly not quite as homogeneous as the preceding quantitative argument on the white substance would suggest. In man, various bundles of fibers have been described in the white substance (e.g., the occipitofrontal bundle) which seem to indicate preferential connections between certain distant cortical regions. Also in smaller animals the homogeneity cannot be absolute, since degeneration experiments (e.g., refs. 2,13) reveal a patchy distribution at least of the callosal associational fibers. Still, it is well possible that the homogeneity is at least approximately realized, and it is interesting to ask the following question: How large must a piece of cortex be in order to be informed on the state of the entire cortex, or alternatively, how large a region of cortex is required in order to send fibers to the whole rest of the cortex? The answer is, obviously, this: Under the supposition of homogeneous connections, the minimal compartment of the cortex which is to provide a fiber for every other such compartment must contain as many pyramidal cells as there are compartments (Fig. 3). Here we suppose that every pyramidal cell provides exactly one associational fiber. In other words, a natural parcelling of the cortex would be into n compartments, each containing n neurons, where n is the square root of N, the total number of pyramidal cells of the cortex. Since N is of the order 10^7 in the mouse, 10^{10} in man, $n = \sqrt{N}$ is about 3,000 in the mouse, 100,000 in man. Dividing the human cortex into 100,000 equal portions, we get compartments of a size about 1 mm, while in the mouse the size would be about 170 μm. Every such "square root compartment" could in principle be informed about the state of every other compartment.

It is interesting to observe that both in man and in the mouse the size of these square root compartments is about the same as that of the dendritic spread of the largest pyramidal cells. If the afferent fibers are well mixed

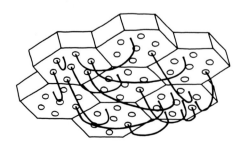

FIG. 3. Illustration of the idea of "square root compartments." In a simple cortex of 49 elements, a subdivision into $\sqrt{49}$ compartments makes it possible for each compartment to send fibers to (and to receive fibers from) each of the other compartments.

within the compartment, every pyramidal cell may have its 10^3 (in the mouse) or 10^4 (in man) inputs chosen from just as many other compartments spread over the whole rest of the cortex. In a way, every pyramidal cell is informed about the state of the entire cortex.

To see the cortical activity as an interplay of $\sqrt{N}$ compartments rather than of N neurons is justified only if within each compartment there is a high correlation of the activities of individual neurons. We may take the discovery of "columns" of neurons with uniform characteristics (14–16,23) in the somatosensory and visual areas as indicating such neighborhood correlations.

A SKELETON CORTEX

The sketch of the mouse cortex I have presented here may be summarized as follows: A set of 10 million neurons of various types are connected together by two sorts of fibers: intracortical, short-range (= a few hundred microns) and corticocortical, long-range connections. All the long-range connections and most of the short-range connections are provided by axons of the numerically prevalent neuron type, the pyramidal cells. Their number, and even more so the number of the fiber connections which they produce, is by several orders of magnitude larger than the number of fibers in the afferent and efferent channels. It should be remembered that this is not true for other "cortex-like" structures, e.g., the optic tectum of the frog, which contains no more neurons than there are afferent fibers (18,20). The large number of cells in the cerebral cortex is related to the wealth of long-range connections in the subcortical white substance. Their number and average length is compatible with the supposition that through them every small region (compartment) of the cortex is connected with every other such region, quite independently of their relative position. Since, on the other hand, the connections within the cortical grey substance must be strongly dependent on the distance (monosynaptic connections are limited to a range of 1 mm or little more), the combination of metric (intracortical, short-range) and ametric (corticocortical, long-range) connections may be an essential feature of the cerebral cortex (24).

To make this clearer, we consider a skeleton cortex with everything left out except pyramidal cells and some of the afferent fibers (Fig. 4). This should be a reasonable simplification, mainly because pyramidal cells are the only elements that are constant constituents of the cortex in all of its variations, and also because they are the neurons which only occur in the cortex. Their most distinguishing feature is the bipartite dendritic tree, with one expansion always near the surface of the cortex (apical dendrites), and another (basal dendrites) which may (isocortex) or may not (hippocampus) be situated at varying depths in the cortex. We have already established that most of the cortical fiber population is provided by the axons

special case 1
olfact.input

general case: Py - Py - connections
long range: A; short range: B

special case 2
other sensory input

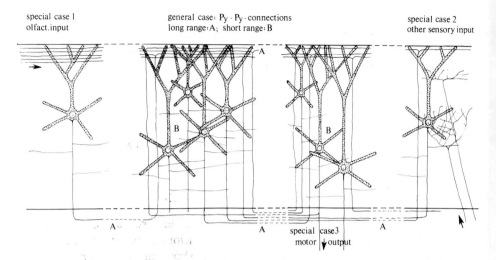

special case 3
motor ↓ output

FIG. 4. The "skeleton cortex" made only of pyramidal cells **(py)** and their connections. **A system:** Apical dendrites, long fibers through the white substance. **B system:** basal dendrites and axon collaterals. The sensory and motor regions are considered special cases of this general scheme.

of the pyramidal cells, which are also bipartite, since their intracortical collaterals enter the system of metric, short-range connections, while the main axons make up the system of ametric, long-range connections. The latter, simplifying a little the data available in the literature [e.g., (2,30)], have their terminations mostly in the first (uppermost) layer of the cortex. On the contrary, the axon collaterals are distributed through the lower layers. It is reasonable to assume, then, that the apical dendrites of a pyramidal cell receive mainly the long-range connections from other pyramidal cells, while the basal dendrites have the axon collaterals of neighboring pyramidal cells as their main input. We may say that each pyramidal cell couples, in its dendritic tree, circuits pertaining to the two systems: A system (apical dendrites, main axons, nonmetrically dependent corticocortical connections) and B system (basal dendrites, axon collaterals, metrically dependent, short-range connections).

This vast system of doubly coupled elements, the pyramidal cells with their A and B connections, is connected with the rest of the nervous system by input and output fibers.

The output poses no problem. It is nothing but a crude version of the state of the cortex itself. Signals leave the cortex via the same sort of fibers that are responsible for the long-range corticocortical connections, the axons of some of the cortical pyramidal cells (e.g., the pyramidal and extrapyramidal motor tracts). In the skeleton cortex, the output is simply a partial description of the activity of the cortical neurons. Whatever logical transformations of the state description of the cortex are made in order to let the result interact with the rest of the brain, they must occur outside of the cortex.

The input is more complicated. There are at least three sorts of input fibers, depending on the geometry of their termination in the cortex. One system of fibers with diffuse terminations throughout the cortical layers has always been assigned ancillary roles, such as the global control of the state of the cortex in arousal or sleep, or the prevention of epileptoid explosions. They are not incorporated in the present picture of the skeleton cortex.

The other two systems are truly input in the conventional meaning. The olfactory input, presumably the oldest in an evolutionary sense, occupies the first layer in a specialized region of the cortex, where it connects with the apical dendrites of pyramidal cells (7). The other sensory inputs, insofar as they could be traced by anatomical or electrophysiological methods (7,11,17,19,22), seem to terminate mainly with rounded telodendria in an intermediate layer of the cortex, and to a lesser extent in the superficial layers.

PHILOSOPHY OF THE SKELETON CORTEX

The following has developed out of an interpretation of the cortex which I have given earlier (4,5). The terminology and also the emphasis has changed somewhat since then.

We consider the cortex as a memory, with the pyramidal cells as the units of the representation. Strongly connected sets of pyramidal cells, much like Hebb's (12) "cell assemblies," represent the things and situations of our perception. We distinguish localized cell assemblies, housed within regions the size of the areas of architectonics, and diffuse cell assemblies, which may be extended over the whole cortex (even bilaterally). The *things* and *situations* are represented by diffuse cell assemblies (in fact they are frequently multisensory), while the localized cell assemblies within the areas represent *aspects* (e.g., visual, acoustic, motor, various linguistic aspects) of the things themselves.

Information about the environment (after an infantile phase in which the connections between the input and the pyramidal cells are established) is incorporated into the cortex by setting up or changing synaptic connections between pyramidal cells. There are two types of information which must be learned: I, which signals often occur together and thus together make up the properties of a thing or situation which it pays to learn, and II, the successions in which the things or situations present themselves. Abstractly, I are the terms and II their (e.g., causal) relations, or: I is the dictionary and II is the syntax. Information of type I must be represented in the brain by the connections of the cells within a cell assembly, that of type II by the connections between one cell assembly and the next.

In this terminology, we can give the following interpretation of the A and B system of the preceding section: Each pyramidal cell is activated by a diffuse cell assembly through its apical dendrite via the long-range afferents to the first layer, and in turn contributes to it through its main axon (A system). It represents that diffuse cell assembly (the corresponding term) within the context of the area in which it is located. Other pyramidal cells in different areas represent the same assembly in different contexts, or if you wish, represent different aspects of the same term. The rules for the successions of terms are laid down in the network of axon collaterals within each area (B system), the evolution of the whole situation being a consequence of the sum of all the rules governing the evolution of the individual aspects of that situation in the various contexts.

The last statement is a hunch based on an argument on symmetry. The information of type I should be incorporated in networks in which reciprocal connections abound, i.e., in which a cell which sends an axon to another cell has a high probability of receiving an axon from the same cell. On the contrary, the information of type II requires more asymmetrical connections, sets of neurons with axons distributed on other sets and these in turn on new sets etc., cascades rather than whirlpools. Now, the network of fibers in the A system is highly symmetric, if we want to believe the quantitative argument which leads to the idea of "compartments," and so is the network of axon collaterals in the B system within each layer. Only in the vertical direction, between layers, the B system provides a cascade network of pyramidal cells, suited to incorporate type II information, since on average the axon collaterals are distributed below the level of the cortex in which the corresponding basal dendrites are located (electrophysiological evidence for this in ref. 1). We may schematically summarize these identifications in the following table:

A system	Diffuse cell assembly	Terms
B system, horiz.	Localized cell assembly	Aspects
B system, vert.	Sequences of cell assembly	Relations between terms (aspects)

An example may illustrate this: We imagine the concept, or term "bird" as being represented by a diffuse cell assembly spread over many areas of the cortex. It embraces many localized cell assemblies representing aspects of the bird, e.g., the image of the bird, the call of the bird, the word bird in various languages. We give the status of cell assembly also to these local representations because they, too, have the property of internal consistency, quite independently of the diffuse cell assembly to which they belong: I may remember that the word "ptica" exists in some language without remembering that it means bird. The evolution of the cell assembly bird, the prediction of what the bird will do next, is a consequence of the evolution of the localized cell assemblies within the areas, representing the vision of a bird taking off, the sound of the call which precedes this, the word sequence "ptica leti" etc.: dynamic properties of the various aspects of the term bird.

MEMORY

If memory is the growth of connections under the influence of activity, the timetable of the development of dendrites, dendritic spines, and axons does not encourage the identification of any of these elements with memory traces. In the mouse, the apical dendrites of pyramidal cells are well developed at birth. The basal dendrites follow soon afterwards (Fig. 5) and are apparently complete around the 10th day of life, when the mouse opens his eyes and begins to explore the world. The dendritic spines also develop

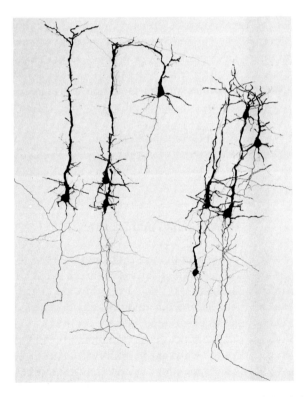

FIG. 5. Camera lucida drawing of pyramidal cells in the cortex of the 4-day-old mouse. The neurons are represented in the arrangement in which they were situated in the preparation. Basal dendrites are shorter than in the adult. Some of the branches of the apical dendrites are also not yet developed. In contrast, the axons with the complete set of axon collaterals are already present.

during the days of emancipation, as soon as the dendritic tree is complete. The axon collaterals are fully developed at birth, except for an increase in length which just keeps up with the increase of the linear dimensions of the cortex during the first 2 weeks of life (29). Thus, the whole equipment of the pyramidal cells is apparently the basis for the establishment of learned connections rather than its effect. It seems that the only likely candidates for memory traces are the synapses, the number of which increases after the macroscopical shape of the neuron is fully established. This whole set of problems is treated more fully in the paper by Schüz (27).

AREAL ARCHITECTONICS

We may summarize the preceding section in the following proposition: the structure of the normal cerebral cortex, as we describe it on the basis of light microscopy, is genetically determined.[2] This must be especially true for the statistical properties of the tissue which form the basis for the subtle distinction of "architectonic areas." Cell layers of different relative thicknesses, differences in the density of perikarya in various layers, differences in their average size, more or less marked columnar arrangement of perikarya, differences in the density, distribution, length, or thickness of myelinated fibers are examples of the statistical parameters which were used, mostly in a physiognomic, nonquantitative way, by the architectonic cartographers.

Therefore, if we want to interpret architectonics, we must think in terms of differences in the readiness of the cerebral cortex to accept information of different kinds in preordained places. We can only sketch a few thoughts in this field.

Hippocampus and Isocortex

This is the most obvious architectonic distinction (Fig. 6). In the hippocampus all perikarya of pyramidal cells are concentrated within a narrow layer. On the contrary, in the rest of the cortex they are distributed throughout the thickness of the cortex from layer II down. The consequence is that in the hippocampus the basal dendrites are all at the same height and, therefore, all have the same chance to be connected to the axon collaterals of their neighbors, depending only on the relative distance. There is ample opportunity for reciprocal connections in the B system, much less for cascaded connections. On the contrary, in the isocortex the staggering of the neurons provides an opportunity for asymmetrical, irreciprocal connections in the B system, as we have already observed.

---

[2] With the possible exception of dendritic spines: see Schüz (27).

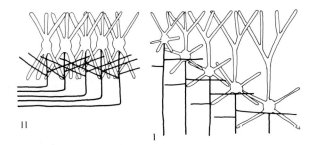

FIG. 6. Two fundamental types of cortex. **H:** Hippocampus with basal dendrites of pyramidal cells collected in one layer, offering the possibility of many reciprocal connections through axon collaterals. **I:** Isocortex, with cell bodies and, hence, basal dendrites of pyramidal cells arranged at different heights in the cortex. This leads to more asymmetrical irreciprocal connections in the vertical direction.

The Strias of Baillarger

Variations in their density are the main markers of the areas in myeloarchitectonics (Fig. 7). The strias are probably nothing but the layers in which myelinated axon collaterals of pyramidal cells are concentrated (3). We do not know why axon collaterals are sometimes myelinated, nor do we know why they are much more heavily myelinated in certain animals (e.g., primates, cat) and in certain places (primary sensory regions, motor areas, certain orbital areas) than in other animals (rodents) and other places (temporal pole, frontal pole, anterior cingulate region). While in the mouse we have seen that there are hardly enough axons to accomodate all the synapses if we suppose that every axon collateral makes a synapse every micron, apparently in other animals there are stretches of isolated conduction. The main variations in the pattern of Baillarger's strias (Fig. 7) can be hypothetically put into relation with variations of the distribution of granular cells and Martinotti cells in different parts of the cortex (4).

The Primary Sensory Areas

In man, the postcentral area 3 (6), the primary acoustic area 41 on Heschl's gyrus and the visual parastriate area 18 have much in common. In the Nissl picture all of them abound in small perikarya, indicating perhaps that they are less involved in the long-range corticocortical traffic than in local operations on the input. The myelin picture of these areas is so typical that it is always possible, by observation at small magnification, to recognize a piece of cortex as belonging to one of them but practically impossible to say which. The characteristic features are: (a) great wealth in myelinated fibers; (b) a strong maximum of myelin density at the level of the inner stria of Baillarger; (c) a narrow maximum of fiber density, the so-called stria of Kaes-Bechterew, at the level of layer II. It is well possible that (b) and (c)

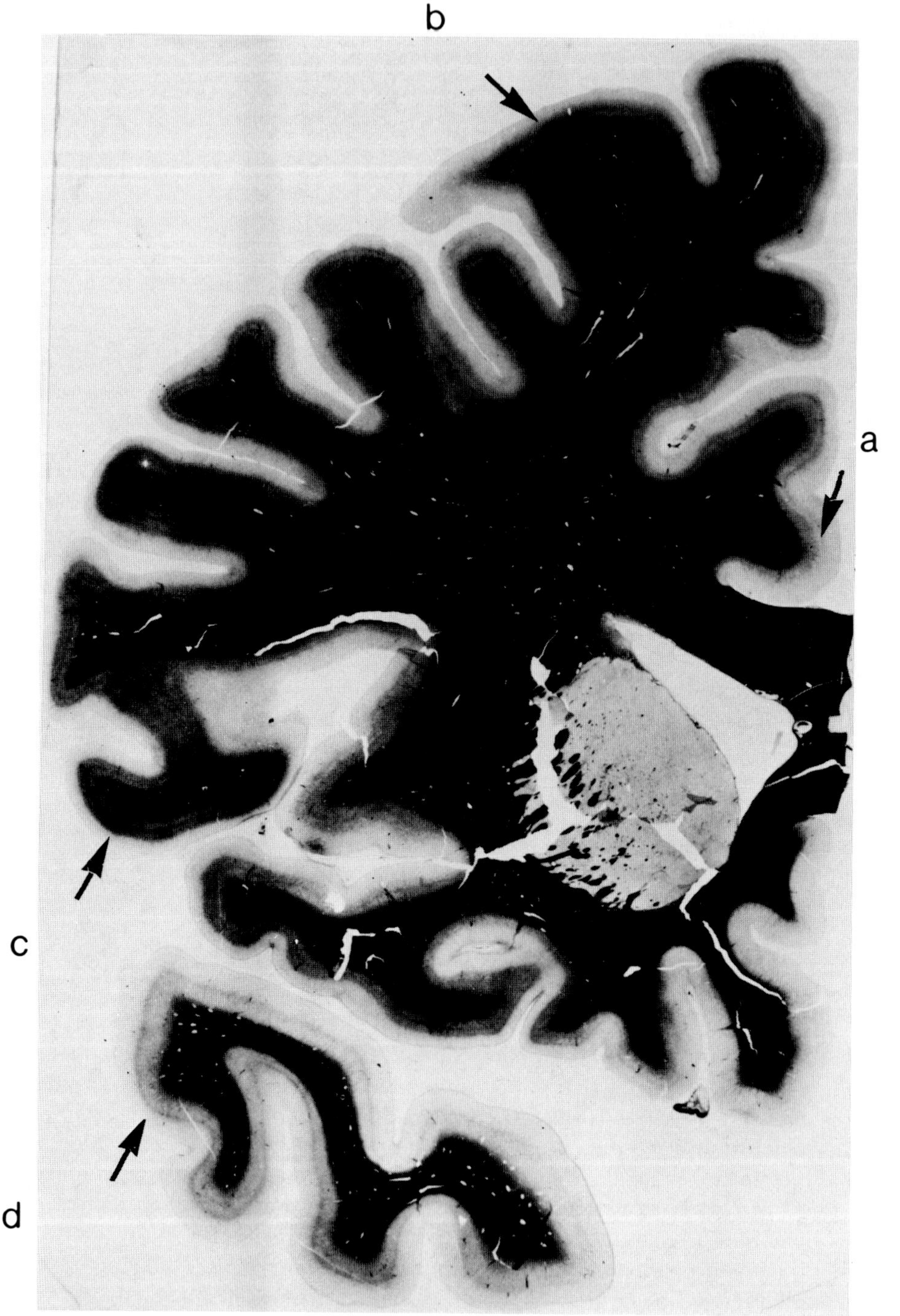
b
a
c
d

are nothing but the macroscopical expression of the presence of numerous myelinated thalamic afferents, but these cannot entirely explain the generally strong myelination of these areas.

Area 17, as is well known, is quite different, especially in the myelin picture, where the stria of Gennari is not comparable to and is not continuous with any of the fiber layers of the other areas. Apparently, there a preprocessing of the visual input occurs, which the other sensory modalities do not require.

Architectonic Variation in the Golgi Picture

Cajal's descriptions of various areas of the cortex have not received the attention they deserve, perhaps because nobody possesses enough Golgi material to be able to confirm and to develop his analysis further. Apart from the presence of various types of stellate and Martinotti cells, the areal variations of the shape of pyramidal cells are impressive in his account.

Areal Distinctions in the Mouse

In the lower (basal) part of the hemisphere the first layer is much thicker, the cell bodies of pyramidal cells tend to be concentrated in a narrower layer and the spread of their apical dendrites is wider. One might interpret this as a transition between the two main cortical types of Fig. 6.

In the pyriform area of the frontobasal hemisphere, where the olfactory tract enters the cortex, pyramidal cells are clearly of two types: pyramidal cells with well-developed dendrites covered with spines, located in the deeper strata, and others with scanty basal dendrites and practically spineless apical dendrites, located more superficially.

Steffen[3] has shown that the length of axon collaterals of pyramidal cells varies in different regions of the hemisphere.

CONCLUSIONS

A real understanding of the areal variation of cortical structure is not possible yet because we do not know what basic cortical computing device

---

[3] Steffen, H. (1975): Quantitative Untersuchungen der Axon-Kollateralen der Pyramidenzellen in der Gehirnrinde der Maus. Master's thesis, University of Tübingen.

FIG. 7. Frontal section through the frontal lobe and the temporal pole of a human left hemisphere, myelin preparation. The arrows indicate areas with evident differences in the myeloarchitectonic picture. **a:** Anterior cingulate region, weak myelination, no stria of Baillarger. **b:** Premotor region, strong myelination of the lower layers of the cortex. **c:** Third frontal convolution (Broca's region), dense stria of Baillarger, almost fused into one and separated from the white substance by a lighter layer. **d:** Temporal pole region, weakly myelinated with only one (the outer) stria of Baillarger.

is thus varied. However, it is possible to develop some general thoughts on the function of the cerebral cortex, starting from the shape of the neuronal elements which are typical for it, the pyramidal cells. When following this procedure, it is comforting to observe that the variations of the structure of the cerebral cortex, where it is applied to different tasks, are mainly variations of the shape and arrangement of these elements.

ACKNOWLEDGMENT

We thank G. Kurz for expert typing and organization, F. Mayer for his extremely careful camera lucida work, D. Stoll for the preparation of the excellent Golgi material, K. Witte for painstaking electron microscopy, and A. Schüz and G. Palm for critical, exhortative, and constructive comments.

REFERENCES

1. Asunuma, H., and Rosen, I. (1972): Functional role of afferent inputs to the monkey motor cortex. *Brain Res.,* 40:3.
2. Benevento, L. A., and Ebner, F. F. (1971): The areas and layers of cortico-cortical terminations in the visual cortex of the virginia opossum. *J. Comp. Neurol.,* 141:157–189.
3. Braitenberg, V. (1962): A note on myeloarchitectonics. *J. Comp. Neurol.,* 118:141–151.
4. Braitenberg, V. (1974): Thoughts on the cerebral cortex. *J. Theor. Biol.,* 46:421–447.
5. Braitenberg, V. (1974): On the representation of objects and their relations in the brain. In: *Lecture Notes in Biomathematics. 4. Physics and Mathematics of the Nervous System,* edited by M. Conrad, W. Güttinger, and M. Dal Cin, pp. 290–298. Springer Verlag: New York.
6. Brodmann, K. (1909): *Vergleichende Lokalisationslehre der Grosshirnrinde in ihren Prinzipien dargestellt auf Grund des Zellenbaus.* J. A. Barth, Leipzig.
7. Cajal, S. R. (1911): *Histologie du Système Nerveux de l'Homme et des Vertébrés.* Paris, Maloine.
8. Colonnier, M. (1964): The tangential organization of the visual cortex. *J. Anat.,* 98:327–344.
9. Cragg, B. G. (1967): The density of synapses and neurones in the motor and visual areas of the cerebral cortex. *J. Anat.,* 101:639–654.
10. Friede, R. L. (1954): Der quantitative Anteil der Glia an der Cortexentwicklung. *Acta Anat.,* 20:290–296.
11. Garey, L. J., and Powell, T. P. S. (1971): An experimental study of the termination of the lateral geniculocortical pathway in the cat and monkey. *Proc. Roy. Soc. Lond.* [*Biol.*], 179:41–63.
12. Hebb, D. O. (1949): *The Organization of Behaviour.* John Wiley & Sons, New York.
13. Heimer, L., Ebner, F. F., and Nauta, W. J. H. (1967): A note on the termination of commissural fibers in the neocortex. *Brain Res.,* 5:171–177.
14. Hubel, D. H., and Wiesel, T. N. (1962): Receptive fields, binocular interaction and functional architecture in the cat's visual cortex. *J. Physiol.* (*Lond.*), 160:106.
15. Hubel, D. H., and Wiesel, T. N. (1965): Receptive fields and function architecture in two non-striate visual areas (18 and 19) of the cat. *J. Neurophysiol.,* 28:229–289.
16. Hubel, D. H., and Wiesel, T. N. (1969): Anatomical demonstration of columns in the monkey striate cortex. *Nature* 221:747–750.
17. Hubel, D. H., and Wiesel, T. N. (1972): Laminar and columnar distribution of geniculocortical fibers in the macaque monkey. *J. Comp. Neurol.,* 146:421–450.
18. Kemali, M., and Braitenberg, V. (1969): *Atlas of the Frog's Brain.* Springer, Heidelberg.
19. Kölliker, A. (1896): *Handbuch der Gewebelehre des Menschen.* Engelmann, Leipzig.

20. Lázár, G., and Székely, G. (1969): Distribution of optic terminals in the different optic centers of the frog. *Brain Res.,* 16:1–14.
21. Lorente de Nó, R. (1949): Cytoarchitecture. In: *Physiology of the Nervous System,* edited by J. F. Fulton, pp. 288–320. University Press, New York-Oxford.
22. Lund, J. S. (1973): Organization of neurons in the visual cortex, area 17, of the monkey (Macaca mulatta). *J. Comp. Neurol.,* 147:455–495.
23. Mountcastle, V. B. (1957): Modality and topographic properties of single neurons of cat's somatic sensory cortex. *J. Neurophysiol.,* 20:408.
24. Palm, G., and Braitenberg, V. (1976): Tentative contributions of neuroanatomy to nerve net theories. In: *Proceedings of the 3rd European Meeting on Cybernetics and Systems Research,* edited by R. Trappl *(in press).*
25. Peters, A., Palay, S. L., and Webster, H. D. F. (1970): *The Fine Structure of the Nervous System.* Harper & Row, New York.
26. Schüz, A. (1976): Pyramidal cells with different densities of dendritic spines in the cortex of the mouse. *Z. Naturforsch.,* 31c:319–323.
27. Schüz, A. (1977): Some facts and hypotheses concerning dendritic spines and learning *(this volume).*
28. Sholl, D. A. (1967): *The Organization of the Cerebral Cortex.* Hafner, New York and London.
29. Steffen, H. (1976): Golgi-stained barrel-neurons in the somatosensory region of the mouse cerebral cortex. *Neurosci. Lett.,* 2:57–59.
30. Tigges, J., Spatz, W. B., and Tigges, M. (1973): Reciprocal point-to-point connections between parastriate and striate cortex in the squirrel monkey (Saimiri). *J. Comp. Neurol.,* 148:481–490.
31. Woolsey, T. A., and van der Loos, H. (1970): The structural organization of layer IV in the somatosensory region (SI) of the mouse cerebral cortex: The description of a cortical field composed of discrete cytoarchitectonic units. *Brain Res.,* 17:205–242.

Author Index

Acuna, C., (56)* 368, 375, *382;*
  (15) 398, 399, 400, *405*
Adams, R. D., (4) 427, *440*
Adey, W. R., (1) 55, *56*
Adinolfi, A. M., (1) 164, *171*
Adrianov, O. S., (1) 320, *333;*
  (1) 414, 418, *424;* (2) 418,
  424; (3) 418, *424;* (4) 418,
  424; (5) 418, *424;* (6) 412,
  424; (7) 412, 418, 420, *424;*
  (8) 415, 416, *424;* (9) 422,
  424; (10) 422, 423, *424;*
  (11) 412, 414, *424;* (12)
  412, *424;* (13) 414, *424;*
  (36) 422, *425*
Aghajanian, G. K., (1) 133,
  134; (2) 165, *171*
Ajmone Marsan, C., (5) 277,
  280; (6) 277, *280;* (7) 277,
  280; (1) 438, *440*
Albe Fessard, D., (1) 394, 395,
  405
Albus, K., (11) 227, *234;* (1)
  363, 365, 367, 373, *380;* (2)
  363, 373, *380;* (47) 373,
  374, *381*
Altman, J., (1) 188, *188;* (2)
  188, *188*
Amassian, V. E., (2) 394, *405*
Anderson, P. J., (6) 177, *189*
Anderson, R. E., (9) 396, 398,
  405
Angevine, J. B., (3) 186, *188*
Annett, M., (1) 250, *255*
Apathy, S. von, (1) 10, *27*
Arbib, M. A., (33) 59, 65, 70,
  76; (34) 79, *97*
Arndt, R., (2) 22, *27*
Arrigoni, O., (4) 183, *188*
Artemenko, D. P., (14) 414,
  416, *424*
Asanuma, H., (2) 55, *56;* (1)
  103, *114;* (1) 444, *464*
Ayala, G. F., (5) 277, *280*

Babuna, C., (17) 187, *189*
Bailey, P., (2) 101, *114*
Baillarger, J.-G.-F., (3) 15, 16,
  27; 357
Balazs, R., (5) 188, *189*
Bar, T., (3) 166, 169, *171;* (4)
  160, 170, *171;* (33) 170,
  173; (34) 166, 168, *173;*
  (35) 160, 170, *173*
Barka, T., (6) 177, *189*

Barlow, H. B., (1) 344, *355*
Batuyev, A. S., (15) 416, *425*
Beaumont, J. G., (2) 249, 254,
  255; (3) 246, *255*
Beisenherz, G., (7) 183, *189*
Benaron, H. B. W., (17) 187,
  189
Benevento, L. A., (3) 365,
  380; (18) 363, 371, 372,
  380; (2) 444, 454, 456, *464*
Benignus, V. A., (1) 309, 313,
  317
Bennett, E. L., (3) 129, *134*
Bental, E., (17) 416, *425*
Berger, H., (3) 393, 400, *405*
Berkley, M., (18) 212, *223*
Berlin, R., (4) 16, *27*
Berry, M., (5) 159, 168, *171*
Besser, L., (5) 22, *27*
Bettinger, L. A., (16) 396, *405*
Betz, V., (6) 14, 20, *27;* (3) 43,
  56; 357
Bignall, K. E., (5) 396, 397,
  405; (18) 420, *425*
Bihari, B., (17) 416, *425*
Bilge, M., (1) 211, *223*
Billings Gagliardi, S. M., (2)
  32, 33, 35, 36, 37, 39, 40,
  41
Bingle, A., (1) 211, *223*
Birsch, H., (16) 396, *405*
Bisconte, J. L., 186
Bishop, E. J., (2) 427, 434,
  436, 438, 439, *440*
Bishop, G. H., (2) 212, *223*
Blakemore, C., (3) 223, *223;*
  (13) 214, 216, *223;* (57)
  221, *225*
Bloom, F. E., (1) 133, *134;* (2)
  165, *171*
Blunt, A. H., (18) 159, 163,
  172
Bogdanski, D. F., (1) 144, *156*
Boggon, R. H., (4) 59, *75*
Bogolepova, I. N., (29) 421,
  425
Boltze, H. J., (7) 183, *189*
Bonin, G. von, (4) 47, *56;* (2)
  101, *114;* (3) 112, *114;* (4)
  103, *114;* (30) 159, *172*
Boothe, R. G., (10) 32, *41;* (5)
  231, *234*
Borenstein, P., (6) 396, *405*
The Boulder Committee, (36)
  161, *173*

Boycott, B. B., (4) 213, *223;*
  (4) 369, *380*
Braak, E., (2) 148, *156*
Braak, H., (5) 99, *114;* (6) 99,
  114; (3) 143, *156;* (4) 137,
  156; (5) 138, *156;* (6) 144,
  156; (7) 140, 141, 142, 143,
  157; (8) 148, *157;* (9) 148,
  149, *157;* (10) 155, *157;*
  (11) 139, *157;* (12) 156, *157*
Braitenberg, V., (3) 444, 461,
  464; (4) 457, 461, *464;* (5)
  457, *464;* (18) 455, *464;*
  (24) 455, *465*
Brazier, M. A. B., 99; (4) 393,
  405
Brodmann, K., (1) 32, *41;* (5)
  43, *56* (1) 59, *75;* (7) 100,
  114; (13) 149, *157;* (5) 358,
  380; 395; (19) 415, *425;* (6)
  461, *464*
Brooks, D., (17) 365, 367, *380*
Brothe, R. G., (49) 363, 369,
  382
Brown, A. G., (2) 337, *355*
Brun, A., (1) 239, *242*
Bucher, T., (7) 183, *189*
Bucy, P. C., (8) 112, *114*
Bullock, T. H., (10) 336, *355*
Bunt, A., (11) 39, *41;* (6) 227,
  229, 230, *234;* (50) 371,
  382
Burton, H., (9) 101, *114;* (31)
  101, *115;* (32) 105, *115*
Buser, P., 395; (5) 396, 397,
  405; (6) 396, *405*

Cadilhac, J., (3) 427, *440;* (12)
  427, *440*
Calvet, J., (1) 276, *279;* (17)
  276, 278, *280;* (1) 281, 299,
  304; (8) 282, *305;* (18) 303,
  305; (2) 331, *333;* (7) 401,
  405; (9) 396, 398, *405;* (18)
  401, *405;* 408; (1) 407, *409;*
  (2) 407, *409*
Calvet, M. C., (1) 276, *279;* (1)
  281, 299, *304;* 331; (2) 331,
  333; (1) 407, *409*
Cammermeyer, J., (1) 120, *127*
Campbell, A. W., (6) 43, *56;*
  (3) 59, *75;* (6) 358, *380*
Carli, G., (9) 342, *355*
Casagrande, V. A., (45) 222,
  225

---

*Numbers in parentheses before page of citation are reference numbers; italicized numbers represent the page on which the reference information appears.

467

Subject Index

475